The Reach of Mind

Essays by

ERICH FROMM
ARON GURWITSCH
EUGENIA HANFMANN
HENRI HÉCAEN
LIPMAN HALPERN
ROLLO MAY
JOSEPH MEIERS
RICARDO B. MORANT
GARDNER MURPHY
PAUL OPPENHEIM
DONALD M. PURDY
WALTHER RIESE
MEYER SCHAPIRO
DAVID SHAKOW
MARIANNE L. SIMMEL
SILVAN TOMKINS
ROBERT ULICH
EGON WEIGL

The Reach of Mind

ESSAYS IN MEMORY OF KURT GOLDSTEIN

Edited by MARIANNE L. SIMMEL

Springer Science+Business Media, LLC

ISBN 978-3-662-39249-2 ISBN 978-3-662-40265-8 (eBook)
DOI 10.1007/978-3-662-40265-8

ORIGINALLY PUBLISHED BY
SPRINGER PUBLISHING COMPANY, INC. IN 1968.
SOFTCOVER REPRINT OF THE HARDCOVER 1ST EDITION 1968

Library of Congress Catalog Card Number: 67–27712

Foreword

Kurt Goldstein's life spanned the whole history of modern psychology. He was born the year before Wundt's official founding of experimental psychology at Leipzig, and only three years after the informal establishment of the first psychological laboratory at the Lawrence Scientific School at Harvard under William James' aegis. He was nine years old when Fechner died, sixteen at Helmholtz' death. He was a student at the Breslau *Gymnasium* while plans were made in G. Stanley Hall's study at Clark University for the establishment of the American Psychological Association, whose seventy-fifth anniversary is being celebrated this year.

Kurt Goldstein's interests, however, spanned far more than psychology. They encompassed all of human endeavor. His earliest inclinations were towards literature and philosophy. When he turned to the study of medicine it was an exchange of a life of contemplation for one of active participation in human affairs, and he envisaged a career of helping human beings in distress. He began by studying the basic substrates of human behavior, and his first publications concern problems of neuroembryology and comparative anatomy. There followed a decade of "fact finding" during which he ranged from anatomy through neurology, psychology and psychiatry, addressing himself to many different disturbances of behavior and the distress they bring in their wake.

A period of consolidation followed when, soon after the outbreak of the First World War, he was called on to organize and direct the *Institut zur Erforschung der Folgeerscheinungen von Hirnverletzungen* at Frankfurt. Now he was responsible for the whole human being of the brain-injured soldiers who came to the institute for treatment and rehabilitation. The very comprehensiveness of the task demanded—and thus created—what came to be formulated much later as the holistic view of the organism. The patients had to be helped to come to terms with the new conditions confronting them, to actualize themselves within the limits imposed by their handicaps, to achieve maximum adequacy vis-à-vis the world. Significant aid in this endeavor depended on the fullest possible understanding of the deficits and alterations wrought by brain injury, and such an understanding could be gained only through intensive analysis of the patients' performances. As the result there began to appear the long series of studies that were to become classics: on sensory and motor deficits consequent to circumscribed cortical lesions; on perception and perceptual alterations;

on tonus and tonus disturbances; and, finally, on language and aphasia whose discussion necessitated a reconsideration of all the so-called higher mental processes.

All along Goldstein had been interested in psychiatric questions, and during the late nineteen-twenties he entered actively into the discussions of the new dynamic psychiatry that had developed in the interim. His first formal statements concerning the holistic approach to biology were made in this context, though its detailed formulation had to await the enforced leisure of exile.

When Goldstein arrived in the United States he was in his mid-fifties; barely spoke the language of the country, with a spectacular career behind him and a recently published *magnum opus* that was not yet available in English. His American colleagues welcomed him with great personal warmth, but his professional and scientific future was uncertain. Yet there was to be a second thirty years' career during which he exerted a major influence on students of neurology, psychiatry and psychology, and on scholars in many other fields. During his last years he returned to his first love—philosophy, literature, and, even if only in passing, problems of aesthetics. And so his intellectual life had come full circle. Though he saw his work as unfinished, he left to us an achievement of rare inner coherence and completion.

The contributors to the present volume represent part of the reach of mind that was Goldstein's, and their initial contact with him dates from different periods of his life and work. They are listed here in alphabetical order.

Erich Fromm is a psychoanalyst, Adjunct Professor at New York University, Extraordinary Professor at the National Autonomous University of Mexico, Director of the Mexican Institute of Psychoanalysis and a Fellow of the William Alanson White Institute of Psychoanalysis, Psychiatry and Psychology. He first met Goldstein in 1918.

Aron Gurwitsch is Professor of Philsophy at the Graduate Faculty of Political and Social Science, New School for Social Research, in New York City. After an early start in mathematics and physics, he came to the Frankfurt Institute in 1921 to immerse himself in psychology under the Gelb-Goldstein aegis. He stayed until 1928, and during that time a close personal friendship developed between him and Goldstein. His later phenomenological writings were much influenced by Goldstein's thinking.

Lipman Halpern is the elected Dean of the Hebrew University Hadassah Medical School where he is also Professor of Clinical Neurology and

Head of the Department of Nervous Diseases. He came to Berlin to work with Goldstein in 1930, and stayed for three years, until both men were expelled by the Hitler regime. They remained friends, and in 1953 Professor Halpern arranged for a visit by Goldstein to the Hebrew University. This was "a festive occasion and Goldstein was the recipient of enthusiastic expressions of the high regard in which he was held, and the Faculty of Philosophy of the Hebrew University presented him with a Scroll of Honor inscribed in both Hebrew and Latin."

Eugenia Hanfmann is Professor of Psychology at Brandeis University. Among her many activities has been the translation and editing of L.S. Vygotsky's *Thought and Language*. Her initial contact with Goldstein via Fritz Heider and Case Lanuti is described in her contribution to this volume. It was the beginning of a close personal and intellectual friendship.

Henri Hécaen is a neurologist, Directeur d'Etudes, Ecole Pratique des Hautes Etudes at the Sorbonne, and on the senior staff of the Centre Neurochirurgical at the Hôpital St. Anne. Goldstein was much interested in Hécaen's work, and especially in his earlier book, *Le Cortex Cérbéral*, published jointly with J. de Ajuriaguerra. Hécaen acknowledges his intellectual debt to Goldstein in his contribution to this volume. The two men met on only a few occasions.

Rollo May is a psychoanalyst, Supervisor and Training Analyst at the William Alanson White Institute of Psychiatry, Psychoanalysis and Psychology, and Adjunct Professor at the Graduate School of Arts and Sciences, New York University. While Dr. May was a graduate student, working on the problem of anxiety, he had a series of discussions with Goldstein from which he came away "not always with agreement, but always with enlargement of my mind and perceptions." They maintained friendly contact through many years.

Joseph Meiers is a psychiatrist in New York City, a consultant at Sydenham (City) Hospital, supervising psychiatrist at the Adler Consultation Center and Mental Hygiene Clinic, and Lecturer in Psychiatry at the New York Institute of Individual Psychology. He studied with Goldstein in Berlin in the early thirties. He became a devoted friend and the compiler of Goldstein bibliographies.

Ricardo B. Morant is Professor and Chairman of the Department of Psychology at Brandeis University. His early acquaintance with Goldstein is described at the beginning of his contribution to this volume. Their discussions continued when Goldstein taught at Brandeis University. Professor Morant commented, "Goldstein's point of view of organismic functioning had a great effect on the development of my own ideas about perception."

Gardner Murphy is a psychologist and Director of Research at the Menninger Foundation in Topeka, Kansas. He describes himself as "a friend and admirer" of Goldstein's. Goldstein often spoke of the warm welcome extended to him by Professor Murphy on his arrival in the United States.

Paul Oppenheim describes himself as a "free-lance philosopher of science." Notwithstanding their different intellectual "styles," a close personal friendship between him and Goldstein developed first in Frankfurt. It was to last for almost fifty years. After both men had come to this country, Goldstein was a guest in the Oppenheim home in Princeton on a number of occasions.

Donald M. Purdy was one of the first to introduce Goldstein to American psychologists with his paper "The Biological Psychology of Kurt Goldstein," published in 1937 in *Character and Personality*. He has been a National Research Council Fellow and a Guggenheim Fellow, and he has taught Psychology at the University of Kansas, at the University of Maine, at the University of Washington and at Mills College. He now lives in New York City.

Walther Riese is Emeritus Associate Professor of Neurology, Psychiatry and History of Medicine at the Medical College of Virginia. He joined Goldstein in Frankfurt in 1917, and the results of their common investigations were reported in a series of papers between 1917 and 1933. They remained in close contact to the end.

Meyer Schapiro is University Professor at Columbia University where he had earlier been Professor of Art History and Archeology. He and Goldstein first met in the nineteen-forties at the Linguistics Circle in New York City. As one of the close friends of Goldstein during his last years, Professor Schapiro spoke at Goldstein's funeral. His moving words were published in *Philosophy and Phenomenological Research* in December 1965.

David Shakow is Senior Research Psychologist at the National Institute of Mental Health, USPHS, where, for many years previously, he was the Chief of the Psychological Laboratory. He first met Goldstein in the mid-thirties, and got to know him well at Harvard in 1938. In the nineteen-forties, while Dr. Shakow was at Worcester State Hospital, he arranged for regular visits, research conferences and seminars by Goldstein, and did much to further personal contacts between Goldstein and American psychologists.

Marianne L. Simmel is Professor of Psychology at Brandeis University and on the staffs of The Massachusetts General Hospital in Boston and The Mount Sinai Hospital in New York City. She first came to Goldstein's laboratory at the Boston Dispensary in 1942, sent by Fritz Heider on a summer's assistantship. She returned the next year, stayed until Goldstein left for New York City, then followed him there. Above all Goldstein taught her how to examine patients and to mistrust all theories, including his own.

Silvan S. Tomkins is Research Professor of Psychology and Director of the Center for Research in Cognition and Affect at the City University of New York. He first encountered Goldstein in 1938 when he served as assistant in a graduate seminar given by Goldstein at the Harvard Psychological Clinic. It did not take long for the two men to develop a lasting friendship.

Robert Ulich is James Bryant Conant Professor of Education Emeritus, Harvard University. He describes his relationship with Goldstein as one of "pure friendship," dating back to a visit in the mid-thirties. Many visits followed that first one, and Professor Ulich recalls with special pleasure a joint evening with Ernst Cassirer.

Egon Weigl is a psychologist, now at the Laboratory of Language Pathology at the German Academy of Sciences in East Berlin. He came as a student to Frankfurt University in the nineteen-twenties, and his doctoral dissertation was supervised jointly by Gelb and Goldstein. During this time and thereafter, he was a frequent guest in Goldstein's house, and became a friend of the whole family. Though there was a twenty-year interval during which they lost touch with each other, they resumed an active correspondence in 1958.

Inevitably only a small group of Goldstein's colleagues, students and friends are represented in the present collection. Many others could have been included. Two individuals must be mentioned in particular, for both had planned to contribute to this volume.

Oliver L. Zangwill, Professor of Experimental Psychology at the University of Cambridge was preparing a paper on ideational apraxia when illness prevented its completion. In a recent letter he wrote: "I would dearly have liked to have paid tribute in this way to a man whose writing taught me so much."

Tilly Edinger, had been Honorary Associate in Vertebrate Paleontology at the Museum of Comparative Zoology, Harvard University when word reached us of her sudden death in May 1967, while this volume was in preparation. She had known Goldstein "almost all my life, except his Königsberg years;" the daughter of Ludwig Edinger, his one-time chief, and a recipient of many honorary degrees for her work on the evolution of the brain, she had a very special place in Goldstein's heart—and he in hers. Her contribution in his memory grew beyond the bounds of a book such as this, and will be published separately in *Senckenbergiana Lethaea* under the title *New Results and Old Errors in Paleoneurology*.

Marianne L. Simmel

Dennisport, Massachusetts
June, 1967

Contents

I

KURT GOLDSTEIN– A LIFE

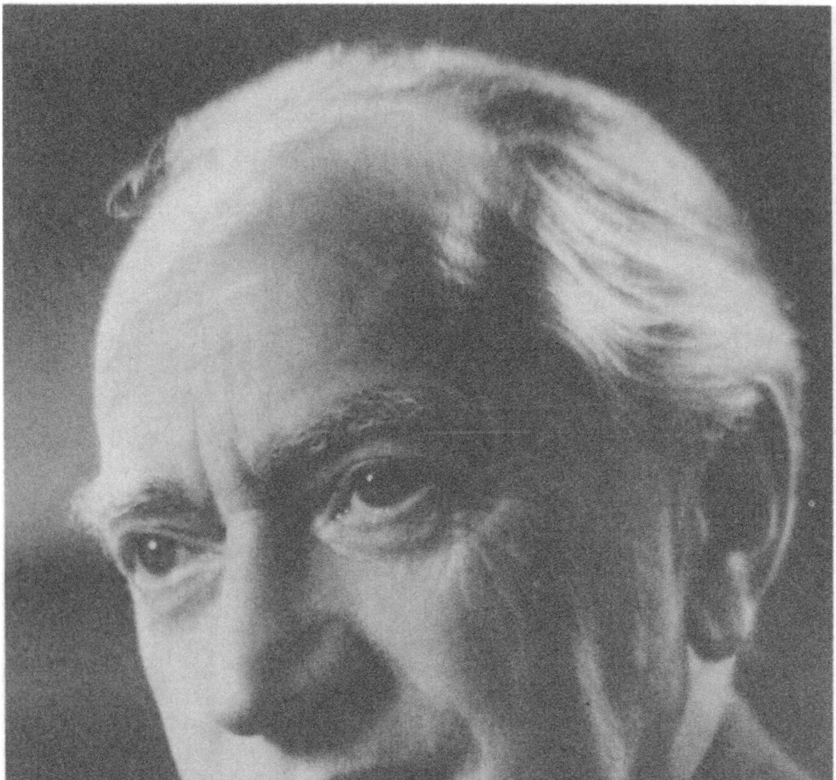

1

Kurt Goldstein 1878—1965

by Marianne L. Simmel
Dennisport, Massachusetts

Kurt Goldstein was born on November 6, 1878, in Kattowitz, a small town in Upper Silesia, the seventh of nine children of an agnostic Jewish family. His father, the prosperous owner of a local lumber yard, had not had much formal education, but had acquired a great respect for scholarship. Thus he saw to it that all his sons obtained advanced university degrees as the proper preparation for life. Goldstein's childhood was spent in a huge house amidst the hustle and bustle of many people. The lumber-yard workmen joined the family for the midday meal; there was a ballroom for festive occasions, just as there were small dark rooms which no one ever entered because they were said to be haunted. There were always visiting aunts or cousins about, among the latter frequently the future philosopher Ernst Cassirer, Goldstein's senior by four years.

In these ebullient surroundings Goldstein grew up a quiet, rather shy boy. He received his early education at the local public school, and soon earned himself the epithet "professor" for always having his nose in a book. He learned to play the cello, and though he did not continue the practice, he retained a special love for cello music throughout his life.

After some years the family moved to Breslau, the local metropolis, and there Goldstein attended the *Humanistische Gymnasium.* Upon graduation he planned to study philosophy, but his father regarded this as a *brotlose Kunst* and sent him instead to work in the business of a relative. Eventually he relented and Goldstein, having had enough of "wrapping up packages" as he later used to describe it, entered Breslau University. He stayed only one semester, then went to Heidelberg to immerse himself in philosophy and literature. The next year saw him back at Breslau, where he now settled down to the study of medicine. At least for the time being he had given up philosophy and, though he knew little of medicine, had resolved to make his life's profession the relief of suffering among the sick. Perhaps it was the old philosophical interest that now drew him especially to the problems of mental diseases.

At that time mental diseases were generally regarded as the result of disorders of the nervous system, and the obvious path to their study lay through neuroanatomy and neurophysiology. Somewhat to his own surprise Goldstein found himself very much attracted to the pathological laboratory, and he later spoke with much enthusiasm about Professor Schaper who had introduced him to neuroembryological work. Karl Wernicke was the chairman of the Psychiatry Department, and he too was much interested in correlations between psychiatric symptomatology and post-mortem findings. He first drew Goldstein's attention to problems of aphasia which were to become a lifelong preoccupation, even though his final formulations differed quite markedly from those of his old teacher.

Goldstein received his M.D. in 1903 with a dissertation on the organization of the posterior column pathways of the spinal cord. In the same year he published four papers on the anatomy and embryonic development of the spinal cord and brain. In 1904 he joined the *Senckenbergische Neurologische Institut* in *Frankfurt am Main,* as assistant to Ludwig Edinger, the man who probably influenced Goldstein's future career more than any other single individual. Subsequently he spent a year in Freiburg with Hoche, then a year in Berlin with Oppenheim. In 1906 he joined the staff of the Psychiatric Clinic of the University of Königsberg, now finally to devote himself to the study and treatment of patients with psychiatric disorders. Initially he met with great disappointment. He found that mental patients were simply relegated to custodial care, without any attempt at treatment. Nor did the prevailing Kraepelinian nosology indicate any conceivable direction for therapy. Goldstein used the opportunity for careful examinations and observations of patients, and published papers on a variety of neurological and psychiatric topics; on motor disturbances, sensory disturbances, the nature of hallucinations, alcoholism, manic depressive states, schizophrenia, etc., as well as studies comparing clinical symptoms and post-mortem findings. One of the earliest of this group of papers is of special interest for psychologists. It was entitled *Merkfähigkeit, Gedächtnis und Assoziation* and published in 1906 in the *Zeitschrift für Psychologie.* It is a discussion of different types of memory deficits created by neurological and psychiatric disturbances, and it foreshadows some of the basic distinctions that underlie present-day differential diagnostic testing. In 1907 he became *Privatdozent* at the University, and delivered his Inaugural Lecture on The Appraisal of Reality During Hallucinatory Experiences.

He stayed in Königsberg until 1914 when he followed Ludwig Edinger's invitation to join him in Frankfurt as first assistant of the Neurological Institute. What both envisioned was Goldstein's return to laboratory investigations in comparative neuroanatomy and neuropathology. But Goldstein had acquired a taste for clinical work and had discovered that clinical investigation could be fruitful. Before long he found himself organizing, under military auspices and with Edinger's encouragement, a hospital and research institute for the study of brain injured soldiers, the famous *Institut zur Erforschung der Folgeerscheinungen von Hirnverletzungen.* He had not forgotten Wernicke's emphasis on the need for intensive psychological studies of the patients, yet he felt that his own preparation was inadequate for such an undertaking, and cast about for an experimentally trained psychologist. He found Adhémar Gelb, his junior by a decade, who had taken a doctorate with Stumpf, and who was to become his closest collaborator and friend.

The Institute developed into a large clinical center for diagnosis, treatment and rehabilitation of neurological and psychiatric military casualties. The early publications deal with the practical problems encountered: there are discussions of bullet injuries to brain, spinal cord and peripheral nerves; papers on war neuroses and hysterical symptoms; articles on the role of the nurse in the rehabilitation program, on expert testimony, on disability benefits, etc. A technical manual entitled *Die Behandlung, Fürsorge und Begutachtung der hirnverletzten Soldaten* appeared in 1919. For Goldstein these were not mere clinical problems: these were the real problems of the human patients, and their solution the only ultimate justification for whatever systematic studies were undertaken.

Advanced students and junior colleagues soon began to join the ongoing research activity. Some of these were psychologists, such as Egon Weigl, now at the German Academy of Sciences in East Berlin, of whom Goldstein always spoke with special warmth. Others came from medicine: Walther Riese, a neurologist and historian of neurology; Frieda Fromm-Reichmann, who was to become one of the pioneers in the psychoanalytic treatment of psychotic patients. Olivia Rosenthal had been an actress and was to work on problems of tactile and auditory localization. Then there was Aron Gurwitsch who travelled from physics and mathematics to philosophy and explored psychology on the way to phenomenology. He later interpreted Goldstein's theory of aphasia in phenomenological terms, and he became a lifelong friend.

The systematic studies can be divided—somewhat arbitrarily, somewhat chronologically and with a good deal of overlap—into four major phases. The earliest studies concerned the relationship between circumscribed cortical injuries and sensory or motor defects, and they foreshadowed the later handbook chapters. Next came the problems of perceptual disturbances and agnosia and, with them, the initiation of the *Psychologische Analysen hirnpathologischer Fälle*, a series of 14 papers, some of them of monograph length, the first appearing in 1918 and the last in 1932. The majority of these dealt with questions of visual perception in patients with damage of the optic tracts or occipital lobes. Here are the studies on the pseudofovea, on the loss of surface colors, on visual agnosia and its influence on tactile recognition and motor functions.

The early and mid-twenties saw an expansion of these problems into the area of cerebellar function and its relation to tonus and tonus disturbances. Among the several papers on this topic is the well-known one on the influence of colors on postural responses.

The same period also saw a consolidation of what had been learned, in the form of major handbook chapters or articles: one on experimental techniques for the study of cutaneous sensations in Abderhalden's *Handbuch der Biologischen Arbeitsmethoden;* another on diseases of the brain and meninges in Mohr's *Handbuch der inneren Medizin.* With Cassirer, Nonne and Pfeiffer, Goldstein undertook to edit the 7th edition of Oppenheim's *Lehrbuch,* and he contributed more than five hundred pages of the final text. A few years later, and perhaps most important of all, there were two long chapters in Bethe's *Handbuch,* one on the cerebellum and one on localization on the cerebral cortex.

Amidst all these studies and preoccupations there had been one that in terms of publication dates—and only in these terms—had lain dormant for almost a decade: the problem of aphasia. Wernicke had first introduced Goldstein to this topic, which was to become perhaps the most enduring preoccupation throughout his life. Goldstein's first paper on aphasia was published in 1906, and another dozen had appeared in print prior to his return to Frankfurt. The monograph *Die transkortikalen Aphasien* had been completed in Königsberg, but appeared only in 1917, dedicated to Edinger. It was a thorough analysis of the psychological processes affected by the various forms of this complex group of aphasic syndromes, a consideration of the correlated anatomical lesions and a discussion of the whole problem of cerebral localization, all based on a survey of the published case material supplemented by Goldstein's own observations. Two or three preliminary papers on amnesic aphasia had followed. Now, eight years and literally hundreds of hours of study later, there appeared the paper on the nature of amnesic aphasia, to be followed in the next several years by a step-by-step analysis of the several and infinitely complex aspects of the whole problem.

The late twenties were to see yet another development of Goldstein's thinking: a growing interest in psychotherapy, a critical examination of Freud's writings, a rejection of much of psychoanalytic concepts and techniques, and an attempt to embody in the larger context of biology whatever he had learned from the neurological and psychiatric patients. A paper published in 1924 on "Analogous mechanisms of symptom formation in neurological and psychiatric illness, with special reference to compulsive symptomatology" had given the first intimation of this direction. In 1927 there appeared an article "On the relationship between psychoanalysis and biology." This was followed by a paper on the nature of anxiety, then, in 1931, by a long handbook chapter "On the plasticity of the organism; based on observations of patients with nervous diseases." Others were to follow even before *The Organism* appeared.

Meanwhile there was an academic career, editorships, societies. On Edinger's death, Goldstein had succeeded him in 1919 as Professor of Neurology at Frankfurt, one of the few universities which, at that time, had a chair in Neurology. Simultaneously he had become director of the Neurological Institute, and he had remained the director of the special institute for the brain injured soldiers. He held various associate editorships; of most interest to psychologists is that he was one of the founding editors of the *Psychologische Forschung* on whose masthead he appeared through volume 17 (1922-1933). In 1927 he became one of the founders of the International Society for Psychotherapy.

In 1930 a larger arena beckoned: A large municipal hospital in Berlin was planning a comprehensive department of neurology, to be housed in a new, specially constructed wing. Goldstein was offered the chairmanship of this department in conjunction with a teaching appointment in Neurology and Psychiatry at the University of Berlin. He accepted after brief hesitation, and with the proviso that he could continue an active association with the Brain Injury Institute in Frankfurt. He settled with high hopes into what was then perhaps the foremost position in his field in Germany, into what should have been his institutional home base for the remainder of his career. Alas, history was not to approve such plans.

Upon Hitler's assumption of power in January 1933, Goldstein was briefly jailed, then released on condition that he leave the country. The Rockefeller Foundation undertook to support him for a year in Amsterdam. It was to be a memorable year: Alone, living in a boarding house, without his family, without any clinical or teaching responsibilities, a period of enforced, uninterrupted leisure which he used to write what was to be his magnum opus, *The Organism*. He dictated the basic draft of this long and complex book in a matter of five or six weeks, leaving his secretary in a state of utter exhaustion. Not so Goldstein. After the day's work he enjoyed evenings of friendly Dutch hospitality and participated in the very active intellectual conviviality of Amsterdam in those years.

Der Aufbau des Organismus was brought out in Holland in 1934 in German. The English translation appeared in this country in 1939, under the title *The Organism: A Holistic Approach to Biology Derived from Pathological Data in Man*, with a foreword by Karl S. Lashley. It has gone through many printings since, has recently been brought out in paperback, and has been translated into many other languages. The book is addressed to biologists in the very broadest sense of the term, which ranges from anatomy and physiology through psychology, neurology, psychiatry and philosophy; it deals with methodological questions as much as, if not more than with facts, and it presents critical assessments of many major theoretical trends of its day and our own.

In 1935 Goldstein arrived in New York City where he settled down to private practice in Neurology and Psychiatry, even though he knew very little English at the beginning. He was appointed Clinical Professor of Neurology and Lecturer in Psychopathology at Columbia University, worked for a time at the Psychiatric Institute on 165th Street and later became chief of the newly organized Laboratory of Neurophysiology at Montefiore Hospital. Here, once again, he was joined by a psychologist, Martin Scheerer, who became an active and devoted collaborator and friend. Together they examined patients, taught medical students and psychologists, directed some Ph.D. dissertations and argued endlessly about problems and manuscripts. Together they published the monograph *Abstract and Concrete Behavior: An Experimental Study with Special Tests*, and assembled the prototypes of the testing materials that have since been distributed by the Psychological Corporation. Another joint monograph, written together with Eva Rothmann—Mrs. Kurt Goldstein in private life—described their intensive studies of an "idiot savant," a mentally defective boy with a phenomenal calender memory. The untimely deaths of first Gelb and then Scheerer, both Goldstein's juniors by many years, were among the few blows of fate to which he never reconciled himself.

During the winter of 1938/39 he was invited by Harvard University to deliver the William James Lectures. They were subsequently published under the title *Human Nature in the Light of Psychopathology*, with a foreword by Gordon W. Allport. The next year, in 1940, he accepted the post of Clinical Professor of Neurology at Tufts College Medical School, a position which, on Leonard Carmichael's suggestion, had been underwritten by the Rockefeller Foundation for five years. Those five years were, I think, very happy years for him. He spent mornings at the laboratory at the Boston Dispensary, afternoons in private practice and at his writing. In addition to a steady stream of articles, he published, in 1942, the book *Aftereffects of Brain Injuries in War, Their Evaluation and Treatment;* and completed major sections of the manuscript of *Language and Language Disturbances,* a treatise on aphasia that was to appear in 1948. For a while he went once a week to Worcester State Hospital where he was welcomed with open arms by David Shakow and the students and staff of the psychological laboratory. Among the work resulting from these visits was the monograph *Case Lanuti: Extreme Concretization of Behavior Due to Damage of the Brain Cortex* which was published in 1944 together with Eugenia Hanfmann and Maria Rickers-Ovsiankina.

He had many friends in Cambridge. Robert Ulich and Aron Gurwitsch were at Harvard. So was the daughter of his old mentor, Tilly Edinger, a paleo-neurologist at the Museum of Comparative Zoology. In Gordon Allport he found an ever-sympathetic ear and sounding board for ideas. And whenever Lashley was in town they would get together. Goldstein felt very close to Lashley, both with regard to their common theoretical orientation and also personally. Although their conversation was always in English, Goldstein used to say about Lashley that he was "so European," and that was why one could discuss problems with him so well. He also enjoyed Mrs. Lashley and appreciated both Lashleys' interest in music—an interest which Goldstein had never lost, even though he generally made little use of it.

These were the years of the Second World War. Goldstein had become an American citizen in 1940, and once a week he examined inductees for the local draft board. He had always been interested in political events, and followed the war news daily from the morning CBS World News Round-Up to Raymond Graham Swing at night. His own history, that of his friends, in fact of his whole generation made for an intensely personal involvement in the progress of the war—and yet, it would be erroneous to say that he was identified with the "American" enterprise. His comment on news of victories was typically: "Das haben die Amerikaner doch eben grossartig gemacht." Not once did I hear him say "we" in this connection. He always felt as a stranger among friendly natives. He was grateful to the country where he and so many others had found asylum first, and then a new home—but it was still a home in exile. When he appreciated things American, or criticized them, it was always as an outsider, a spectator. His English was never effortless, and he was not unaware of the restrictions which an English-language situation imposed on him: he became more circumspect, less critical, and he felt he could not really pursue a discussion to its limits. Nor was it only the language. It was the American experience that he lacked. In part, I think, it was also a difference of generations. Most of the "Americans" of his acquaintance were a generation or two younger, and the difference in experience was historical as much as geographical. For example, he would often comment on the lack of tradition on this side of the Atlantic. I remember once replying that all the tradition in the world would not help anyone to even the tiniest hamburger, be it here or in Europe. His immediate reply was "Ach was," followed by "The younger generation thinks only of its stomach," and, finally by "You are probably right, and that is just what is so awful." I never could argue him out of that final adjective.

In 1945 the Tufts appointment came to an end. Goldstein was 67 years old, and, by the rules of academic life, should have retired. This was as unthinkable for him temperamentally as it was impossible financially. He returned to New York City to private practice and various teaching activities. For a few years he taught at City College and at the Graduate Faculty of the New School for Social Research; then, in his late seventies, he began to commute once a week to Brandeis University. During these years he developed a new love and enthusiasm: his American students. He never tired of talking about "his" City College students, and later the graduate students at Brandeis: how intelligent they were, how genuinely interested in the problems, how hard working, how they would not settle for the easy answers.

In 1958 the larger world joined in the celebration of Goldstein's eightieth birthday. Several generations of students and friends assembled to present him with a collection of manuscripts especially collected for the occasion. Two groups of these were subsequently published in two special Goldstein Anniversary issues of the *Journal of Individual Psychology* and the *American Journal of Psychotherapy;* the remainder appeared in various specialty journals. The Hebrew University sent a beautiful scroll, composed in his honor, and the University of Frankfurt awarded him the *Doctor Honoris Causa.*

Goldstein's final years were often lonely. In 1960 Mrs. Goldstein died. Thereafter a cousin kept house for him with great devotion. His oldest daughter and her family moved to be near him, and he came to depend on their company. He enjoyed sharing his thoughts with his daughter and son-in-law, and was pleased when both obtained advanced degrees in psychology. He had published well over 300 articles and books, and for many years his writings had influenced the international community of scholars: from the early nineteen-twenties when his observations and theories of aphasia had had a profound impact on the British neurologist Sir Henry Head, to the post-World War II and recent publications by Maurice Merleau-Ponty who presented Goldstein's ideas to French philosophers and psychologists. Yet he continued to write. A draft for his autobiographical contribution to volume V of *The History of Psychology in Autobiography* was completed in the spring of 1965. Withall, he complained of tiring easily, and he felt himself getting old. Many of the friends of his own generation had died, as had so many younger ones: first Adhémar Gelb; then Kurt Koffka, whom he had gotten to know well in the thirties; then Max Wertheimer, whose colleague he had been at Frankfurt; then Ernst Cassirer, the cousin who shared his interests and thoughts, and who had been the first to call attention to the philosophical significance of Goldstein's work; then Albert Einstein, an old friend; then Karl S. Lashley, the "American" friend; then Martin Scheerer; and finally Heinz Werner, of whom he had become very fond, although they had never been personally close. Even so, he was surrounded until the end by a number of friends who were intellectually attached and personally devoted to him, and with whom he remained in constant contact. One of these must be especially mentioned: Meyer Schapiro, the art historian, whose wisdom and humanity he shared. Other friends, New Yorkers or out-of-towners, would call him more or less frequently, and then witness the battle between his joy of their having called and his acute distaste for the telephone.

He fell ill while staying with friends in Vermont. A stroke soon after his return to New York City left him paralyzed on the right side and unable to speak. Having studied aphasia all of his life, and in unsurpassed depth, he now indicated by gestures that he was unable to speak, and he took his paralyzed arm in his left hand and let it drop to indicate his inability to move it. He died three weeks later, on September 19, 1965, in New York City.

Reprinted with minor changes and corrections from the *Journal of the History of the Behavioral Sciences*, 1966, *2*, 185–191, by permission.

2

Kurt Goldstein

by Robert Ulich
Cambridge, Massachusetts

It is often difficult to determine which sources of influence have molded one's own thinking, but I believe that my conception of education has been deeply affected by Kurt Goldstein's writings on the psychophysical nature of man.

Nothing, however, has contributed more to the sense of inner community between Kurt Goldstein and me than the intimate conversations in our homes and on our walks in the woods of New Hampshire where my late wife and I had rented a cottage in the neighborhood of Mt. Monadnock.

It was there that Goldstein revealed to me the deeper motives which had brought about his understanding of humanity and its place in the universe. So far as I know he was not influenced by any institutional form of religion. Being a Jew was for him more a destiny than a mission. But he certainly was a profoundly religious man. Although his scientific conscience would never have allowed him to mingle philosophical speculation with empirical investigation, he, like Albert Einstein, could not cease wondering about the gigantic phenomenon of life.

He looked at the mystery of individual being as embedded in the greater mystery of the totality of Being. The visible and comprehensible in the cosmos of things pointed, so he thought, at the invisible and incomprehensible sources of the creation, and he fully accepted the dictum of Goethe (who was to him the consummation of wisdom) that we should courageously explore the explorable but stand in awe before the inexplorable.

Kurt Goldstein once referred admiringly to the young Goethe's essay *Über den Granit* (1783) from which I quote a few lines in somewhat free translation:

> I am not afraid of the reproach that a mere fancy for self-contradiction has caused me to pass from the investigation of the human heart, that youngest, most sensitive, agile, changing and so easily broken part of the creation[1] to the oldest, firmest, deepest and most unperturbable son of nature [i.e., granite]. For one will probably

[1] Goethe refers here to his *Leiden des Jungen Werther* of the year 1774, and other products of his *Sturm und Drang.*

> admit that all natural things are most intimately related to each other and that the searching mind refuses to be excluded from anything within its reach.
>
> So one will, I hope, allow me, who has suffered and still suffers from so many storms and rapid commotions in his own heart and the heart of others—one will, I trust, grant me the sublime peace which we receive from immersing into the solitude and quiet greatness of nature [knowing that the rock of granite on which we rest connects us with the center of the earth].

Kurt Goldstein often quoted the mature Goethe's philosophical poems, which he knew by heart:

> Was wär' ein Gott, der nur von aussen stiesse,
> Im Kreis das All am Finger laufen liesse,
> Ihm ziemt's, die Welt im Innern zu bewegen,
> Natur in Sich, Sich in Natur zu hegen,
> So dass, was in ihm lebt und webt und ist,
> Nie Seine Kraft, nie Seinen Geist vermisst.

Which reads, again freely translated:

> What kind of God!—pushing the world from outside,
> Letting it spin in circles round His finger!
> He wants the Cosmic All to be His dwelling.
> Diffused and clad in Universal Being,
> He wishes that whatever grows and strives
> Would feel that from his spirit all derives.

Once he remarked about the *Farbenlehre:* "Obviously, Goethe was scientifically wrong, but ultimately he was right in his protest against Newton's mechanical picture of the world. The future may show that both were right."[2]

Kurt Goldstein was a "mystic," if we understand mysticism not in the vulgar sense, as another kind of superstition and undisciplined intuition, but in the sense of the reverential attitude of the disciplined mind which realizes the limits of the human intellect and feels at the same time the power of the Great Unknown within and around it.

[2] A short paper by Kurt Goldstein on Goethe's Methods of Scientific Inquiry bears out Professor Ulich's remarks and may be of interest to the reader. It was published in German under the title: "Bemerkung zum Vortrag von Prof. Otto Meyerhof: Ueber Goethe's Methoden der Naturforschung," in *Proceed. Rudolf Virchow Med. Soc., N.Y.*, 1949, *9*, 110–112.—*Editor.*

It was this awareness of the metaphysical in life that rendered Goldstein suspect to minor minds who still adhered to atomistic forms of behaviorism and who wondered suspiciously about his many-sided interests, which extended from medical research to psychology and philosophy. What was he really, they asked: a physician, a psychologist, or a philosopher? Patient and kind though he was in his ordinary life (his soft Silesian accent was characteristic of his personality) he was angry at those of his colleagues and students who believed they had a monopoly on true scholarship because they identified "research" (with the accent on the first syllable) with absence of imagination. At least I can find no other reason for the opinion that it was difficult "to get along with that German professor."

At the time of his Brandeis lectures in the middle of the 1950's, Kurt Goldstein stayed at my home in Cambridge. During our long breakfast—we both disliked a hurried beginning of the day—he contemplated his own life. It had been an unusually productive life, but also one of grief and disappointment. The forced emigration had wounded him beyond recovery, not only personally, but also as a reflection of the dark abyss in the depth of humanity. He spoke of the eternal human problems of sin and guilt which appeared in every man's life, and of the incapacity of even those closest to one another to help in times of distress.

When I saw Kurt Goldstein the last time in his New York home, I felt in him, as I could see it in every painting and piece of furniture, the influence and loving care of a highly cultured woman, his cousin, Mrs. Falk. We sat around the well-bedecked table, drank an excellent Mosel wine and talked about old friends and their interests. I left him, feeling inspired at having been in the presence of a great man, a man whose insight and mature serenity had enabled him to combine into a noble synthesis the many antitheses of human existence. Goethe, so it seemed to me, had returned to him. I heard later that he often asked his cousin to read to him from Goethe's works.

Soon thereafter he was struck by the illness from which he never recovered.

3

Kurt Goldstein—The Man and His Work

by Walther Riese

Glen Allen, Virginia

The man whose memory we are celebrating made a place for himself in the history of neurology. The history of neurology can be divided into three epochs. At its inception neurology was purely clinical, and the result of a slow process extending over centuries. It was directed towards the isolation and description of great clinical pictures, such as epilepsy, apoplexy, paralysis agitans, etc.; but it remained a chapter of the general doctrine of diseases which in its turn became internal medicine. The second epoch fell at the end of the nineteenth century and the first third of the twentieth century. Neurology at that time was strongly neuro-anatomical and neuropathological. An avenue to a new foundation of neurology on an anatomical basis seemed to be opened by Vesalius in the sixteenth century and certainly by the so-called school of neuropathologists of the eighteenth century. But the establishment of this new foundation suffered a surprising retardation until it became a reality rather suddenly and rapidly in the nineteenth century. The great French clinicians of the 19th century intended no more than to *complete* the clinical picture by anatomical findings in order to obtain a total picture of a given disease. But at the turn of the century the tendency to *interpret*, if not to *explain*, nervous diseases by structural changes became increasingly evident. Anatomy usurped the leading role in the doctrine of diseases which henceforth appeared to be deprived of their dynamics and their chronological features. This view reflected a crude mechanics of a distorted life, leaving room for *organized* structures but not for *organizing* principles. We seem to have entered a third epoch, a neurosurgical one, a legitimate offspring of the second epoch but showing a strong tendency to make therapeutical use of neuro-anatomical data. Since the life processes appear to this generation to be sufficiently explained by the system of centers and pathways, the destruction of nodal points and the severance of connections or associations were expected to produce changes in vital and nervous processes, i.e., dysfunction and disease, but, strangely enough, also the opposite, i.e., improvement or even cure.

None of the three epochs can be understood correctly without a thorough evaluation of the medical, cultural and social foundations of the respective era, the educational standard, the intellectual structure and needs of physician and patient. The legacy left to posterity by the third epoch might be an impersonal, anonymous and interchangeable disease picture and a therapeutical procedure, often applying drastic and precarious means, a procedure not always supported by an insight previously obtained into the working of the method applied, though this insight has remained the prerequisite of an intelligible and intelligent cure since the days of the Greeks.

Goldstein's neurological efforts and achievements fell mainly in the second of the three epochs here distinguished. He himself has made more than one contribution to neuroanatomy, comparative neurology and neuropathology, enlarging considerably our factual knowledge in these areas. Above all, his studies on the development of the *corpus callosum*, i.e., the great structure connecting the two cerebral hemispheres, the brain of the *Teleostei*, and the atrophy of the *substantia nigra* in post-encephalitic Parkinsonism must be cited in this connection. But his work on the doctrine of *cerebral localization* exceeds all other investigations of this kind. Very soon and very vigorously Goldstein opposed the overstressing of the anatomical viewpoint in cerebral localization. He did this at a time when neuroanatomy celebrated true triumphs in clinical fields and even in physiological psychology. Goldstein denied neither the significance of structures nor the possibility of cerebral localization. He only wanted to relegate both to their proper fields and keep both within their own limits. He was searching for a constructive formula of those functions which are accessible to cerebral representation and localization. His thought was constantly dominated by the idea of a total, unitary function of all nervous events—indeed of all organic events. This prevented him from localizing more than the most elementary primitive functions of motion and sensation (his "periphery of the brain"). In a sense, this view was anticipated by his early work on hallucinations. Though at that time he considered hallucination still as a regionally-determined disorder, he postulated, in addition to the activity of the sensory centers, an extensive involvement of the cerebral cortex. Similarly, he believed it to be impossible to derive the judgment of reality solely from a quantitative criterion of perception. This judgment, he said, rests instead on the awareness of a correspondence within the total and actually available field of perception; it is, he concluded, a critical function of the entire psyche. There was a time in his career when he was convinced that the *Gestalttheorie* was the answer to his problems and, particularly, to the problem of cerebral localization. But ultimately he found his own formula. Cerebral activity, he said, is always a total one, but always with ever-changing regional accents, in accordance with the needed and more or less activated structures, an ever-changing play of *figures* and *backgrounds*. Goldstein was one of the first and the few to adopt and to defend vigorously C. von Monakow's revision of the traditional version of cerebral localization. C. von Monakow rejected a localization of functions and allowed no more than a localization of symptoms, i.e., disturbed functions. He advanced the thesis that every attempt to localize successive events, particularly the so-called "superior" activities (language, purposeful acts, gnosis) is condemned to failure, because of the *history* of cerebral functions and the universality of excitations affecting necessarily the entire brain in the course of this history (chronogenetic localization). In Goldstein's interpretation it is the *actual* situation which dominates the cerebral picture. Goldstein did not consider the study of the history of nervous function to be his task. In his view, the driving forces of normal and abnormal cerebral events are the actual situation, its demands, their relation to the possibilities still remaining to the individual and his attempts to solve the problems set before him, even though these may overpower him and elicit "catastrophic reactions." The structures and the regional factor contribute to the figure that stands out against the background of the total excitation.

It is the ever-changing or alternating, thus the dynamic nature of nervous function, which is expressed by Goldstein in terms of the figure-background process. The terms have been borrowed from visual experience, more specifically from the famous figure designed by Rubin for the demonstration of the alternation phenomenon (we see now a white vase on a black background, now two black faces on a white background). Goldstein introduced this phenomenon as a dynamic model of nervous function at a time when the static view in the purely spatial terms of centers, tracts, and connections was still uncontested; he most obviously and most courageously challenged the conventional and traditional teaching and learning in this area of neurology. But he was far from denying factual evidence. That a functional disorder, i.e., a symptom (such as aphasia, apraxia, agnosia, etc.) can be correlated with a regional cerebral lesion is indeed a fact. But these observations, though countless in number, justify no more than a cerebral localization of symptoms, which Goldstein admitted; they do not justify a localization of the undisturbed functions, which Goldstein rejected. The observational material which the neurologist and neuropathologist have in front of them, are individuals suffering from disordered functions, and, in the event of death and autopsy, their brains. Conclusions reached from these observations must be in terms of the material explored. But nobody ever was able to test in an intact individual the cerebral localization of undisturbed language which is more than just inarticulate sounds uttered by an individual on regional electrical stimulation of his cerebral cortex. It seems justified to assume, Goldstein concluded—with caution—that to each performance corresponds excitation of definite structures in the cortex, not at a circumscribed area, but widespread over the whole cortex. This is what Goldstein saved from a shipwrecked cerebral localization.

Goldstein tried to ascribe a still greater scope to the alternating reactions just mentioned. Not only did he believe alternating reactions to be frequent in patients with mental diseases; above all, he interpreted them as the detachment of a part of the organism from the rest or, in significantly Goldsteinian terms, as *actions in isolation*. With this distinctive feature he reached his own definition of the concept of "primitive," deprived by him of all phylogenetic or developmental criteria. He challenged the view held by Lévy-Bruhl and others, according to which the behavior of primitive people shows an inferior mentality—an expression of a prelogical stage of mind. People in primitive societies may not be inferior, Goldstein concluded; their behavior may correspond to what he has characterized as concrete behavior. It was Goldstein's principle of investigation and interpretation to reach out for the greatest possible application of experiential data which to most of his contemporaries remained lifeless singularities buried in the closed workshop of their craft. This is the reason why there was often little difference between Goldstein's professional and his conversational language, and perhaps even between Goldstein, the scientist and Goldstein, the man. In his last letter addressed to me, he wrote that his memory was failing, and that he remembered only the pleasant things of his life; and further, that he considered this selective recollection to be in full conformity with his "theory." When I asked him to be a little more specific as to that part of his "theory" to which he was referring, it was already too late. The statement thus stands as a sort of a scholar's last will in terms of the closed career of his scientific mind; as so frequently in a last will, the deeper meaning lies hidden behind the words and may be explored in the future.

It is primarily from his observations of brain-injured persons that Goldstein derived the criteria of disease. More specifically, the condition which he called "catastrophic condition," taught him "the essential characteristics" of being sick: first, disordered behavior which makes the individual unable to use his capacities and so to come to terms with the demands of his environment; second, anxiety. Disordered behavior and anxiety, he said, are the objective and subjective expressions of the situation of danger in which the organism is when it is no longer able to actualize its essential capacities, i.e., to "exist." It is this "hindrance of self-actualization" which became the target of the intense psychotherapy advocated and practised by one of Goldstein's early and most distinguished associates, the late Dr. Frieda Fromm-Reichmann.

There are implied in Goldstein's view of cerebral localization constituents which characterize his attitude, his observational and experimental results in other fundamental problems of neurology. Again, his tendency toward holistic views must be cited. It was this holistic view which led him to reject any isolated event in an organism living under natural conditions. The final result was his rejection of the reflex as a useful model of neural processes; this meant no less than the rejection of the foundation of the neurology of his generation. Audaciously, he attacked the traditional hierarchy of reflexes, their complex constitution out of elements, their coupling, switching, shunting, facilitation and inhibition, a terminology reflecting the laboratory of the experimental physicist rather than the observation of the physiologist. Goldstein later applied this interpretation to psychoanalysis, which he saw as resting on a similar isolating and decomposing procedure, and as revealing a tendency to construct human behavior and fate out of isolated types of behavior—the so-called complexes, that were increasing in number, just as the almost countless isolated reflexes in neurology. His investigations of the so-called "induced tonus phenomena" furnished new material to support his holistic views. Inspired by Sherrington's discovery of "decerebrate rigidity" and the analysis of the posture of an animal decerebrated by a section at the midbrain level, Magnus and his associates had described a number of new reflexes which could be elicited from parts of the body at rest, or in motion, and which determined an appropriate distribution of the involuntary tension, or tonic innervation, of remote parts of the body. The posture, falling, righting, and locomotion of an animal thus prepared seemed to result from these reflexes which became known as tonic neck reflexes, righting reflexes and postural reflexes. Goldstein demonstrated these reflex actions in the intact human subject. Moreover, he was able to show that in these reflexes the relation between stimulating and stimulated organ is reversible. Their release is possible from both sides, thus indicating a reciprocal influence. But is this result, one must ask, still compatible with the traditional diagrammatic scheme, according to which stimulation and reaction occupy the two fixed extreme positions of the reflex arc and which, as a rule, are not interchangeable? Goldstein here opened an avenue to a *rational* interpretation of the organism, which rests on the interdependence and the reciprocity of the parts. The activity of each part is influenced by that of every other part, and vice versa. (It is true that Goldstein himself did not draw this conclusion). Thus we come to understand Goldstein's skeptical attitude towards a hierarchical order within the organism and the whole chain of living beings.

Things are quite different in experimental and pathological conditions. We then have to face an organ reduced by artificial or natural means and an isolated incident. Goldstein described the mode of function of the central nervous system in experimental or pathological conditions as *dedifferentiation*. By this expression as well as by his emphasis on the difference between the immediate effects of injury (loss of function) and the altered mode of functions of the preserved (now isolated) parts, he acknowledged, though unwittingly, Hughlings Jackson's legacy. Jackson established increasing differentiation as an essential criterion of evolution, loss of differentiation as a criterion of dissolution, or the reverse of evolution. Jackson also set forth the basic difference between negative and positive symptoms. Goldstein listed the following criteria of dedifferentiation:

1) A raised threshold; 2) reduced responsiveness to stimulation; and 3) defective power to differentiate between qualities. He listed the following effects of isolation: 1) Forced responsiveness; 2) abnormal dependency upon the quality of the stimulus; 3) extension of the stimulus effect with respect to space and time; and 4) the phenomenon of alternation between opposite reactions.

Goldstein did not accept the assumption of a disinhibited activity of the isolated parts; in this, he deviated from Jackson and the English neurological tradition. The Babinski sign was not considered by Goldstein as a disinhibited, phylogenetically old reflex, but as a reversal of the conditions of excitability. The Babinski phenomenon is a rudiment of a flight reaction whose first phase it represents. Similarly, the automatisms of the legs seen in transverse lesions of the spinal cord, are not "walking movements," but indications of the lowered stability of the figure formation. It is an essential element of Goldstein's doctrine of method to avoid conclusions drawn from external resemblances which are often misleading. An observational or experimental result does not gain its true importance until all conditions under which the result is obtained are known and appreciated. To this end, the most careful recording and evaluation of even the most insignificant detail are needed; this might be called the Hippocratic element in Goldstein's doctrine of method; no prejudice, no cherished theory should be allowed to interfere with this principle. A patient seems to solve the task set before him; actually he failed because surreptitiously he solved another task, or he solved the task in a way different from the way he was supposed to solve it.[1] No more conclusive evidence of the truth of this observation could be offered than the analysis of the famous patient Schn. who suffered from visual agnosia, resulting from an injury to the occipital areas. On superficial observation he did not seem to offer any disorder of visual recognition. Only on patient and repeated examination, extending over years, did it become evident that he did not reach recognition by visual means but by the most minute movements of his head, which allowed him to invent and to elaborate a system of rapid and imperceptible tracings of visual objects. These tracings served as a *detour* by means of which he reached a kinetic and perfect gnosis. The traditional explanation of an isolated loss of visual representations was no longer workable; the assumption of a rearrangement and reform of the whole gnostic system was unavoidable. Goldstein later demonstrated that such rearrangements occur only when the defect is a total one; in a sense, the totally injured individual is better off than the partially injured one. This is particularly obvious in the formation of a new fovea of best vision in total hemianopia. Anatomically speaking, the new fovea is located in the periphery of the retina, thus strengthening the view that structures do not invariably correspond to related functions. It is not enough simply to state the result of a given examination: data are ambiguous, they derive their significance from the way or detour by which they are obtained. This leads to the necessity to define the relation between a given task and the patient tested. An individual suffering from the inability to perform purposeful movements (apraxia) may not be able to purse his lips. But he may whistle a song without any difficulty.

The difference of the result lies in the difference of the procedure by which, in the first case, a consciously isolated, meaningless, and purposeless act is performed, whereas in the second case, a meaningful and integrated act is intended.

Similar observations had been made by H. Jackson on the aphasic patient who, depending on the particular situation, does or does not have a given word at his command. Jackson was satisfied with the explanation that in aphasia, emotional or inferior speech may be preserved, though intellectual or propositional speech is seriously affected. This interpretation is significant of the spirit of the nineteenth century inasmuch as it traces the difference in result to the difference in *segments* of function. In Goldstein's view, it is always the *total* situation, the task to be solved, in brief, it

[1] He called this the "fallacy of effects."

is life which determines the effect, and which is always the manifestation of the whole individual. This, however, does not justify a retreat from the essential task of determining with precision how the patient as a whole behaves under changing conditions, and how he solved the problem at stake. Only after reaching a complete understanding of the always total and never aimless behavior of the patient, may his behavior be explained. It is in this area that Goldstein's observations of brain-injured soldiers of the first World War reached their full significance. Again, the fruitfulness and novelty of his method came to the fore. It was the nature of his observational material, but also Goldstein's individual structure and affinity, which let him face the task as a psychological one; he undertook it in close cooperation with Gelb, a psychologist of stature. Disregarding the conventional and paralyzing separation of organic processes from so-called "functional" ones, Goldstein approached the psychological and psychopathological analysis of the functions and types of behavior of brain-injured individuals. Nobody had done it before him.

It is true that Goldstein, on one occasion, cited his own teacher, Karl Wernicke, as his forerunner. Wernicke, Goldstein said, "tried to understand the symptoms of the patients psychologically and to combine this understanding with the findings of their brains." But in reading Wernicke's original texts, one learns that, after having drawn an anatomical blueprint of aphasia, Wernicke tried to deduce from his diagrammatic scheme the various types of speech defects resulting from brain lesions. This was the point of departure for Freud's critical study on aphasia, that masterpiece of neurological thought by an author—at that time still a neuropathologist and in his early years—who, as he confessed himself, had no personal observation on aphasia to offer. What distinguished Wernicke's approach from that of Freud and, above all, of Goldstein, was that Wernicke used the anatomical findings as first principles of the interpretation of aphasia, a procedure very different from that of Goldstein. It may have been Goldstein's devotion to his teacher which induced him, generous as he was, to claim Wernicke as his forerunner. But it makes all the difference whether one merely combines anatomy with symptomatology, as did Wernicke, or whether one studies and interprets the nature and genesis of aphasia on its own grounds and in its own terms. These must be those of language and thought, not those of cerebral tissue, which can neither speak, nor understand, nor write, in brief, which cannot communicate, language being the most refined and noble means of communication.

If Goldstein had done no more than to apply psychological methods and analyses to severe organic injuries, he would have secured his place in the history of experiential sciences.

It was customary—and may still be—to abdicate functional or psychological analysis as soon as destruction reached beyond microscopical size. Should it be true, as the late V. von Weizsäcker once asked, that in the final analysis the difference between "functional" and "organic" threatens to be no more than a difference in magnification? It is true that Goldstein never gave up the traditional difference between "functional" and "organic." But it remains equally true, that as an interviewer, he never allowed himself to be overwhelmed or disarmed by anatomical findings suspected or demonstrated; and he never forgot that he addressed an individual, not a brain. He could have quoted Descartes, who once replied to one of his opponents: "One thing is certain: I know myself as a thought, and I positively do not know myself as a brain." Goldstein even reached the conclusion that many phenomena essential for psychotherapy can be seen more clearly in organic patients than in those with functional nervous diseases.

The atmosphere in Goldstein's Frankfurt hospital for brain-injured soldiers resembled that in family life. Patients, physicians, relatives, friends, and many citizens actively participated in the realization and maintenance of a serene and relaxed outlook. It is true, this could be suddenly and transitorily disrupted when, on the occasion of a celebration or a festivity, an epileptic attack or an explosive irritation of a patient painfully brought home to us the human misery we were witnessing and assisting.

At the time when Goldstein tried to explore the laws presiding over the functions and vital manifestations of brain-injured individuals, and to understand them psychologically, even psychoanalysis shrank from an analysis of organically damaged individuals. It is true that ultimately psychoanalysis is an offspring of the heroic era of neurology and its classifications. It was only later that P. Schilder had the courage to offer a psychoanalysis of general paresis. The historian can trace the origins of psychoanalysis to Paris. For a long time Vienna remained reluctant, to say the least, to accept that disturbing Freudian thought which had slowly matured ever since his attending the famous Tuesday lectures of Charcot.

Of all aspects of behavior displayed by individuals suffering from cerebral disease or injuries, it was language which attracted Goldstein's greatest interest in his early days. He published a great number of articles and monographs on the subject. I cannot trace here in detail the lines along which his view on disordered language or aphasia developed and matured.

The final result was reached by the analysis of amnesic aphasia and the inability of the patients to name colors; no other tool was needed than the well-known woolen skeins of Holmgren.

In the history of aphasia Goldstein stands in the forefront of those who reject explanations in terms of the so-called "elementary functions" (such as visual, acoustic, kinetic representations or images), their hypothetical anatomical substrata and their equally hypothetical associations. Like some of his predecessors, Goldstein was convinced that aphasia is the result of a fundamental and most general disorder. But unlike Trousseau and Pierre Marie, who were satisfied with the assumption of a rather vague intellectual disorder, Goldstein strove for a more precise definition of this disorder. Language, he said, is one of the essential characteristics of human nature, inasmuch as it is tied to man's highest capacity, the capacity for abstract behavior. He also called it categorical behavior, or the objectifying attitude, or even voluntary behavior. In the abstract attitude we are not directed toward an individual object but toward a category, of which that object represents itself only as an accidental example and representative. To this behavior Goldstein opposed the immediate concrete attitude, a more primitive type of behavior, in which the action is directly determined by momentary sense impressions, in which the individual is directed toward the concrete thing in its particular uniqueness, and in which words are used less as representative of categories than as individual properties, which, like other properties, belong to the object in question. Due to the cortical lesion, the (amnesic) aphasic is able to assume only the more concrete, the more realistic attitude . Not only speech, but also his general behavior is characterized by a greater concreteness, seen ultimately by Goldstein as a predominance of acting over thinking.

There can be no doubt that Goldstein's interpretation of aphasia is the most general ever conceived. He believed speech defects resulting from brain lesions reflect in a particular field the basic disturbances found in brain lesions at large, such as the inability to assume "a mental set" voluntarily, or to take initiative; the inability to distinguish in a given situation between essential and non-essential factors, or to understand the situation as a whole; the inability to shift voluntarily from one aspect of a situation to another; and, subsequently, the rigidity so significant of brain-injured persons who are stereotyped, compulsive and abnormally bound to stimuli from without and within; their inability to detach themselves from a given stimulus and to react simultaneously to two different stimuli, or to make a choice between them; consequently, their loss of freedom, the priority given by them to purely formal and external rather than inner principles of classification and order, their anxiety when facing emptiness, the incomplete demarcation of such individuals from their surrounding world, their inability to do anything which necessitates detaching the ego from the outer world, or from inner experiences. It was Goldstein's conviction that the same basic disorder may explain syndromes generally considered as different entities, such as aphasia, apraxia, agnosia, lack of orientation and attention, dementia, and even apparent lack of emotional response. To repeat, in still more generous terms, the basic disorder is defined by him as a more concrete attitude and opposed to a more abstract or categorical one. Goldstein was impressed by patients suffering from amnesic aphasia who named the color of a given object not simply blue, but sky-blue; not simply red, but blood-red; and who were unable to sort out woolen skeins according to the *category* of the name. Goldstein concluded that in these patients the name of the color was in indissoluble union with the object itself, and that the patient was no longer able to reach the name by *abstract* and purely *conceptual* thought. The world of the brain-injured patient, he concluded, has become a more individualized and a more intuitive one; the patient falls back on a more concrete attitude; has left the highest and specifically human level of abstract thought. To reach this conclusion, no more was needed than to listen carefully to the patient's answers.

But Goldstein did not want to consider the two types of behavior thus distinguished as the effects of two separate capacities; they are rather, he said, two levels of the capacity of the human being. Human existence presupposes the influence of both capacity levels. The abstract attitude must prepare the condition in which an individual can perform a demanded task. A task can never be performed with concrete behavior alone. The participation of one or the other approach in a performance differs according to the different significance of one or the other approach for the fulfilment of the task.[2]

If I were to formulate, in general terms, the significance of Goldstein's scientific career, achievements and teaching, I would be tempted to say that it was not so much a specific and limited result or doctrine, though these are not lacking, but his scientific enthusiasm, the continuity of labor and approach which stand out against a background of the most diversified subjects and tasks set before him in the changing conditions of his life; the changing academic and scientific climates in which he had to work; the

[2] *cf.* Riese, W. Type, evolution and localization of aphasia following neurosurgical relief in a 60 year old scientist affected by paralysis agitans. *Confinia Neurologica*, 1949, *9*, 216–225.

several changes of the structure of society during his life time; the rise and fall of doctrines of nervous function, human behavior and man's place on earth and in the universe. He never remained neutral or aloof from the mêlée of ideas. But he was nobody's unconditional follower or apologist. Instead, he tried to identify his own inner world *vis-à-vis* the tenets and terminologies of the great doctrines of his era, whether Gestaltpsychology, Psychoanalysis, Phenomenology or Existentialism. He always remained in close contact with the spirit, the voice and the demands of his time and of the young generation.

When subjecting a patient to an examination, he intended to forget all more-or-less dogmatic interpretations, allowing himself to be impressed and guided solely by an unprejudiced observation. He seemed to mark a new first start in the history of the patient and his disease. In a sense, his approach was deliberately naive, setting the patient in the limelight and shifting to the examiner the role of a teachable audience. The uninformed witness or unfriendly reader might misinterpret this approach and suspect that, under these circumstances, the examiner is the unavowed victim of the patient's graciousness or dishonest tendencies. There is no panacea for this suspicion other than to test the graciousness and the general trustworthiness of the patient, the examiner's self-evaluation, and, finally, the inner evidence of the patient's responses and reactions.

With these concluding statements I have reached one of the most earnest efforts made by Goldstein, the physician, i.e., never to allow the technical and professionalistic factor to overshadow the human figure of his patient. In spite of his scientific enthusiasm and the never-relaxing search for objective truth, it was always man who was in the center of his endeavor, man in health and disease, in wealth and poverty, in war and peace.

Two mutually contradictory processes of thought emerge from Goldstein's analysis of the organism: first, those of isolated activities versus the activity of the whole, and, second, those of concrete versus abstract behavior. The organism thus appears as a kind of higher truth that comprehends both and in which these contradictory processes merge themselves. Goldstein did not intend to project this thought process on its historical matrix; nor did he want to express this thought in the technical terms of a twofold dialectic. In his most revealing *Notes on the Development of my Concepts*[3] he nevertheless admitted the influence of philosophic ideas, particularly those of Kant, Ernst Cassirer and Edmund Husserl. He thought that it is not possible simply to carry over facts or concepts

[3] *cf.* Goldstein, K. Notes on the development of my concepts. *J. indiv. Psychol.*, 1959, *15*, 5–14.

from one field of knowledge to another; but he acknowledged with great satisfaction the acceptance of his views by some of Husserl's eminent adherents such as Aron Gurwitsch, Alfred Schütz and Maurice Merleau-Ponty.

A final word on Goldstein as a teacher. His was not the self-set task to introduce the beginner, step-by-step, to the elementary data of neurology, be they observational or experimental ones. His students and his associates had to be prepared from the very outset to face the *problems* arising from the situation in which the physician finds himself when interviewing and examining a patient, when testing the reactions of his nervous system, the functional disorders, the regional lesions and their pathological nature. The student learned neurology *in statu nascendi et crescendi*. Faithfully continuing the line of thought of one of his own teachers, Ludwig Edinger, Goldstein believed the writing of a scientific paper to be the safest road to conquering an as yet unfamiliar ground, affirming thereby the old truth: *docendo discimur*. Goldstein's method, his militant attitude towards all problems in front of him, his freedom from dependence upon paralyzing traditions, the rapidity with which he seized, examined, accepted or rejected new pathways and viewpoints—all these factors demanded from his students and associates the presence and almost constant activation of qualities and virtues which were bound to limit the number of his disciples. But nobody could escape the deep impression left by the passion of his investigation and his discourse.

This address was delivered at a meeting honoring the memory of Kurt Goldstein on March 27, 1966, at the New School for Social Research in New York City, N.Y.

4

Personal Impressions of Kurt Goldstein

by Gardner Murphy

Topeka, Kansas

I think of Kurt Goldstein as a presence; a genial and generous paternal figure; a prophetic figure; the realization of an ideal; or, in Aristotelian guise, a form working through an unstructured medium and giving it meaning; the embodiment of a way of conceiving the individual organism, and through it the life process upon the face of the earth. One needs the whole of Kurt Goldstein's life to see the entelechy, the self-actualization, the dialectic stages in the process of achieving full meaning.

The story of the vivid, imaginative, Central European Jewish boy who loved ideas whether from history, philosophy, natural science, or medicine is a familiar one. He was the realization of a type, even, we may say, without invidious distinctions, a Jewish intellectual type. Like Max Wertheimer with whom he can well be compared, he saw big meanings which gave a context for little meanings; like Fechner he contrasted seeing from below and seeing from above, but unlike Fechner, he was more and more drawn to the seeing from above. He could find no real place for the process of compounding the little until it makes the big. This, I think, was one of the reasons why, though the embodiment of an evolutionary age, he had no real traffic with the randomness of variation, selection, and adaptation. He could see adaptation only in terms of the fulfillment of an inherent pressure of the organism upon reality.

This, I think, is the meaning of the world-renowned studies of Gelb and Goldstein, which brought out the ultimate psychological character of brain damage in studies of men with skull and brain injuries from the battlefields of World War I. It was Goldstein's vision of wholeness that showed the *reconstitution* of the visual field. When, for example, the physical basis for a particular visual response had been shot away, the result was not a form loss, the removal of a detail because its physical basis was gone. On the contrary, there had to be a kind of normal vision. If the fovea as an anatomical and functional unit was no longer available, there had to be a "pseudo-fovea." If a stimulus fell partly upon a microptic region, partly upon a normally functioning region, the object would be seen as a whole in reduced form, but still in its normal guise; or if circumstances allowed, the whole object would be seen in its full normal size. The object would not be seen half in microptic, half in normal size, whatever the anatomical "demands" of the situation might be. What Gelb and Goldstein demonstrated was a unit character of visual response, a tendency of the brain to give a definition with the full meanings of the integral activity of the central nervous system itself. Indeed, going beyond what was then being discovered in British neurology by Henry Head and his collaborators, and what was being discovered by Max Wertheimer and his colleagues in experimental psychology, the reality was stated a bit more imaginatively in terms of a function not of the brain as such, not of the whole central nervous system as such, but the *organism* in its full integrity. A man as a man still has to see in holistic terms.

This led, of course, to philosophical issues of a sort already broached by vitalists on the one hand, and phenomenologists on the other hand. It raised questions about the real, or at least assumed necessity for working "parts" to be put together. It seemed to assume some sort of resolution of the whole-part problem. This was the problem solved by the Gestalt psychology of Wertheimer, Koffka, and Köhler in terms of the doctrine of "membership character," according to which the small is seen in the light of the large. It also implied some ideas not so remote from the holism of Smuts, the creativity doctrine of Bergson, the self-fulfillment of Driesch, and many other anti-atomistic doctrines of the early twentieth century. It would be petty to raise the question of whether Kurt Goldstein stood first chronologically or logically among the proponents of holistic thinking, for the essential fact is that he went *all the way*. He went as far as human thought in the era could allow. He went so far as to challenge Darwinian evolution on the one hand, and the whole scientific method of part-whole analysis on the other. The empirical data from the head-wounded subjects offered simply the embodiment of an idea which was taking shape in Goldstein's mind, and which continued to take shape in the next two decades until embodied—in his year as a refugee in Amsterdam, 1935—in his extraordinary book: *The Organism.*

This is, in a sense, a definitive book. It represents the deliberate driving of an idea to its limits. It allows no derivation of wholes from parts at any point. When he stood at the brink—the same brink at which Kurt Lewin stood when he decided that there *must* be parts somewhere, somehow—Goldstein took the alternative that there are no parts. There are just living organisms and their functions, their entelechies, their purposes, their modalities of living.

Changing again to a new intellectual habitat and climate, and arriving upon American shores among tens of thousands of intellectual refugees, he found himself welcomed by those who understood both the broad philosophy of his approach, and the specific neurological skills which he embodied. He was welcomed, for example, at The City College of New York, and at Brandeis University, and at one hospital after another, in which he showed the perceptual-cognitive reconstruction of life by the brain-damaged, and in the clinical settings in which, in collaboration with Martin Scheerer, he devised tests showing levels of intellectual operation depending upon the level of brain function. The Goldstein-Scheerer tests made clear to the clinically initiated the reduction from an abstract level of thought to a concrete level—for example, in a matching of colors—which indicated not a piece-by-piece loss of intellectual power, not a fragmentation, but a basic difference in the modality of the response. What appeared then in the patient who had lost his way in the floors and elevators of the hospital, appeared likewise in the response to the test situation. It was the brain-damaged man of World War I who held the lamp for the hospital and clinic examiners of the 'forties and 'fifties. The volume: *Human Nature in the Light of Psychopathology* which emerged was not a human nature with something missing; rather it was a human nature reduced by dire circumstance to a somewhat less fully human way of functioning.

To the question "What is man?" the reply must be given in terms of the fullness, and this must mean that perception, cognition, memory, and indeed motive, emotion, and personality must all share in the holistic redefinition. There is a place here for basic biotypes, a place for the understanding of different modalities of biological organization. Not that one is better than another; not that types lend themselves to an evaluative hierarchy; but rather, very simply, that some are more fully human because they are capable of more complete actualization of intrinsic humanity.

This formulation of the issue makes more clear, perhaps, why the great holistic leaders of the era—Wertheimer and Goldstein—could not quite fully agree. Wertheimer had pushed the study of perception as far as it could go in the direction of a new definition of the whole-part relationship, but throughout his years he clung to a cognitive conception of personality. This can be seen in his last book on *Productive Thinking*, in which there is an almost complete orientation to cognitive issues with hardly even an awareness of psychoanalytic and other dynamic interpretations of the thought process. It was only in his pupils, Arnheim and Wolff, that Wertheimer's Gestalt approaches to personality began to be developed experimentally, and ingenious as these are, they do not redefine the interrelations between cognition and the life of motivation. After all, it is expressive behavior that the Arnheim and Wolff studies emphasize, not the ultimate or inherent unity of personality as such. From an American point of view the difference, however, between the Wertheimer approach and the Goldstein approach seems much less impressive than the basic similarities, and the American psychologist can only regret that in Wertheimer's last years there was no full flowering of communication between Wertheimer and Goldstein.

Wertheimer died in 1943. Goldstein, allowed another two decades of life, became assimilated more and more intimately into American neurological, psychiatric, biological, psychological, group process; perhaps most of all, he became a living presence among psychologists who were interested in the ultimate structural and functional questions of man and environment. Psychologists had witnessed through the whole career of K. S. Lashley the renaissance of a belief in wholeness of central nervous system function, as against the localization theory of the late nineteenth century, and for them the persistent problems of "cerebral localization" made the Lashley emphasis a cardinal touchstone for modernness of thinking. It was in the doctrine of "equipotentiality" that Lashley had first defined such a holistic definition of brain function. Goldstein was understood in the frame of reference given by Lashley, just as Lashley had been understood by a number of German psychologists within the framework of German philosophy. Without quibbling about differences, it may properly be stressed that Lashley's trend of thought and Goldstein's trend of thought seemed to the rising generation of American psychologists, during the 'thirties and 'forties, to be almost equivalent. Something was gained and something lost by this almost literal equating of Goldstein and Lashley. But in the long run it was a gain, for it represented a new and vital way of viewing organisms, a view "from above." It was a view in which life, instead of being interpreted from beneath in terms of supposed physical and chemical processes of accretion and blind interaction, somehow sets the stage upon which physical and chemical realities can occur. The data are not all in, and the holistic biology is not yet written. Kurt Goldstein, however, had the courage and the vision to push the conception just as far as he knew how to push it. With charm, grace, and power he conveyed this message of the totality of life, and the life sciences of today need an ever-deeper understanding of this prophetic message.

II

ACTION

5

Suggestions for a Typology of the Apraxias

by HENRI HÉCAEN

Paris, France

Whatever the future of neuropsychology may hold, the work of Kurt Goldstein will always represent a major historical step in its development. The essence of his general thesis, as distilled in time, is part of our common heritage; many no longer even think to attribute to the original author the paternity of notions that now seem self-evident. Every chapter of our discipline continues to bear the marks of Kurt Goldstein's ideas. To be sure, his most famous investigations centered on specific topics, such as the aphasias and the agnosias; yet, there is no area in our field where some work of his did not leave its imprint. Thus, it seems entirely appropriate to dedicate to his memory a study of the apraxias.

In fact, we need only recall his presentations of an anatomico-clinical case of unilateral left ideomotor apraxia which constituted one of the first verifications of Liepmann's thesis (10); or his analysis of abstract and concrete motor performances in a patient with Pick's Disease published jointly with Katz; nor have we forgotten his brief but suggestive remarks in the book of 1948 on the defects of gesture and pantomime in aphasic patients.

HISTORICAL INTRODUCTION

The history of apraxia actually begins only with Liepmann's paper (19) on the case of the *Regierungsrat M.T.*, a case soon to become famous. Liepmann's precise description of the clinical disturbances of motor behavior led him to distinguish clearly the apractic syndrome from, on the one hand, defects of object manipulation due to impairment of their recognition and, on the other hand, from the incoherent gesticulations of the demented. He took the old term *apraxia*, utilized until then for faulty manipulation of objects due to gnostic disturbances, and added the qualifying adjective to coin the new term *motor apraxia*. However, Liepmann's paper contained more than clinical observations. The post-mortem examination of the patient's brain had shown lesions of the left hemisphere and the corpus callosum, and these formed the basis for a discussion of the problem of localization.

Following that publication, Bonhoeffer (2), Pick (25), Kleist (15) and, on repeated occasions, Liepmann himself (20) returned to the problem of the defects of motor performance and described various additional clinical aspects. Finally, in 1908, Liepmann (20) accomplished a synthesis of the clinical, anatomical and psychopathological aspects of apraxia and its different forms. For him, apraxia was a single, unitary disorder, an impairment of the mechanism of the voluntary act. Symptomatic variations resulted from the fact that this mechanism could be disturbed at different psychological levels. He distinguished three forms of apraxia:

1) *Melo-kinetic Apraxia*—described by Kleist as *innervatorische Apraxie*, resembling almost a simple paretic disorder and representing the loss of kinetic memory of one limb. It resulted from a lesion of the cerebral motor area which, were it more severe, would produce paralysis.

2) *Bilateral Ideomotor Apraxia*—corresponding to what Liepmann had originally called motor apraxia—was the result of the isolation of the *sensorium commune*, i.e., the parietal region of the left hemisphere, from the area of execution of the same hemisphere. If the lesion was in the corpus callosum and isolated only the right executive zone, ideomotor apraxia was limited to the left limbs.

3) *Ideational Apraxia*—corresponding to the disturbances described by Pick (25)—defects of the utilization of the most common objects even though these were recognized by the patient and named correctly. In this form the kinetics of the limbs were said to be intact, while the ideational progress of the act was disrupted. The syndrome resulted from left hemisphere lesions that were more diffuse and more posteriorly located than those giving rise to ideomotor apraxia.

And yet, for Liepmann, the whole memory of the complex act could not be limited to a circumscribed zone of the cortex, the central or parietal convolution; visual, tactile, kinesthetic and even acoustic elements must participate in the global memory image. A circumscribed focus of the lesion could thus hardly cause the loss of a motor memory.

This anatomico-clinical synthesis found rapid acceptance. It provided the inspiration for subsequent studies on the pathology of motor performance. Only von Monakow (22) and his student Brun (4) refused to grant any localization for the apraxias and proposed a purely descriptive classification.

After 1918 the problem was taken up again repeatedly: First within the framework of the physiological theory of Sittig (29), for whom apraxia was close to paralysis, with all the intermediaries existing between these two extremes of motor impairment; then as part of the attempt to unify gnostic and practic disorders (Poppelreuter (27), Foix (8), Morlaas (23), Schilder (28), Lhermitte (17, 18), Grünbaum (12)); and, finally, by the isolation of a new clinical aspect. In 1920 Kleist and Strauss (30) described constructive apraxia and related it to left posterior parietal lesions. In 1949 Russell Brain (3) isolated apraxia for dressing, and in 1950 and 1951 McFie, Piercy and Zangwill (21), on the one hand, and Hécaen, Ajuriaguerra and Massonet (13), on the other hand, described visuo-constructive defects due to lesions of the right hemisphere. In 1958 Denny-Brown (7) distinguished formally, on the basis of behavioral studies, between conceptual apraxias and kinetic apraxias; the latter are unilateral, and are the result of a rupture of the normal equilibrium between withdrawal and contact reactions; depending on the lesion, whether it is parietal or frontal, one of these two types of reaction predominates on one side of the body and interferes with the correct execution of gestures.

CLINICAL DEFINITION OF THE VARIETIES OF APRAXIA

Recent investigations have led us to a more systematic view of the various forms of impairment of motor action. They can be ordered according to their modes of appearance and associated clinical symptoms, an order that also corresponds to the anatomico-clinical findings, i.e., the hemispheric lateralization of the lesion.

In the first place, we retain only the four great classes of defective motor performance: 1) *Ideomotor Apraxia;* 2) *Ideational Apraxia;* 3) *Constructive Apraxia;* and 4) *Apraxia for Dressing.* All these meet Déjérine's (5) somewhat negatively stated criteria of apractic phenomena; that is, impairment of motor action in an individual whose executive apparatus is intact (i.e., absence of paralysis, ataxia or choreoathetosis) and who retains the understanding of the action to be performed (i.e., absence of gnostic disturbances and global intellectual defects). We do not include here melo-kinetic apraxia, bucco-linguo-facial apraxia, unilateral apraxias and apraxia of trunk movements or gait. On the one hand, these are often difficult to distinguish from defects of motor or psychomotor origin and, on the other hand, they do not appear to be correlated with the hemispheric lateralization of the lesion.

Ideomotor apraxia

The impairment is limited to simple acts while the ideational plan necessary for the production of complex activities is preserved. Complex actions can be executed while their constitutive elements are disturbed.

This practic disorder manifests itself either in the absence of response, or by diffuse, amorphous, synkinetic movements which are abrupt, disorganized and poorly aimed, either *qua* movements, or through confusion of two different movements, or by simple repetitive iteration of the previously executed movement.

Ideomotor apraxia is generally bilateral. But in Liepmann's famous case only the right extremities were affected, a condition that appears to be very rare. Contrariwise, Liepmann himself had stressed the frequency of unilateral left ideomotor apraxia, and we recall that Kurt Goldstein published an anatomico-clinical observation of typical unilateral left apraxia. This type of apraxia poses special problems to which we shall return presently.

Ideational apraxia

The picture is characterized by impairment of the logical and harmonious sequence of the several elementary movements that make up a complex act, though each movement by itself is executed correctly. As a disturbance of the action-to-be-accomplished, ideational apraxia is not limited to particular body segments; on the contrary, it is a defect of the sequential integration of the activities of the several segments.

The relationship between ideomotor and ideational apraxia is still not altogether clear. In fact, while ideomotor apraxia is seen typically by itself, without accompanying ideational apraxia, the reverse situation appears more questionable. The series we published in 1960 (1) contained eight cases of ideational apraxia as against 47 cases of ideomotor apraxia, and in Liepmann's series, published in 1908, there had been six cases of ideational apraxia to 24 cases of ideomotor apraxia. In our series we had three cases of ideational apraxia without ideomotor apraxia, if indeed this is how they should be described. Actually their disturbance consisted only of an impairment of the coordinated movements of the two hands.

We must emphasize also that other clinical symptoms associated with these two types of apraxia are similar, although they appear more frequently and with greater severity in ideational apraxia: aphasia, constructive apraxia, finger agnosia, and spatial agnosias.

The anatomical findings to be discussed below are also in favor of Liepmann's original conception, as well as that of Kleist (16). Evidently the main difference between ideomotor and ideational apraxia is primarily one of the severity of the defect. Denny-Brown (6) also does not separate the two types clearly; he regards both as signs of a conceptual impairment, the loss of propositional utilization of objects. But, secondarily, Liepmann (20) drew a distinction: in ideomotor apraxia the dissociation between the sensorimotor components of an action can still be transcended by the control of the ideational concept, while in ideational apraxia the ideational concept itself is disturbed. Thus Liepmann envisages ideational apraxia predominantly as a special difficulty of general psychological functions; for Foix (8), however, it remains an entity unto itself, independent both of ideomotor apraxia and of global psychological impairment. Morlaas (23) admits that the disorder is not one of execution and considers it a variety of agnosia: the agnosia of utilization of objects. Though the patient can name the object and can even give a verbal description of its use, he is incapable of evoking the motor acts necessary for that use. Zangwill (31) partially agrees with this thesis, but does not exclude defects of motor execution altogether. According to him, manual dexterity is always disturbed in ideomotor apraxia.

The relationship between ideomotor and ideational apraxia may now be restated as follows: in the most severe forms ideational apraxia is superimposed on ideomotor apraxia not because the movements required for the manipulation of objects are more complex, but because the defect is so profound that even the presence and manipulation of concrete objects can no longer bring to bear their normal facilitating influence on the movements. This is a useful formulation provided we introduce one further distinction among motor disturbances in ideomotor apraxia: that which exists between impairment of symbolic or expressive gestures on the one hand, and, on the other hand, defective "demonstration" of the utilization of an object in its absence.

Constructive apraxia

Described first by Poppelreuter (27) and so named by Kleist and Strauss, this is the most frequent form of apraxia.

Following its isolation by Kleist and Strauss (30), constructive apraxia had been related, until recently, to left parietal lesions. However, the studies of McFie, Piercy and Zangwill (21) and Hécaen, Ajuriaguerra and Massonet (13) demonstrated definitively that disorders of constructive performance are encountered also in patients with lesions of the right hemisphere where, for whatever reason, their frequency of appearance and severity are even greater than in patients with left-sided lesions.

Of course the symptomatic setting within which constructive apraxia manifests itself varies with the hemispheric localization of the lesion. If the lesion is in the left hemisphere, constructive apraxia is associated most typically with disturbances of language, while with right-sided lesions we find it associated with sensory and spatial impairment. Furthermore, it seems that there are qualitative differences in the constructive performances of patients with right- and left-sided lesions—though this is still a somewhat open question. In left-sided lesions we have noted a simplification of the structure of the patient's drawing by comparison with the model, an improvement of his drawing when he carefully attends to the model, and a beneficial effect of practice. In the drawings of patients with right-sided lesions we have observed larger numbers of unrecognizable details, errors of spatial organization of parts, errors of proportions, a diagonal orientation of the design and, finally, frequent neglect of the left side in the spontaneous design as well as in copying.

In the light of these observations, various authors posit a visual-spatial defect as the basis of the apraxias incident upon right-sided lesions, and what is essentially an impairment of programming or execution for the apraxias that occur with left-sided lesions.

Apraxia for dressing

This is characterized by the disorganization of the act of dressing only, in the absence of ideational or ideomotor apraxia.

Apraxia for dressing is found in the same context of symptoms as constructive apraxia in patients with right-sided lesions, i.e., sensory and spatial defects. It occurs, however, less frequently than do the other visuo-constructive defects, the proportions being about 1:4. Most probably we are dealing here with an order of vulnerability of two activities that are otherwise almost always associated, in which dressing tends to resist disorganization better than do the constructive performances.

ANATOMICO-CLINICAL SYNTHESIS

We can now attempt a synthesis on the anatomico-clinical level. In terms of the performance fields affected, and their accompanying symptomatology, the several types of disturbances of action can be divided into two major groups corresponding to the hemispheric lateralization of the lesions. There remains a third, more heterogeneous group which can be related to anterior and callosal lesions.

Apraxias secondary to post-rolandic lesions of the left hemisphere

Here belong bilateral ideomotor apraxia, ideational apraxia—in our series these two varieties have never been observed in right-handed patients with right-sided lesions—and one aspect of constructive apraxia. These three clinical types have been described either as conceptual defects, as defects of execution, or as defects of programming of motor action. Lesions of the posterior area of the left hemisphere, i.e., of the supramarginal and the angular gyrus, seem to play a specific role in the mechanism of these disorders, especially in constructive apraxia. On the basis of our anatomico-clinical findings, frontal lesions can be excluded in the determination of these three types of apraxia. However, we have found statistically significant correlations between the presence of constructive aphasia and involvement of the parietal lobe, either alone or in combination with other areas. Altogether, it seems that more massive lesions of greater extent are necessary in order for ideational apraxia to make its appearance.

Apraxias secondary to post-rolandic lesions of the right hemisphere

Here belong the constructive apraxias with spatial disorganization and apraxia for dressing. The effect of the total amount of destruction is much more marked in this hemisphere than in the left. A relative equipotentiality of the three posterior lobes seems also to have been retained, even though in our anatomico-clinical material the role of parietal lesions becomes a statistically significant factor in the production of visuo-constructive impairment.

Apraxias secondary to frontal and callosal lesions

We must consider first the impairment of praxis due to anterior lesions. Here apraxia of limb movements is always unilateral and is often seen in conjunction with tonic disorders, such as forced grasping, in which case all kinds of movements are contaminated by these abnormal reactions. Analogous to the frontal apraxia, we find, with parietal lesions, a kinetic "repellent" apraxia which is also unilateral and characterized by predominant reactions of withdrawal and avoidance. These two types of "apraxia" manifest themselves on the side contralateral to the cerebral lesion, irrespective of which hemisphere is involved, i.e., without hemisphere preference. Melo-kinetic or innervation apraxia is said to be due to contralateral lesions of the motor cortex. Actually, one could easily regard them as simple motor defects. Apraxia for voluntary mouth-tongue-face movements with preservation of automatic and reflex movements of the same structures seems related to lesions of the *rolandicop erculum*, especially, but not exclusively, to left opercular lesions, which explains its frequent association with expressive aphasia.

From the beginning, Liepmann regarded callosal lesions as determinants of left unilateral ideomotor apraxia. Once the commissure was destroyed, the zone of motor execution of the right hemisphere no longer received from the left zone of motor execution the necessary coordinating influences that ultimately stem from the left sensorium. This thesis subsequently fell into disrepute, but has recently been revived by N. Geschwind (9) who accounts for the experimental findings on split-brain preparations in terms of the role of the corpus callosum in the transfer of training.

With perhaps the exception of mouth-tongue-facial apraxia we can eliminate the apraxias of frontal and callosal origin on account of their many variations described above: the unilateral character of the disturbance, the lack of specificity of the defect, the absence of hemispheric lateralization of the lesion. We shall omit them from our general discussion, thus following the example of Denny-Brown (6), who separates them altogether from the bilateral apraxias and regards them essentially as symptoms of a disequilibrium between two types of motor reactions that are normally in equilibrium.

CLASSIFICATION OF PRACTIC DISTURBANCES

The anatomico-clinical findings already indicate certain distinctions between several types of motor acts, each belonging to a particular sphere of activity. We must also mention another dissociation wrought by pathology: the disorganization of the system of finger communication in deaf-mutes with lesions of the "language area," a disturbance that occurs in the absence of ideo-motor or ideational apraxia.

The studies of Goodglass and Kaplan (11) provide further evidence concerning the specificity of practic disturbances as compared with general defects of communication. These authors addressed themselves to the following questions: 1) Is apraxia a central impairment of communication? 2) Is apraxia a specific disturbance of movement? 3) Is the impairment of gesture related to a non-specific intellectual defect? They investigated the motor performances of patients with cerebral lesions, with and without aphasia, in quantitative terms, studying so-called natural expressive gestures, conventional gestures, simple pantomime, i.e., description and utilization of objects, and complex narrative pantomime. Though the defects of gesture were found to be more severe in the aphasic group, there was no direct relationship between the degree of impairment of gesture and that of language. By comparison with the control group it appeared that the essential disturbance of the aphasic subjects was related to improvement of the performance under conditions of imitation. This would imply an impairment of the execution of movements rather than a simple defect of formulation. However, within the control group, the performance of gestures by patients with right-sided lesions was much superior to that of patients with left-sided lesions, despite similarities of general intellectual deficit. From these findings Goodglass and Kaplan conclude that the impairment of gesture must be considered a practic impairment related to a left-side lesion rather than as an aspect of a central defect of communication. Nonetheless, it must be remembered that a direct relationship exists between gestural impairment and intellectual deficit, irrespective of the presence or absence of aphasia.

It should be emphasized that these results distinguish between simple and complex narrative pantomime on the one hand, and expressive and conventional gestures on the other hand. Furthermore, we must note that real manipulation of objects was not impaired in those patients who showed defects of simple pantomime, i.e., the manipulation of objects not actually present.

Utilizing various criteria we have searched for the common denominator of the several classifications that have been suggested, in the hope that such agreement as we could find among them might serve as a basis for isolating the modalities of gestural behavior and its perturbations. A first approximation is suggested by the clinical and behavioral findings as well as by the usual descriptions of gesture. These yield the inventory of different types of gestures which is given below, and which can provide a foundation for subsequent, less empirically oriented discussions.

I. *Gestures Displayed in the Absence of Objects*

A. Codified gestures supplementing language, e.g., the manual language of deaf-mutes, the language of artificial gestures.

B. Gestures which accompany spoken language.

C. Conventional symbolic gestures, e.g., the sign of the cross, the military salute, etc.

D. More or less conventional expressive gestures, e.g., menacing gestures, gestures indicating the presence of a bad odor, etc.

E. Descriptive gestures:

1. gestures related to one's own body:
    - (a) gestures that do not involve the utilization of an object, e.g., twirling the ends of one's moustache, smoothing down one's hair, etc.
    - (b) gestures involving the use of an object, e.g., smoking, eating, combing one's hair, placing a ring on one's finger, etc.
2. gestures that simulate the use of objects:
    - (a) non-sequential acts, e.g., turning a key in its lock, cutting with scissors, etc.
    - (b) gestures requiring the cooperation of the two hands and consisting of sequences of different acts, e.g., driving a nail with a hammer, sharpening a pencil, lighting a match.

II. *Acts of Manipulation of Real Objects*

A. Acts which do not directly pertain to one's own body:

1. simple acts, e.g., the manipulation of a pair of scissors, a watering can, a key, etc.
2. actions consisting of a sequence of acts, e.g., lighting a candle, putting a letter into an envelope.

B. Actions with respect to one's own body:

1. simple acts, e.g., putting on one's spectacles, or combing one's hair.
2. actions consisting of a sequence of acts, e.g., dressing oneself.

III. *Acts of Graphic Representation and Construction*

This inventory of gestures and acts may serve as a starting point. Let us remember, however, that while certain of the actions listed above may be disturbed in isolation by pathology, the disorganization of others occurs only as part of a picture of multiple deficits. Furthermore, we can now attempt a classification based on a logical distinction of signs and symbols such as has been proposed by Pierce (26), and whose wider significance has been underlined by Jakobson (14).

1. *Symbolic Gestures*

(a) strictly codified and systematically organized.

(b) conventional, less rigorously defined symbolism, with a link of artificial contiguity between signifier and signified.

2. *Iconic Gestures*

Mimicry, more or less codified expressive reactions, hence the necessity to speak of iconic symbols. The link between signifier and signified is one of similarity.

3. *Indexical Gestures*

Acts that describe the utilization of objects; the link between signifier and signified being one of real contiguity.

With Jakobson we hasten to emphasize that this tripartite division of signs rests more on the hierarchy of their properties than on the properties themselves. This explains, for example, the necessity to speak of iconic symbols. But a description of gestures must also take account of their simultaneous or successive character. Thus, successiveness marks substitutive gestural language which belongs to the manipulative acts performed in the presence or absence of the object to be manipulated. By contrast, simultaneity characterizes above all conventional symbolic gestures and the majority of expressive gestures. Thus, we can add a new dimension to the preceding classification.

Characteristic of Sign	*Temporal Aspect*
1. Symbolic Gestures	
(a) codified system, language substitute	successiveness
(b) conventional symbols	simultaneity (for the most part)
2. Iconic Expressive Gestures	simultaneity
3. Indexical Gestures	
(a) descriptive of the utilization of objects	
1. simple	simultaneity
2. sequential	successiveness
(b) manipulation of real objects	
1. simple	simultaneity
2. sequential	successiveness

This temporal dichotomy cuts across the preceding classification. Of course, this temporal aspect is not the only interloper; there is also a spatial aspect that should be considered. Finally, another distinction must be retained, that of the relationship of the response to the stimulus eliciting it: is the action executed on verbal demand, in imitation of the visually perceived action of the experimenter, is it a reproduction of a movement imposed on the passive subject, i.e., kinesthetically perceived, or is it a descriptive gesture following visual or auditory presentation of the object?

We cannot really be surprised that pathology does not offer us rigorous distinctions between the different types of gestures and acts. Add to this that the clinical findings reported all too often lack sufficient detail. Basically we are dealing only with more or less rapidly made observations, not with true experiments and systematic controls.

A review of fifty-two case histories of patients with ideational or ideomotor apraxia reveals certain typical associations or dissociations, the significance of which has, however, not yet been tested statistically. There appears to be a strong tendency for the simultaneous presence or absence of ideational praxis involving a sequence of acts, i.e., manipulation of real objects, and ideomotor praxis for gestures simulating the manipulation of objects which also necessitates sequentially organized acts. Another association, less clear than the preceding, is that of conventional symbolic gestures and expressive gestures (iconic symbols) with acts simulating the manipulation of objects not requiring sequential organization, i.e., of simultaneous acts.

Conversely, there appears to be a clear dissociation between conventional symbolic gestures and acts simulating the manipulation of objects that require sequential organization of the components.

Another point must be noted with respect to the stimulus. Apraxia may be present only in response to the verbal command, while the acts in question are well executed in imitation. Here then, symbolic and expressive gestures fail to be elicited, yet the acts of manipulation of objects, be they present or absent, are properly executed. This is the inverse of the observation made by Goodglass and Kaplan (11). We must note also that the same apraxic patients often fail to recognize otherwise well-known emblems, and generally show some intellectual deficit.

We might add that in patients with unilateral apraxia we have always found disturbances of all types of gestures and acts, irrespective of the stimulus employed to elicit them. This constitutes one more argument for the peculiar character of these unilateral disturbances as compared with the bilateral practic disorders.

We can now classify the disturbances of gestures and acts according to several different criteria:

I. *Disturbances Classified According to the Sphere of Activity Involved.*

1. Impairment of the manipulation of objects (ideational apraxia).
2. Disturbances of dressing (apraxia of dressing).
3. Defects of purposeful gestures, be they symbolic or expressive (ideomotor apraxia).
4. Impairment of activities involving spatial representation (constructive apraxia).

II. *Disturbances Classified According to the Affected Body Part.*

1. Segmental apraxias (innervation apraxia).
2. Unilateral apraxia (kinetic apraxia, repellent or magnetic apraxia).
3. Mouth-tongue-facial apraxia.
4. Apraxia of trunk movements and of the lower extremities (trunk-feet apraxia, apraxia of gait).
5. Bilateral apraxia.

III. *Disturbances Classified According to the System of Communication Affected.*

1. Impairment of gestures substituting for language (aphasia of deaf-mutes).
2. Defects of gestures accompanying language (including, perhaps, disturbances of intonation).
3. Disturbances of conventional symbolic gestures.

4. Disturbances of more or less conventionalized iconic gestures (this and the preceding group corresponding to ideomotor apraxia).

5. Impairment of indexical acts, descriptive gestures with manipulation of real objects (ideational apraxia), or simulation of such acts in the absence of real objects (ideomotor apraxia).

IV. *Disturbances Classified According to the Stimulus Eliciting the Response.*

1. Impairment of the response to verbal command.
2. Impairment of imitation of a visual model.
3. Disturbance of repetition in response to a kinesthetic stimulus.
4. Impairment of the response to auditory stimulation, e.g., the characteristic noise of an object.
5. Impairment of the response to visual stimulation, i.e., to a pictured object.

STAGES IN THE DEVELOPMENT OF GESTURE AND ACTION AND THE PROBLEM OF APRAXIA

The foregoing attempts to systematize the disturbances of gesture and action, based, as they are, on anatomico-clinical, behavioral and semiotic criteria, must now be related to the results of genetic studies. Let us find out whether investigations of the development of gesture and action reveal separate stages that suggest a similar dissociation of intentional activities. To be sure, the developmental history and its moments of integration will not reproduce identically those of its disintegration; yet, it may reveal certain basic processes that could all too easily escape our attention were we to concern ourselves only with the behavior of adults.

We refer here to Piaget's studies (24), based largely on his personal observations. Piaget demonstrates the appearance of coordinated systems of movements whose integration is the product of either a newly-discovered result or of an intention. The acquisition of these systems depends both on the subject's past experience and on internal processes of equilibration which, as a result of the attending integration, become more stable and regular. Two kinds of coordination can be distinguished: first, internal coordinations, the mechanism by which, for instance, several partial movements are integrated to produce a unitary act. Here it does not matter whether the partial movements had previously existed in isolation, or whether they became progressively differentiated in the course of their ongoing coordination. The second type may be described as more external coordinations of two or more self-contained acts now brought together to form a new act of a higher order.

Piaget begins his study of the development of action at the sensorimotor stage that precedes the appearance of language. The schema of an action "is the general structure of that action which remains constant throughout its repetition, becomes consolidated through exercise and is applied to different situations in their ever varying settings" (24, p. 552).

At the first stage there is only consolidation and generalization of the reflex schema. With the beginning of the second stage new acquisitions result from the incorporation of new elements into the initial circular reflex, and we can speak thus of praxis. In the next stage new schemata are produced through the coordination of vision and prehension. Exploratory behavior manifests itself during the fourth stage, a stage that is characterized by the external coordination of previously independent schemata of action. During the fifth stage, appearing at the beginning of the second year, the coordination of separate schemata is accompanied by a differentiation of these same schemata as a function of experience, i.e., behavior now begins to accommodate itself to unforeseen events.

The sixth stage is marked by the internalization of what had previously been external coordinations of schemata, and by the active invention of new means. This stage coincides with the appearance of symbolic activities.

Piaget emphasizes that this development cannot be explained in terms of simple cumulative associations. We must recognize here processes of assimilation. He defines assimilation as a process of integration whose result is a schema, and which can be analyzed into three aspects, each depending upon the others: functional or reproductive association (repetition and, through repetition, consolidation of the action), associative recognition (discrimination of objects as a result of an existing schema), and associative generalization (extension of the schema). The internal coordination of schemata thus corresponds to the product of cumulative associations, while their external coordination depends on reciprocal assimilations.

Once these processes of assimilation are recognized, the problem of the relationship between practic coordinations and intelligence *per se* disappears: sensorimotor intelligence, which may be defined as the subordination of means to ends, is nothing but the coordination of these very same acts. Between the ages of one and one-half and two years "symbolic functions" emerge along with the acquisition of the socially determined systems of signs among which language is the most important one. Whereas signifier and signified had remained undifferentiated heretofore, they now become separated. Consequently, representation becomes possible and appears, together with differentiated imitation and virtual images (through interiorized imitation). This is the stage of representative thought, of which two different aspects must be distinguished. The first, the figural aspect, relates only to configurations and excludes all transformations. Piaget acknowledges the role of accommodation (the adjustment to the object) during the transition between sensorimotor and representational stages. For him the progress of imitation presages symbolic functions, and he comes to regard the mental image as simply the interiorization of imitation. There follows, however, a second aspect, the operational aspect, consisting of all those activities that transform the object and directly prolong the action. An operation is not the representation of a transformation, but a transformation of the object which can be executed symbolically but which cannot be reduced to a figure or a symbol. An operation is thus defined as an interiorized or interiorizable action which is reversible and, as an operational structure, integrated according to the laws that characterize the relevant system.

In the preoperational stage (between the ages of two and seven or eight years) operations are gradually built up, but as yet they lack logical reversibility and group structure. From ages seven or eight to twelve years concrete operations appear. This is a stage of concrete manipulations unaccompanied by verbal formalization. It indicates the uninterrupted transition between practical and symbolic intelligence, and leads Piaget to the conclusion that we must continue to stress the profound functional identity of practic and gnostic operations.

Piaget's presentation is of very special interest to our studies, for he envisages the possible similarities between the several developmental stages and the various types of disorganization of action and gesture produced by pathology. Addressing himself to the tripartite classification of apraxia by Ajuriaguerra, Hécaen and Angelergues (1), he acknowledges the similarity between their three categories of disturbances and his own three developmental levels. To the sensori-kinetic apraxias, characterized by disturbances of the sensorimotor synthesis (melo-kinetic apraxia, repellent or magnetic apraxias) corresponds the sensorimotor stage. To the somato-spatial apractognosias—characterized by the disorganization of the relationships between body and space, and manifesting themselves as a disturbance in the spatial organization of action (visuo-constructive deficits of patients with right-sided lesions, apraxia for dressing)—there corresponds the stage intermediate between elementary sensorimotor behavior and symbolic behavior. The beginning of the latter, according to Piaget, is in imitative functions that guarantee the transition between sensorimotor and symbolic behavior. Finally, to the apraxias of symbolic action—which we now prefer to define as apraxias of programming and which comprise ideational, ideomotor and constructive apraxias due to left-sided lesion—to these corresponds the representational stage with its two aspects, the figural and the operational aspects. Now Piaget poses the following question: does the disturbance consist of an alteration of the operations themselves, or is it an alteration of the symbolic image of the action, or even of the verbalization subserving its representation; in other words, is the disturbance one of the representation of the act, the (symbolic) design, or is it a disturbance of the execution of the (symbolized) act?

The present synthesis permits us to regard the several types of disorganization as a hierarchic series rather than as formally separate entities. We shall try to respond to Piaget's question by comparing his systematization with our above analysis. Though our answer must, for the time being, remain provisional, it is at least capable of being subjected to empirical verification.

For all practical purposes the stage of sensorimotor coordinations corresponds well to the sensorimotor apraxias such as melo-kinetic apraxia, or unilateral limb-kinetic apraxia, i.e., those that approach paretic motor deficits or tonic disturbances. At a higher level the somato-spatial apraxias (visuo-constructive apraxia in patients with right-sided lesions, apraxia for dressing) transcend the level of simple sensorimotor coordinations but do not extend beyond deficits of integration of spatial qualities of the divers sensory avenues: thus, we find disorganization of action in relation to corporeal or extra-corporeal space, and hence the justification of the term apractognosia to describe these disorders.

As to the group of apraxias that correspond to Piaget's stage of representation, we may have to deal with two separate aspects. This appears to be true even if we eliminate the disorders of the systems of codified gestures which are a formalized language and can substitute for it, e.g., the finger language of deaf-mutes, as well as the gestures which normally accompany spoken language and seem to constitute analogues of the dysprosodies. Still, the remaining practic disturbances that make up the representational disturbances concern at least two different capacities of action, each having acquired relative independence of the linguistic system—though this is not to deny the organizing role of that system in the course of development. The first sub-group is that of disturbances of the language of gesture, that is to say, of a system of codification belonging to a given socio-cultural group, even though it is not formalized. It corresponds to the figural aspect of the representational stage and consists of the ideomotor apraxias with disturbances of symbolic and expressive (iconic) gestures. The second sub-group is represented by the disturbance of propositional utilization of objects, or disorders of programming of sequential actions, and corresponds to the operational aspect of this stage. Ideational apraxia (disturbances of manipulation of real objects) is a disturbance at the level of the concrete operations, while ideomotor apraxia of gestures (describing the utilization of objects) is a striking alteration at a stage intermediate between the preceding and a higher level of systematization and interiorization; this disturbance manifests itself in constructive apraxia of programming.

Thus we have attempted to classify the various disturbances of gesture and action according to behavioral criteria, according to 1) the clinical context in which they manifest themselves; 2) the seat of the lesion giving rise to the defect; 3) the level of the resulting disorganization; and 4) the changes in different systems of communication which they manifest. By taking into account the points of view of genetic psychology and semiotic studies we have tried to elaborate a means of analysis of these disturbances that is more precise, more systematic, and, methodologically less ambiguous than previous attempts have been. Yet, at no time have we offered definitive classifications. We regard our suggestions as hypotheses whose models stem from other areas of scientific research. The most important task is still before us: that of verification of our hypotheses by subjecting patients with cortical lesions to a battery of tests designed to explore their practic performances along the lines of our typology. Only in this way can we verify or reject the validity of our typology, as we discover the associations and dissociations wrought by pathology and come to understand the evolving mechanisms underlying the disturbances. The very definition of this task would have been impossible but for the experience of the clinicians who, by means of observation and the anatomico-clinical method, prepared the way, by establishing the formal difference between the disturbances of the act of dressing and those of object manipulation or expressive gestures, between defects of voluntary mouth-face-tongue movements and those of the extremities, between disorders of systems of gestures as substitutes for language and other systems that are relatively independent of language. Even with regard to the defects of constructive activity (drawing, etc.) the clinicians recognized the likelihood of two distinct aspects: one in which difficulties of spatial integration predominate, and another that may best be described as a disorder of programming of action.

Nevertheless, the problem of dissociation and isolation of types must not be allowed to mask the unity of disturbances of gesture and action that are clinically grouped under the name of apraxia.

Motor, sensory or general intellectual disorders undoubtedly influence practic functions, not only as elements favoring the appearance of the apraxias, but also by contributing certain peculiar aspects to these disturbances. However, neither motor, psychomotor, nor gnostic disorders, nor states of confusion or dementia produce, by themselves, the disturbances of gesture and action that have been classically defined as apraxia. The patient suffering from visual object agnosia will utilize the object correctly as soon as he has recognized it, e.g., through tactile exploration, and he can demonstrate its utilization; despite a hemiparetic motor defect he can express himself through gestures—be they ever so clumsy; the incoherence of gestures and actions of the demented or the confused has no more resemblance to apraxia than the psychomotor automatisms of the epileptic or the bizarre gesticulations of the catatonic.

We must maintain here the same distinction as that which exists between the incoherent language of the demented, the verbal automatisms of the epileptic, the dysarthric disturbances due to subcortical lesions, the neologisms of the schizophrenic and the language disturbances of the aphasic.

SUMMARY

Following a review of the anatomico-clinical synthesis published by Liepmann in 1908 and the additional varieties of apractic symptomatology that have been described since, we suggested an initial classification which emphasized the role of the hemispheric lateralization of the lesion in the determination of the clinical aspects of apraxia.

With that as a starting point, and a "naive" description of the gestures and actions affected, we proceeded to a first approximation of a typology on these clinical and behavioral grounds. Subsequently we went on to a semiotic approach inspired by the general division of signs (Pierce, 26, Jakobson, 14) to elaborate a classification which, while less empirically based, yet took account of the temporal characteristics of the different types of praxes, i.e., their dependence on simultaneity or successiveness. Finally we pointed out that the disorders of gesture and action may manifest themselves as a function of the stimulus (verbal, visual, etc.).

Utilizing these various criteria (the sphere of activity, the parts of the body affected, the system of communication involved, the type of stimulus to which the patient responds) we have drawn up a multidimensional classification. When we compared that with Piaget's elaboration of the development of action and gesture in the child, we found a good deal of agreement between his classification and ours.

The typology we have suggested should furnish a useful matrix for the study of practic disorders in terms of which the earlier, relatively unsystematic observations may be assessed. Confirmation or rejection of its validity can only be obtained by systematic application of a battery of tests exploring the various types of gesture and action here postulated.

REFERENCES

1. Ajuriaguerra, J. de, Hécaen, H., and Angelergues, R. Les Apraxies; Variétés cliniques et latéralisation lésionnelle. *Rev. Neurol.*, 1960, *102*, 566–594.
2. Bonhoeffer, K. Casuistische Beiträge zur Aphasielehre. II. Ein Fall von Apraxie und sogenannter transcorticaler sensorischer Aphasie. *Arch. f. Psychiat.*, 1903, *37*, 800–825.
3. Brain, R. Visual disorientation with special reference to the lesions of the right cerebral hemisphere. *Brain*, 1941, *64*, 244–272.
4. Brun, R. Klinische und anatomische Studien über Apraxie. *Schweiz. Arch. Neurol. Psychiat.*, 1921, *9*, 29–74; 1922, *10*, 185–210.
5. Déjérine, J. *Sémiologie des affections du système nerveux.* Paris: Masson et Cie, 1914.
6. Denny-Brown, D. The nature of apraxia. *J. nerv. ment. Dis.*, 1938, *126*, 9–33.
7. Denny-Brown, D., and Chambers, R. A. The parietal lobe and behavior. *Res. Publ. Ass. nerv. ment. Dis.*, 1958, *36*, 35–117.
8. Foix, C. Contribution à l'étude de l'apraxie idéo-motrice. *Rev. Neur.*, 1916, *1*, 285–298.
9. Geschwind, N. Disconnexion syndromes in animals and man. *Brain*, 1965, *88*, 237–294; 585–644.
10. Goldstein, K. Der makroskopische Hirnbefund in meinem Falle von linksseitiger motorischer Apraxie. *Neurol. Centralbl.*, 1909, *28*, 898–906.
11. Goodglass, H., and Kaplan, E. Disturbance of gesture and pantomime in aphasia. *Brain*, 1963, *86*, 703–720.
12. Grünbaum, A. Aphasie und Motorik. *Z. ges. Neurol. Psychiat.*, 1933, *130*, 385–412.
13. Hécaen, H., Ajuriaguerra, J. de, and Massonnet, J. Les troubles visuo-constructifs par lésions pariéto-occipitale droite. Rôle des perturbations vestibulaires. *Encéphale*, 1951, *1*, 122–179.
14. Jakobson, R. On visual and auditory signs. *Phonetica*, 1964, *2*, 216–220.
15. Kleist, K. Gehirnpathologische und lokalisatorische Ergebnisse. 4. Mitteilung über motorische Aphasien. *J. f. Psychol. Neurol.*, 1930, *40*, 338–346.
16. Kleist, K. *Gehirnpathologie.* Leipzig: Barth, 1934.
17. Lhermitte, J., Levy, G., and Kyriaco, N. Les perturbations dans la représentation spatiale chez les apraxiques. A propos de deux cas cliniques d'apraxie. *Rev. Neurol.*, 1925, 586–600.
18. Lhermitte, J., Massary, J. de, and Kyriaco, N. Le rôle de la pensée spatiale dans l'apraxie. *Rev. Neurol.*, 1928, *11*, 895–903.
19. Liepmann, H. Das Krankheitsbild der Apraxie (motorische Asymbolie). *Monatsschr. f. Psychol.*, 1900, *8*, 15–44; 102–132; 182–197.

20. Liepmann, H. *Drei Aufsätze aus dem Apraxiegebiet.* Berlin: Karger, 1908.
21. McFie, J., Piercy, M. F., and Zangwill, O. L. Visual spatial agnosia associated with lesions of the right cerebral hemisphere. *Brain,* 1950, *73,* 167–190.
22. Monakow, C. von, *Gehirnpathologie.* Vienna: Halder, 1905.
23. Morlaas, J. *Contribution à l'étude de l'apraxie.* Dissertation, Paris, 1928. A. Legrand (Ed.).
24. Piaget, J. Les praxies chez l'enfant. *Rev. Neurol.,* 1960, *102,* 551–565.
25. Pick, A. Studien über motorische Apraxie und ihr nahestehenden Erscheinungen. Leipzig: Deuticke, 1905.
26. Pierce, C. S. Speculative grammar. In: *Collected Papers,* Vol. II. Cambridge, Mass.: Harvard University Press. 1932. Cited by R. Jakobson.
27. Poppelreuter, W. *Die psychischen Schädigungen durch Kopfschuss,* Vol. 1, Chapter 4: Die Optische Apraxie. Leipzig: Voss, 1917.
28. Schilder, P. *The Image and Appearance of the Human Body.* London: Routledge and Kegan Paul, 1935.
29. Sittig, O. Über Apraxie. Eine klinische Studie. *Abhand. aus d. Neurol., Psychiatr., Psychol., u.i. Grenzgebt.,* 1931, *63,* 1–248. Berlin: Karger.
30. Strauss, H. Über konstruktive Apraxie. *Monatsschr. f. Psychol.,* 1924, *56,* 65–124.
31. Zangwill, O. L. Le problème de l'apraxie idéatoire. *Rev. Neurol.,* 1960, *102,* 595–603.

From the Centre Neurochirurgical de l'Hôpital Sainte-Anne, Paris. R.C.P. No. 41 of the Centre National des Recherches Scientifiques, with the aid of the Institut National de la Santé et de la Recherche Médicale. Translated from the French by Marianne L. Simmel.

III

SPACE

6

Factors Influencing Adaptation to Rotated Visual Fields: The Role of Meaning

by RICARDO B. MORANT
Wellesley, Massachusetts

I first became acquainted with Kurt Goldstein's work, and with the man himself, through one of his great admirers, Heinz Werner. These two men shared a dual interest in language and perception and, though dealing with different populations of subjects, they came to many conclusions in common. Goldstein's stress on holistic functioning had had a great impact on Werner and his colleague, Seymour Wapner, especially on their thinking about perception. In the early fifties, when I was a graduate student at Clark University and working on the sensory-tonic theory of perception, I became impressed by Goldstein's concept of the integrity of the organism. His studies of perceptual disturbances in cerebellar patients, his emphasis on the equalization tendencies of the organism, his research and his ideas, formed an important part of all our theoretical discussions. My interest in space perception—an area which interested Goldstein very much—dates back to those days. In the present paper I shall deal with the influence of one variable in particular which intrigued him: meaning.

Various factors have been shown to influence adaptation to rotated visual fields. Some years ago Gibson (2) demonstrated that the inspection of a tilted line leads to an apparent displacement of a vertical line which is subsequently viewed. If the inspection line is tilted less than 45° clockwise off the vertical axis, a true vertical line later appears tilted counter-clockwise; a clockwise tilt is required in order for it to look vertical. If the inspection line is tilted more than 45° off the vertical axis, the true vertical line later appears tilted clockwise; in order to look vertical, it requires a counter-clockwise tilt. Gibson attributed this change in the position of the apparent vertical to the axis toward which adaptation takes place. When the line is tilted less than 45° from vertical, adaptation is toward the vertical axis. When the line is tilted more than 45° from vertical, adaptation is toward the horizontal axis.

The general rule is that tilted lines adapt toward the axis or norm to which they are closest. The direction in which a vertical line is affected depends on whether adaptation has been to the vertical or horizontal axis. If the vertical and horizontal axes of space are dependent on each other—if adaptation consists of a general reorientation of visual space—then adaptation toward the horizontal should affect a vertical test-line as much as adaptation toward the vertical though, of course, in opposite direction.

Figure 1 shows the after-effects for a vertical test-line. The abscissa represents the preset tilt of the inspection-line from vertical (0°) through horizontal (90°). The ordinate represents the average position of the test line accepted by the subjects as vertical after they have viewed one or the other of the several tilted inspection lines. This is not exactly the function that one might expect from Gibson's formulation, but it is close enough for our purposes. The apparent discrepancies have been discussed in a recent paper by Morant and Harris (7) who collected these data. In the experiments to be reported below we shall deal only with that part of the curve which extends from 15° to 75°.

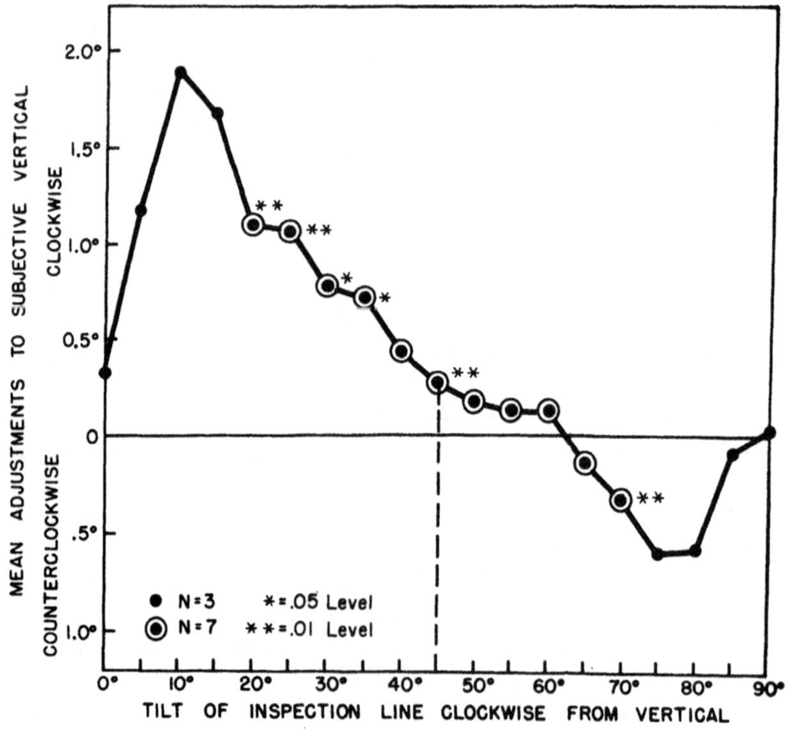

Figure 1. Subjective vertical as a function of inspection tilt.

In various recently published studies prisms have been used to rotate the entire visual field. The results of these studies are in some respects similar to those reported by Gibson and, in other respects, quite different. In the first place, if the subjects wearing prisms are allowed to walk around, the effects are much larger. In the Gibson condition, when the subject sits and inspects a tilted line, the effects are on the order of .5° to 2°, whereas in the prism tilt conditions with subjects walking about, the effects can run up to 6° or 7°. Active motion, as Richard Held (3) has demonstrated, is an important variable in some of these prism situations. Another factor which has been shown to be important—the factor to be examined in this paper—pertains to the kind of inspection field that is used. It turns out that if an isolated line or field of lines is viewed through prisms, it does not seem to make much difference whether the subject is walking or sitting; the results so obtained are quite similar to those reported by Gibson. However, if the inspection field is composed of tilted objects rather than lines, a different result occurs.

The findings shown in Figure 2 have been reported by Morant and Beller (6). We had subjects inspect either a field of lines in an otherwise dark room, or in a more "natural" scene (the halls and classrooms of a school building) while they wore prisms which rotated the perceived world 15°, 45° or 75°. After inspecting one or another of these displays, sometimes while walking and sometimes while sitting, the subject's judgment of the apparent vertical was measured. In the line conditions (the bottom two curves) we get essentially the kind of function predicted by Gibson. The direction of adaptation is toward the vertical or toward the horizontal axis, depending upon whether the inspection field is closer to one or to the other. That is, the 15° and 75° tilts yield after-effects in opposite directions. This is not what occurs when the inspection field consists of objects. In that case, the 15° and 75° tilts yield after-effects in the same direction. Irrespective of the degree of tilt, the adaptation is always toward the vertical axis. Since the differences in results obtained between walking and sitting are not relevant to our discussion, they will not be discussed further.

Why should such different effects be produced by object and line fields? The answer is implicit in the considerations which led us to set up the study in the first place. Normally our visual field is composed of *meaningful* visual configurations, of objects that have specifiable orientations or past histories of experienced positions. For example, walls are normally vertical; floors are normally horizontal, etc. We thought that, unlike isolated lines which adapt toward the nearest axis, perception of a field of naturalistic

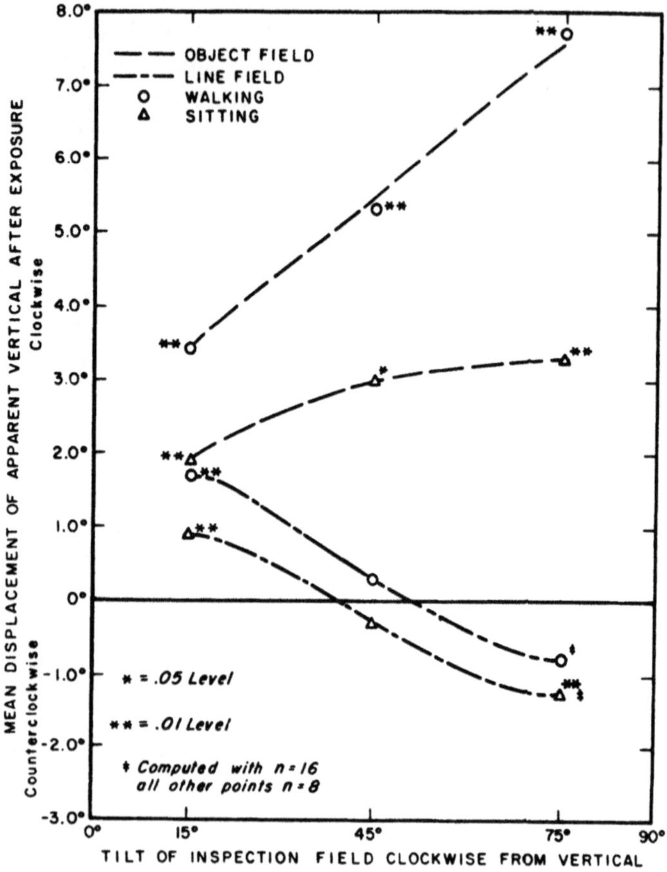

Figure 2. Adaptation to object field vs. line field; subjects sitting vs. walking.

objects would adapt so as to right itself; that is, so as to have the objects come closer to their normal orientation. Figure 2 shows that this is precisely what happens.

However, a simpler explanation of these results is possible—one that does not involve us in such a high order concept as meaning. The two stimulus conditions—the line and object fields—have different geometrical properties. Short of an analysis of the object field condition which exhaustively evaluates the distribution of vertical, horizontal and diagonal lines at various prism tilts, we have no way of concluding that the difference between the object and line field conditions is not due to purely geometrical differences. The sum total of all the stimuli in the object field conditions might be such as to lead to verticality in both the 15° and 75° conditions.

The difference between the two possible explanations is critical. What may be at issue is the paradigm of Gestalt psychology that perception is reducible to an analysis of contour processes (see Köhler and Wallach, 5). As I have drawn the distinction, *figures* can be described simply in terms of their geometry, that is in terms of their contours. An analysis of the contours of *objects* is not sufficient to describe them. Reference to the viewer is required, i.e., an experiential factor must be invoked in order to describe the meaning of objects.

In order to distinguish between the two possible explanations, we need a visual inspection field whose object properties can be changed without changing its geometry: a field which can, on the one hand, appear to be composed of a series of isolated lines and, with a change in attitude of the observer, be seen as an object—a form with a history of preferred position. *A priori* such an object need not be three-dimensional; a two-dimensional meaningful representation that has been encountered in the subject's past in a specific orientation satisfies our requirements as well as any three-dimensional real object. Since three-dimensional displays are more difficult to handle in the laboratory, we have chosen two-dimensional displays: outline drawings which can be seen either as patterns of lines or as representations of meaningful objects. Experiments I and II served to establish the fact that two-dimensional representations of objects do indeed give rise to righting effects; in that sense these experiments are merely preliminary to our main argument.

In all experiments which follow, mechanically rather than prismatically rotated visual configurations were used. The studies were conducted by Miss Gretchen Gibbs.

EXPERIMENT I

A magazine picture of a sailboating scene, with predominantly vertical and horizontal contours, was attached to a disk and rotated in the plane perpendicular to the subject's line of sight. The subject viewed the picture through a reduction screen. The tilt of the picture was the independent variable. The dependent variable was the adjustment of the picture to the apparent vertical.

Fifteen college students served as subjects. The picture was preset at a given inspection tilt. The subject inspected the scene through the reduction screen for one minute and then closed his eyes while the experimenter set the picture to objective vertical. Thereafter he opened his eyes and adjusted the picture so that it appeared vertical to him. This procedure was followed twice for each of five different degrees of tilt of the picture: 15°, 30°, 45°, 60°, and 75°, presented in one of five different random orders. Two control readings were taken for each subject just prior to each inspection condition.

The results are shown in Figure 3. In brief, all significant adaptation after-effects are toward the vertical, irrespective of the degree of tilt of the inspection field. The 75° inspection condition is not significantly different from zero. Thus, our findings are unlike those of experiments using isolated lines as inspection figures (2, 7) and, at least as far as the direction is concerned, entirely comparable to the results of the subjects who viewed the school corridor through prisms. One important difference should be noted, however. In the prism situation, the size of the after-effect is positively related to the degree of tilt; Ebenholtz has recently confirmed this (1). The inverse is true here. The after-effect decreases as a function of the inspection tilt. We shall see as we go on that this pattern is constant in the whole series of studies to be reported.

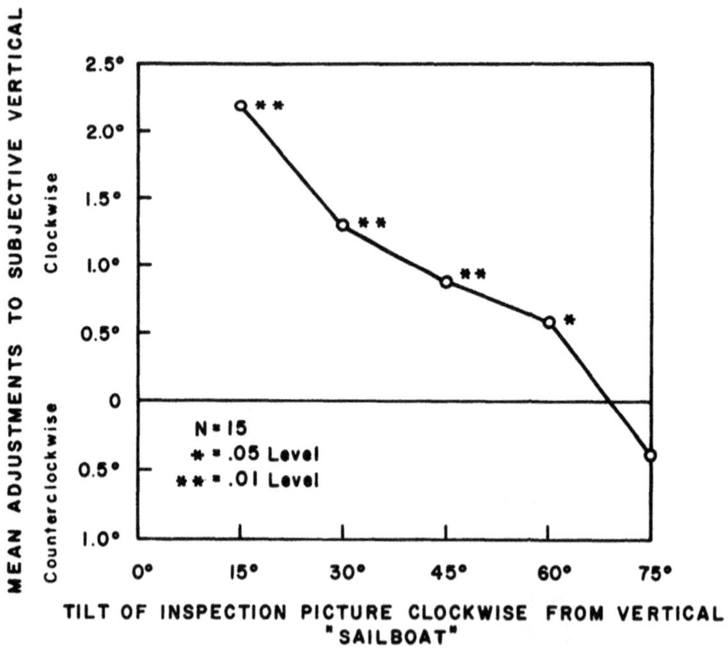

Figure 3. Results of Experiment I. Test figure same as inspection figure—"Sailboat."

EXPERIMENT II

The results of a second experiment using ten different subjects were essentially the same as those of the first. Unlike the first experiment, in which the sailboat picture was used both for inspection and test, in the second experiment the sailboat picture was used for inspection, but a straight line was used for the test. One half of the time, the line was presented at vertical and the subject asked to adjust it to subjective verticality; the rest of the time it was set at horizontal and the subjects adjusted it to subjective horizontality. As can be seen from Figure 4, the results are similar to those presented in the last figure. The effects for the vertical and horizontal axes are remarkably close.

Both these experiments demonstrate that two-dimensional meaningful displays give essentially the same unidirectional after-effect as three-dimensional inspection figures, and that the effect is demonstrable with mechanically rotated representational fields.

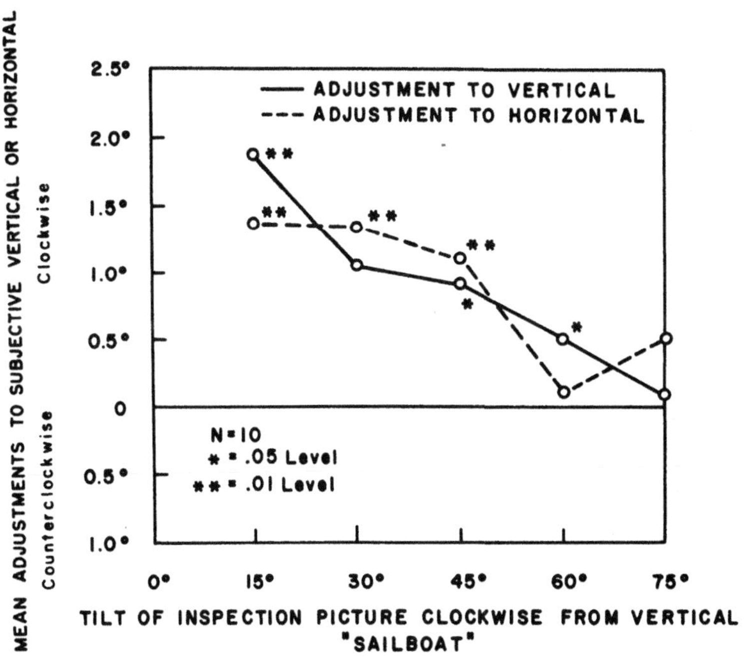

Figure 4. Experiment II: Inspection figure: "Sailboat"; test figure: single line.

EXPERIMENT III

Basically, the same method as in Experiment I was used with ten subjects, and a new, critical inspection figure as shown in Figure 5. Again, the figure was inspected at the various degrees of tilt; the subject's task after each inspection was to adjust the figure to the vertical. Not unexpectedly, the results are essentially similar to those originally reported by Gibson. When the configuration is tilted less than 45°, adaptation is in one direction; when greater than 45°, it is in the opposite direction.

Having completed the first half of the study, subjects were now asked to see the figure not as a cross and unrelated line, but as the number "4". Systematic questioning established the fact that none of the subjects had seen it as the number "4" in the first part of the experiment. Figure 6 presents the results for BEFORE and AFTER seeing the configuration as the number "4".

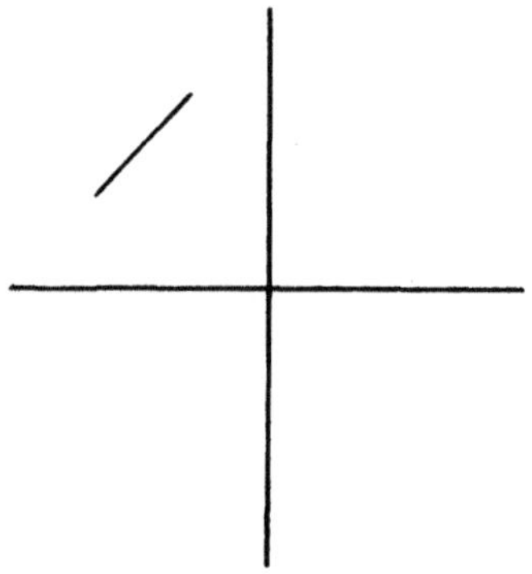

Figure 5. Inspection figure and test figure for Experiments III and VI.

When the configuration was seen as a pair of crossed lines with an unrelated diagonal, adaptation was toward the vertical in the less than 45° tilts and towards the horizontal in the greater than 45° tilts. When it was seen as a "4", adaptation was always such as to right the number; there was no difference in direction between the less than and greater than 45° tilts. The two curves representing BEFORE and AFTER differ significantly from one another.

EXPERIMENT IV

It was not possible in Experiment III to balance out the order of presentation of the configuration. Once the configuration is seen as the

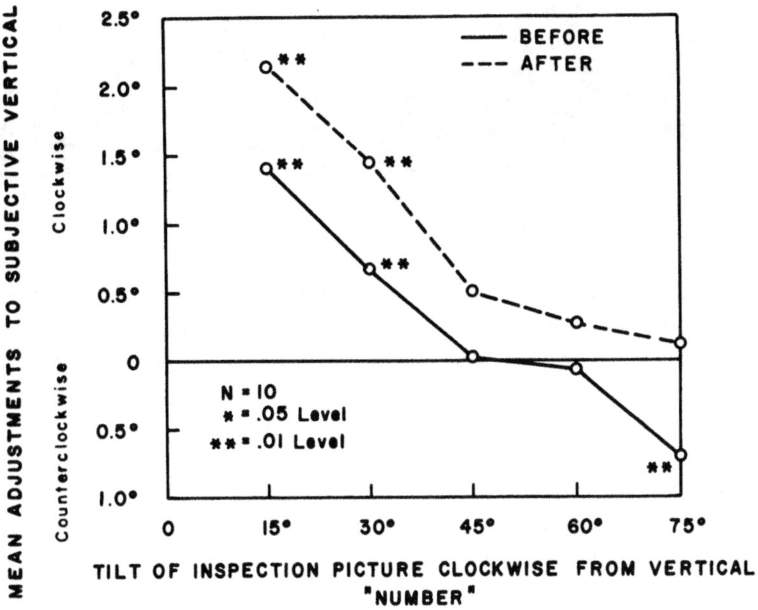

Figure 6. Experiment III. Figure 5 seen as a line pattern on inspection and test (BEFORE); then seen as "4" on inspection and test (AFTER).

number "4," it can no longer be assumed that the subject will be able to see it naively as a series of tilted lines. Thus, the meaning of the configuration and the order of presentation are confounded. In a control experiment a group of new subjects were tested only with the configuration seen as the number "4". The results were congruent with those of Experiment III, i.e., the AFTER results in Figure 6.

EXPERIMENT V

The purpose of this experiment was simply to test the generality of the previously obtained effects. Another configuration was selected which could also be seen as figure or as object; it is shown in Figure 7a.[1] This figure can be seen as a group of four strangely shaped white figures on a black ground (Figure 7a), or as the word FLY on a white background. Figure 7b facilitates the latter organization for the reader. Figure 7b was not used in any of our experiments.

[1] This figure has been adapted from one oroginally published in Warner Brown and Howard C. Gilhousen, *College Psychology*, 1950, pp. 330 & 332. Reprinted by permission of Prentice-Hall, Inc., Englewood Cliffs, New Jersey.

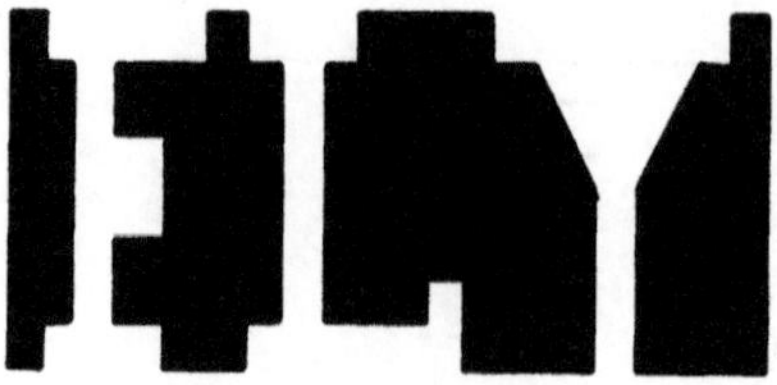

Figure 7a. Inspection and test figure for Experiment V.

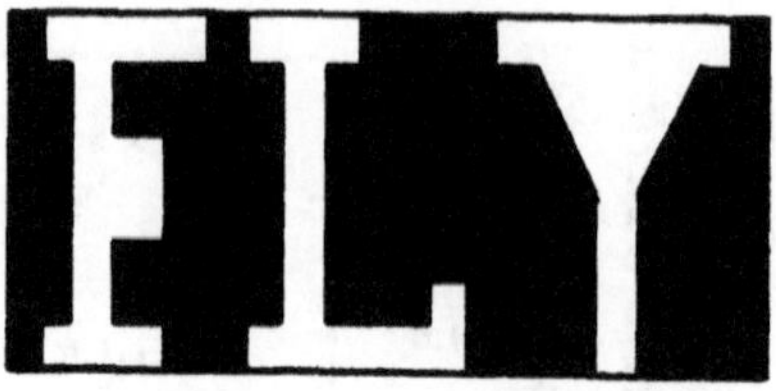

Figure 7b. Demonstration figure (not used in any experiment).

Of thirteen subjects shown the Figure 7a, three recognized the word spontaneously and were dismissed. The remaining subjects were shown the configuration at two degrees of tilt: 15° and 75° clockwise from vertical. Adaptation was measured in the usual fashion. Subsequently the subjects were assisted in seeing the configuration as the word FLY. As soon as they had seen the word clearly, they were retested at the same two degrees of tilt. The results are presented in Figure 8.

When the configuration is seen as four strange figures (the BEFORE condition), adaptation occurs toward the nearest axis; toward the vertical

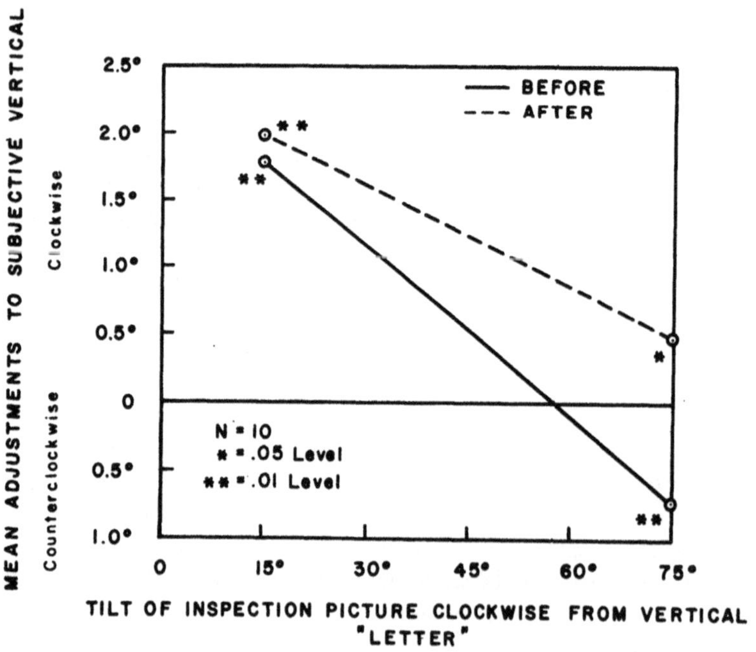

Figure 8. Experiment V: Figure 7a seen as a meaningless configuration on inspection and test (BEFORE); then as FLY on inspection and test (AFTER).

in the 15° condition and toward the horizontal in the 75° condition. Both after-effects are significantly different from zero in opposite directions. When the configuration is seen as the word FLY, adaptation is such as to right it. Again, both after-effects are significantly different from zero, but this time both are in the same direction.

EXPERIMENT VI

Can we conclude that we have demonstrated our point—that meaning affects the perception of form? There is one objection, it seems to me, that could be raised to these experiments. In our original prism situation with lines on the one hand and an object-filled view on the other, we put forward the possible criticism that the difference in results could be attributed solely to the fact that different stimulus fields were used in the line and object conditions. We attempted to counter this possible criticism through the use of identical physical stimuli for both figure and object. But are the stimuli really identical in both conditions in the "4" and FLY experiments? Geographically, to borrow Koffka's term, it would seem that the answer is "yes," it is the same physical stimulus. Behaviorally—since that is our independent variable in these experiments—the answer is "no." The stimulus has a different specifiable normal orientation when seen as figure or object. But it may be that in a very real sense, because of the changed behavioral environment, the geographical situation elicits a different response. Having once induced the set to see the configuration as an object we do not then immediately measure an after-effect. The whole technique consists in having the subject inspect the stimulus with this new set. The point is that the character of the inspection may be different before and after the "meaningful object" set is given. Specifically, different eye movement patterns might occur under the two conditions. In that case, the difference in direction of adaptation could be most parsimoniously attributed to differences in the retinal flow pattern and not to changed meaning *per se*.

Various techniques suggest themselves to resolve the problem, for example, stopping the image on the eye through reflecting mirrors or through a stalk contact lense arrangement, or more simply, by using after-images. We have not done these studies. We have tried to circumvent the difficulty in another direct way—by having the subject systematically move his eyes in exactly the same pattern in both the figure and object conditions, thus keeping the retinal flow pattern constant.

With ten new subjects we used the stimulus pattern of Figure 5 that had served in Experiment III. The subjects were trained to move their eyes to four different points in the configuration in a given pattern to the beat of a metronome. Two angles of tilt were used—15° and 75°. Again, after the first half of the experiment was finished, the subjects were shown that the configuration was actually the number "4". They were then retested with the same pattern of eye movements. Figure 9 presents the results.

The results of the BEFORE condition are similar to those we have reported thus far. The after-effects are significantly different from zero and in the opposite direction for the 15° and 75° tilts. The AFTER condition is not quite so clear. It does not differ from zero; that is, the effects are at the level of chance. Nevertheless, the fact that the average is actually in a non-righting direction is somewhat troublesome. (The two 75° conditions are significantly different from one another although the two 15° conditions are not.)

The difficulty is not hard to find. Subjects spontaneously report that it is difficult to hold the configuration as a "4" while moving the eyes. The "4" quality tends to drop out during the movements, particularly at the 75° tilt. But something even more interesting tends to occur at the 75°

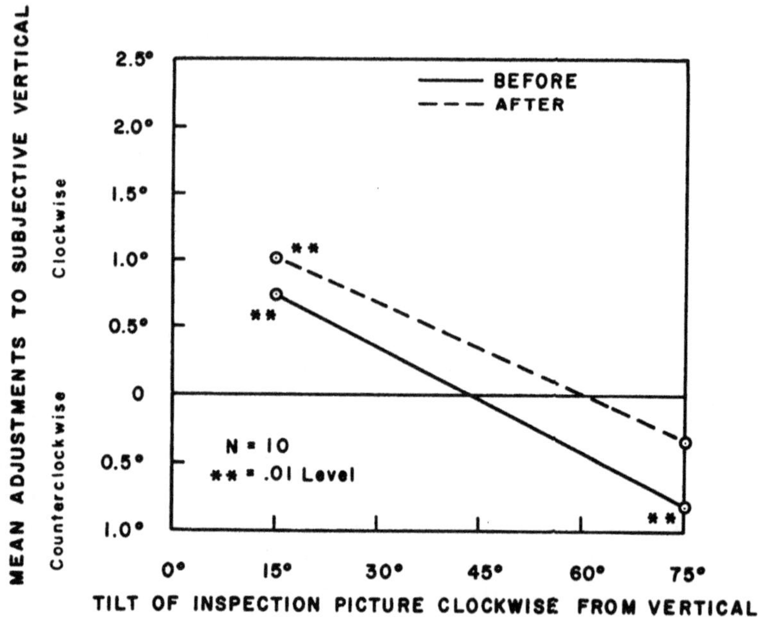

Figure 9. Experiment VI: Figure 5 for inspection and test; forced eye movements during inspection. BEFORE and AFTER as above.

tilt—something we had not encountered before we introduced eye movements.

At the 75° tilt, the left facing number "4" is occasionally seen as a right facing number "4." Another look at Figure 5 may help us in visualizing how this can occur. If we imagine the figure rotated 90°, we can see that it would represent a right facing "4". This is what was sometimes seen at the 75° tilt with the enforced eye movements. Of course, we would expect adaptation to occur in opposite directions depending upon the direction the "4" was seen to be facing.

We have conducted other experiments on this problem utilizing other techniques. I shall forego their discussion here, except to say that the results are congruent with those of the experiments reported above.

DISCUSSION

What have we demonstrated? If we follow Köhler and assume that form perception is isomorphic with a brain field, and that the properties of the brain field can be studied through perceptual displacement effects, then we have shown that meaning affects form perception. We have shown, to use Goldstein's phrase, that the perception of form is not stimulus-bound. Something besides the contour affects form.

The question becomes somewhat harder to answer outside of Köhler's Gestalt model. It is clear that the subject has responded differently to the stimulus array in our two conditions; but does that in itself tell us that the raw sensation of form has been different? Is it not possible that the sensation is identical in the two conditions but that something else—say, the memory traces made contact with—are different? When the subject sees the configuration as a cross and a diagonal, a different memory trace is activated than when he sees it as the number "4". The same stimulus array elicits two different memory traces according to the set taken (in this case the meaning given) by the observer. Phrasing the question this way, however, lands us onto one or the other of the horns of a dilemma. Do we distinguish between sensation and perception and undo what we have learned from Gestalt psychology? Shall we begin asking once again whether or not our subjects are making the object error? And if we don't draw a sharp distinction between sensation and perception, don't we risk broadening the definition of perception to include all of the cognitive processes? If we do that, there is no problem in demonstrating that meaning affects perception. Indeed, the problem would be to determine what does not. The "New Look" psychology of a few years back taught us what Cervantes and Shakespeare and Stendhal already knew so well—that values, needs, passions, hopes, etc., all determine how man perceives the world in this broad sense of the term "perceives."

This is not the time to review the New Look, the Functionalist, demonstrations. Mary Henle (4), Carroll Pratt (8), Hans Wallach (9), Carl Zuckerman and Irvin Rock (10), among others, have done just that. They have shown us that the supposedly perceptual effects were really effects of memory, or selection, or response, or just plain differences in how sloppy or inattentive different subjects were willing to be. The danger inherent in this broad definition of perception is that we confuse perception itself with the result of the perceptual process; in other words, we confound perception and its interpretation. More importantly, however, such a broad definition makes us wonder how we manage to communicate with one another at all, if what we perceive is determined by so many individually different factors. I assume that outside of learned conferences, agreement is the rule and autism the exception.

Where are we left then? On the one hand, it is Gestalt psychology which draws the distinction between the geographical and the behavioral environment. On the other hand, it is also Gestalt psychology that stresses the autochthonous laws—that minimizes the effect of experience (for that is all that meaning is) on perception. Something has to give. I should like to suggest the following formulation.

Whenever organization of any sort occurs, meaning of a sort must also occur. But we can distinguish various stages of organization. The most basic is the separation of the figure from the background. By this, I refer to the experience when looking into the void, that it is occupied, that there is something there. The second is the organization of simple figures into more complex ones. A field of dots organizes itself perceptually into rows, columns, diagonals, etc. The third is the organization of these patterns into objects, that is, into configurations with specific directional valences of various sorts. The organization of objects into a scene, and the organization of scenes into a situation are each of a farther and higher order.

At which of these levels have the effects which we have been reporting occurred? I want to be conservative and assume that it is at what I have herein labelled the third level—that of the organization of patterns into objects—the level at which organization, I think, is disturbed in cases of visual agnosia. My reason for wanting to be conservative is that it is difficult to imagine that it could occur at an earlier level, for that would mean that experience profoundly affects the basic organization of stimuli into forms. The ability of the brain-damaged and the schizophrenic, of the child and lower animal to function perceptually in the world, argues against this, it seems to me.

Thus our experiments can be interpreted in either one of two ways. Either interpretation has, I think, important theoretical implications for Gestalt theory. First, we can assume that we have demonstrated that meaning affects the basic organization of stimuli into forms. This may be so, but it strikes me as somewhat radical. If we pass up this interpretation of our results, then the second alternative follows: Our experiments demonstrate that adaptation and displacement effects are determined not by the properties of the projection field created, but rather by the properties of the memory traces which they give rise to. Adaptation is determined by the memory trace invoked by the sensory process, rather than by the sensory process *per se.*

In either case there is a broader implication—a basic methodological one—and that is, that a perceptual theory predicated on the analysis of contour processes may not be similar to one predicated on an analysis of objects as its basic datum. Goldstein, I am sure, would have insisted that we live in a world of objects, not of contours.

REFERENCES

1. Ebenholtz, S. M. Adaptation to a rotated visual field as a function of degree of optical tilt and exposure time. *J. exp. Psychol.*, 1966, *72*, 629–634.
2. Gibson, J. J. Adaptation, after-effect, and contrast in the perception of tilted lines. II. Simultaneous contrast and the areal restriction of the after-effect. *J. exp. Psychol.*, 1937, *20*, 553–569.
3. Held, R. Movement-produced stimulation is important in prism-induced after-effects: a reply to Hochberg. *Percep. Mot. Skills*, 1963, *16*, 764.
4. Henle, M. An experimental investigation of past experience as a determinant of visual form perception. *J. exp. Psychol.*, 1942, *30*, 1–22.
5. Köhler, W., and Wallach, H. Figural after-effects: an investigation of visual processes. *Proc. Amer. phil. Soc.*, 1944, *88*, 269–357.
6. Morant, R. B., and Beller, H. K. Adaptation to prismatically rotated visual fields. *Science*, 1965, *148*, 530–531.
7. Morant, R. B., and Harris, J. R. Two different after-effects of exposure to visual tilts. *Amer. J. Psychol.*, 1965, *78*, 218–226.
8. Pratt, C. C. The role of past experience in visual perception. *J. Psychol.*, 1950, *30*, 85–107.
9. Wallach, H. Some considerations concerning the relation between perception and cognition. *J. Pers.*, 1949, *18*, 6–13.
10. Zuckerman, C. B., and Rock, I. A reappraisal of the roles of past experience and innate organizing processes in visual perception. *Psychol. Bull.*, 1957, *54*, 269–296.

Presented at the Kurt Goldstein Memorial Meeting, held at the 37th Annual Meeting of the Eastern Psychological Association on April 1, 1966, in New York City. This investigation was supported by Research Grant M-3658 from the National Institute of Mental Health, U.S. Public Health Service.

7

Studies on the Inductive Influence of Head Posture on Various Functions in Unilateral Disequilibrium

by LIPMAN HALPERN

Jerusalem, Israel

Dedicated to the memory of Kurt Goldstein,
father of the concept of induced tonus phenomena.

Until now, the significance of head posture has been considered chiefly from the symptomatological point of view. It is common knowledge that changes in head posture occur in general disturbances, such as meningeal or muscular disorders, or as a corrective posture in local lesions producing dysfunctions such as diplopia, homonymous hemianopsia or unilateral positional vertigo. Deviation of the head also occurs with posterior fossa tumors and may for some time be its only sign. A few year ago, F. A. Mettler (22) summarized our present knowledge concerning deviation of the head, analyzing the various structures whose involvement may cause abnormal head posture.

The classical investigations of R. Magnus (21) enriched our knowledge with a new fundamental concept, showing that head posture not only undergoes passive changes but can, under certain conditions, exert an active influence. In his experiments on animals he demonstrated that turning the head to one side caused extension of the "facial" and flexion of the "occipital" limbs. Tonic neck reflexes were later observed also in the human being under pathological conditions. They appear, with certain variations, particularly in diffuse cerebral disorders of traumatic or inflamatory origin, as well as in tumors of the deep structures of the brain in children and adults alike.

The discovery of the tonic neck reflexes disclosed first the existence of an extended motor relationship between different parts of the body. It revealed further the important fact that head posture not only influences the tone and position of the extremities under pathological conditions, but is certainly effective under normal conditions too.

Once these findings were generally accepted, scientific interest in the significance of head posture in general—and specifically in human beings—seemed to have exhausted itself until K. Goldstein (1, 2, 3, 4, 5) postulated his concept of the phenomena of induced tonus. His interesting observations on "the tendency to optimal behavior" in man, within which framework he also dealt with the problem of head posture appear, however, not to have received adequate consideration. Further studies and observations have demonstrated very convincingly the biological significance of head posture and its systematic dynamic effect on the organism under pathological conditions. These experiences were gathered mainly from patients with systematized, unilateral disturbances of equilibrium within the symptom complex of the sensorimotor induction syndrome.

CLINICAL BACKGROUND

The syndrome of sensorimotor induction in unilateral disequilibrium (6, 7, 8, 9, 10, 11) is characterized by the fact that changes in postural pattern may induce changes in various functions of the organism. It must be stressed that, in speaking of unilateral disequilibrium, we are not referring to the symptomatology of discoordination, the constituents of which, such as nystagmus, ataxic pointing, adiadochokinesis and tremor, are characteristic chiefly of cerebellar lesions. The unilateral disequilibrium referred to here is related primarily to the syndrome of displacement, which, from the clinical point of view, is altogether different from the syndrome of discoordination. The unilateral disequilibrium of the displacement type should be considered as essentially of vestibular origin. It stems from faulty perception of the vertical and horizontal planes in space, and results in a lateral deviation of the trunk and of the homolateral extremities outwards and downwards. It is remarkable that this basically postural displacement is actually transferred inductively to other perceptual spheres and produces ipsilateral displacements in the optic, tactile and kinaesthetic fields as well. These phenomena of unilateral sensorimotor displacement form the first and primary group of symptoms of our syndrome. Furthermore, the unilateral, pathological deficit in postural balance may cause extensive disturbing effects on other functions of the organism. The disturbances thus produced represent a second and secondary group of symptoms of the syndrome, and they manifest themselves in a qualitative and quantitative dedifferentiation of function. All these disturbances can be improved or aggravated systematically by specially contrived conditions. Among the latter belong passive changes of head position which produce systematic alterations that exercise a corrective or aggravating influence, depending on the side to which the head is inclined or turned.

THE SYSTEMATIC EFFECT OF HEAD POSITION ON VARIOUS FUNCTIONS

In patients with unilateral disequilibrium the spontaneous posture of the head is of special interest. In some, the spontaneous posture of the head is not visibly different from the normal. In those patients, however, in whom unilateral disequilibrium constitutes the basis of the sensorimotor induction syndrome, deviation of head posture is observed almost invariably at the height of the disease. Such patients keep the head inclined to one side, without being aware of it. In any given patient the deviation becomes more or less pronounced in the course of time, and depending on the characteristics of the disease. In certain cases the abnormal position of the head appears only when the patient closes his eyes. An already existing spontaneous deviation of the head is aggravated by eye closure. The direction of the deviation is generally to the side of the disequilibrium, and only in some severe cases to the opposite side. Sometimes, during the course of the disease, a change of head deviation from the homolateral to the contralateral side occurs. In these patients the new head position is maintained with great constancy. If the patient's head is turned passively to the extreme right or left while his eyes are closed, and he is then asked to turn it back to the midline, he invariably returns it to the previously held spontaneous position, i.e., he stops short of the midline, or goes beyond it, depending on the direction towards which the head had been turned originally. In some of these patients, an involuntary, automatic movement of the head occurs occasionally, of which they are not aware. That is, the head, having been turned passively to the contralateral side, returns in a series of jerking movements to its abnormal spontaneous position. All these facts indicate that the changed head posture of these patients constitutes a meaningful phenomenon, the biological importance of which has been verified by systematic investigations.

As described above, in the foreground of the clinical picture is the disturbed body posture that manifests itself in a unilateral disequilibrium of the displacement type. The disturbance consists of the aforementioned inclination of the head, usually to the side of the disequilibrium, of a downward and outward deviation of the homolateral arm and leg, of a tendency to fall to the homolateral side, and of past-walking to the same side. These disorders are most conspicuous when visual control is eliminated and they occur without the patient's awareness.

Furthermore, it can be shown that changing the spontaneous head posture, in the sense of a stronger inclination or rotation of the head to one or the other side, may produce either a correction or an aggravation of the already existing disequilibrium. The specific effect varies from patient to patient. In some patients displacement of the head to the homolateral side produces an aggravating influence, while a corrective result is achieved by displacing the head to the contralateral side. In other patients, exactly

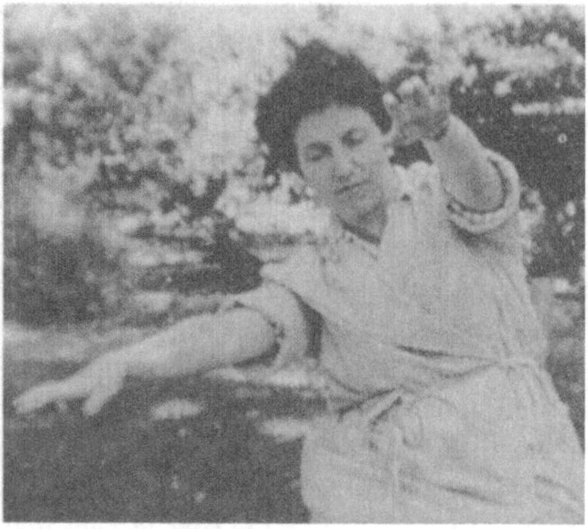

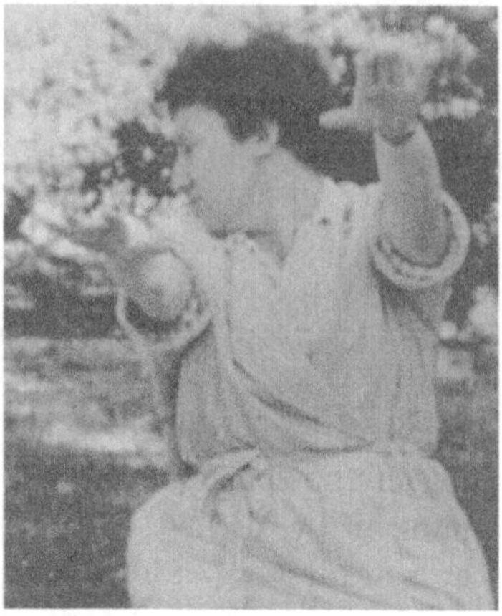

the reverse occurs. The effect itself has a systematic character which can be demonstrated best in the pathological tendency to fall to one side and the spontaneous descent and deviation of the homolateral arm. The displacement of the head to one side corrects these tendencies, while its displacement to the opposite side aggravates them, as can be seen in Figures 1, 2 and 3.

It is of interest that in some patients the converse effect has been observed, i.e., displacement of the arm induces automatic turning of the head to the homolateral side.

While the inductive influence of head posture on the disturbed equilibrium represents a mutual, inter-motor relationship, further examination in these patients reveals that this influence also affects sensory functions. As already mentioned, unilateral displacement in the postural sphere induces homolateral, sensory displacements in the visual, kinesthetic and tactile spheres. The sensory disturbances manifest themselves in unilateral distortion of the perception of the coordinates of space. Using only the homolateral eye, patients show a visual displacement of the vertical and horizontal coordinates and distortion of the perception and drawing of geometrical figures. In the tactile sphere, a small rod, placed vertically or horizontally on the homolateral side of the chest is perceived as being correspondingly tilted. In the kinesthetic field, the displacement becomes evident when the patient, with his eyes closed, is asked to hold a rod vertically or horizontally in the homolateral hand. It has also been found that just as changing the spontaneous head posture corrects or aggravates the disequilibrium, so does it influence these sensory displacements. It is worth adding that the deviation of the visual perception of the horizontal

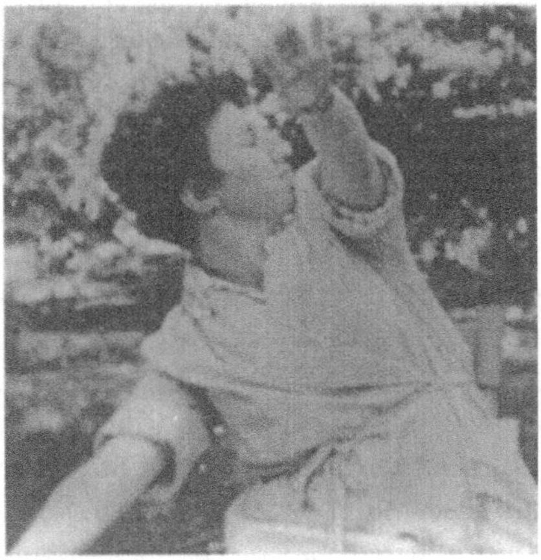

Figure 1. Spontaneous inclination of the body to the right and deviation of the right arm in a patient with a right-sided sensorimotor induction syndrome.

Figure 2. Passive turning of the head to the right corrects the inclination of the body and deviation of the arm.

Figure 3. Passive turning of the head to the left aggravates the inclination of the body and deviation of the right arm.

sometimes also affects the patient's handwriting. When he is asked to write with only the homolateral eye open, the line of writing deviates, unbeknownst to the patient. This deviation of the line of writing which appears with the spontaneous deviation of the head, disappears when the head is turned to the side which produces a correction of the disequilibrium. The induced corrective effect of altering the spontaneous head posture also affects distortions of drawings of geometrical figures.

The systematic effect of altered head posture concerns not only the constant and primary phenomena of sensorimotor displacement, but, as already mentioned, leads also to secondary quantitative and qualitative alterations of various functions. The quantitative alterations of sensory perception are most pronounced in the visual and tactile spheres, and they manifest themselves in unilateral micropsia or macropsia, and in unilateral microstereognosis or macrostereognosis. Characteristically, these two kinds of impaired perception of size present themselves homolaterally, appearing in that eye or hand which corresponds to the side of the disequilibrium.

Unilateral micropsia is associated with ipsilateral microstereognosis and unilateral macropsia with ipsilateral macrostereognosis. With the homolateral hand the same patients also overestimate or underestimate weights and distances. These disturbances, too, are systematically influenced by altering the spontaneous head posture. When the head is turned to the side producing the aggravating effect on the disequilibrium these disturbances visibly increase, while they decrease or totally disappear when the head is turned to the corrective side. It is surprising that this systematic effect concerns not only estimation of weight and distance, the performance of which requires the motor use of the homolateral hand, but also the purely sensory perception of size by the visual and tactile organs.

The systematic effect of head posture also extends to a much wider range of qualitative disturbances. (13, 14, 15). In patients with unilateral disequilibrium showing the features of the sensorimotor induction syndrome, there sometimes exists a hearing impairment of the homolateral ear. As expected, we found that altering the spontaneous head posture is apt not to exercise a corrective effect on this static impairment of the acoustic function. However, altering the spontaneous head posture in patients with normal hearing produces a measureable impairment of acoustic perception, which manifests itself only in that ear which corresponds to the side of the disequilibrium, as seen in Figure 4. Still more evident is the systematic effect of head posture on visual functions. Sometimes patients complain spontaneously of blurred vision, and examination usually shows impaired visual functions in the homolateral eye. Such monocularly impaired vision is the combined result of a number of disturbances. To these belong—as described earlier by V. v. Weizsäcker (24, 25), K. Goldstein, K. Goldstein and W. Jablonsky (3), F. H. Quadfasel (23), and by ourselves—the above-mentioned monocular displacements in the perception of the coordinates of space. There exist frequently also a homolateral, dynamic visual field constriction, a change in refraction, fusion of closely dotted lines when seen with the homolateral eye, altered perception of visual size and impaired discrimination of colors. It is of interest that this unilateral impairment of visual function which results from summation of the single disturbances can be systematically influenced by passive turning of the head, just as the single disturbances can be so influenced. Turning the head to the side which produces a corrective effect on the disequilibrium reduces or annuls the disturbances, while turning the head to the aggravating side increases or even provokes them.

A patient with a right-sided syndrome of sensorimotor induction, including monocular displacement of visual coordinates, may serve as an illustration of this condition (12). The patient was unaware that she kept her head inclined to the right. The deviation was about 10° and was present on repeated examination. The head could be moved freely, actively and passively, and in all directions. When the head was turned passively to the left, the patient stated that this position was disagreeable and uncomfortable; with the head turned passively to the right she felt relatively well. If, while the patient's eyes were closed, the head was passively rotated, first to the right and then to the left, and she was thereafter asked

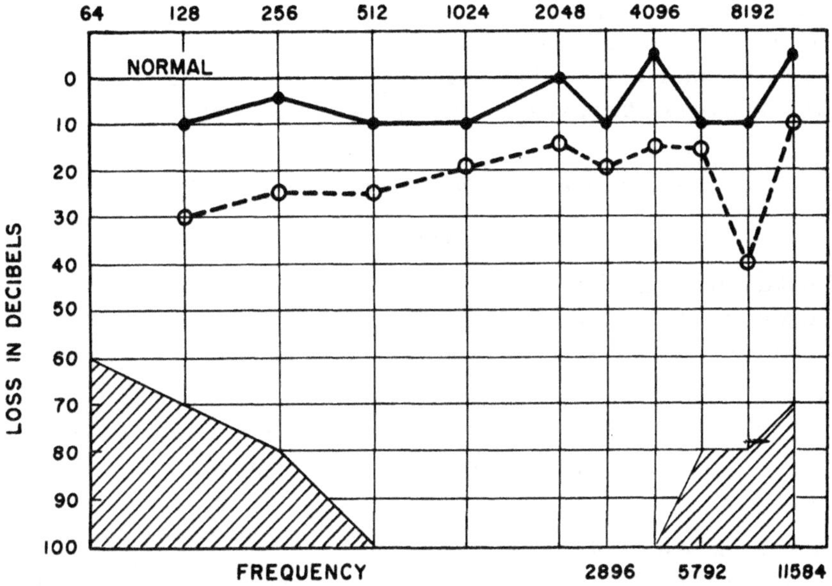

Figure 4. Influence of head position on auditory thresholds in a patient with a left-sided sensorimotor induction syndrome. Inclination of the head to the extreme left (broken line in graph) causes a left-sided impairment of hearing averaging 10 to 20 db at all frequencies. Shaded area is beyond maximum limits of audiometer.

to place it in the midline, the head always ended up spontaneously inclined to the right.

As to visual disturbances, the patient complained of considerable difficulty when reading. Sometimes small print could be read without effort, while at other times even large print could not be made out. The letters blended into one another and gave her the impression of being superimposed. Sometimes, even if the print was relatively small, a letter, a word or even a whole line obtruded itself strikingly, as if it were printed in another typeface. Repeated ophthalmological examination, while the head was kept in the spontaneous position, showed the following results: The eyes moved freely in all directions. There was no diplopia or nystagmus, neither spontaneous nor on fixation. The pupils reacted promptly to light and to convergence. On the left side there was slight exophthalmos. The media were clear. Special examination of vision gave the following results: Right eye 6/12 – 6/9? Left eye 6/18, cyl. 0,5 Ax. 90°, 6/12? The eye tension, the fundi and the visual fields were normal on both sides.

Examination with Stilling's color plates showed normal results with the exception of plates 27 and 56.

To determine the possible influence of a change in head position on visual functions, the patient's visual acuity was examined repeatedly.

Visual Acuity in Various Positions of the Head

First Examination

Spontaneous inclination of the head to the right
Right eye: 6/12 to 6/9 + 1.25 6/6?
Left eye: 6/18 cyl. – 0.5 90° 6/12?

Extreme inclination of the head to the right
Right eye: 6/6 (the patient states that the letters appear to be much clearer than with spontaneous inclination).
Left eye: 6/12 – 6/9?

Extreme inclination of the head to the left
Right eye: 6/9 (the patient sees everything very indistinctly and faded, the letters fuse together).
Left eye: 6/18 (reading faulty; the patient complains of blurred vision).

Second Examination

Spontaneous inclination of the head to the right
Right eye: 6/12 – 6/9? + 6/6 (the patient sees the letters distinctly).
Left eye: 6/6?

Extreme inclination of the head to the right
Right eye: 6/12 – 6/9 + 1 6/6 (the letters are very distinct).
Left eye: 6/6? (the letters are distinct).

Extreme inclination of the head to the left
Right eye: 6/12 – 6/9? + 1 6/6? (the letters are faded).
Left eye: 6/9 (the letters are very faded and unclear).

Third Examination

Spontaneous inclination of the head to the right
Right eye: 6/12 ? + 1.0 6/6 ?
Left eye: 6/9? – 6/6??

Extreme inclination of the head to the right
Right eye: 6/12 + 1.0 6/6.
Left eye: 6/6?

Extreme inclination of the head to the left
Right eye: 6/12 + 1 6/6?? (the numbers extend sideways and become faded).
Left eye: 6/12 − 6/9 ? (the numbers are still more faded, the 8 looks duplicated, as if printed one upon the other).

Comparison of the results for the three head positions showed that, despite some variations, inclination of the head to the right improved, while inclination to the left reduced the visual acuity.

The influence of head posture on color perception was examined under the same conditions, as the patient herself had become doubtful about her identification of various colors.

Color Perception in Various Positions of the Head

Spontaneous inclination of the head to the right
Binocular: The numbers 56 and 27 are not recognized.
Right eye: All plates are seen much clearer and are easily recognized.
Left eye: The numbers 56 and 27 are not recognized. 39, 42 and 48 are recognized with difficulty.

Inclination of the head to the extreme right
Binocular: All numbers including 56 and 27 are easily recognized.
Right eye: All numbers are recognized at once.
Left eye: 56 and 27 are not recognized, 68 only slowly.

Inclination of the head to the extreme left
Binocular: The numbers 56, 27, 97, 25, 68, 75 and 89 are not recognized.
Right eye: Recognition of numbers is delayed.
Left eye: Recognition is generally retarded. The numbers 56, 27, 97, 34 and 68 are not recognized at all.

These results illustrate the same influence of head posture on the perception of color as on visual acuity: inclination of the head to the right corrected color perception, while inclination to the left impaired it.

Head posture in these patients also influences the dedifferentiation of sensibility that appears frequently on the side of the body with disequilibrium. The disturbance, which by its very nature is a secondarily induced impairment, affects the qualities of superficial sensibility and occasionally also those of deep sensibility. An important aspect of these disturbances is the extreme variation in their degree, as is the case with all secondarily induced disturbances in these patients. They depend obviously on the severity of the basic pathological condition, and are accordingly more or less conspicuous. We have shown that these secondary disturbances of sensibility, as demonstrated by tests of two-point discrimination and vibratory perception, are also systematically influenced by head posture (17, 18).

With regard to two-point discrimination, the perceptual dedifferentiation which takes place here manifests itself spontaneously in a way analogous to the fusion tendency in the visual sphere. A series of closely spaced tactile stimuli, as produced, for instance, by pressing a comb on the homolateral side of the body, is perceived by these patients as a continuous line. Investigation revealed that this disturbance of two-point discrimination is systematically influenced by altered head posture. The results of these investigations are illustrated below in two patients with the sensorimotor induction syndrome.

In the first patient, with a left-sided syndrome, turning of the head to the left produced a systematic aggravation of all disturbances. The same effect was obtained for two-point discrimination, as shown in Table 1.

TABLE 1. THE EFFECT OF VARIATION OF HEAD POSITION ON TWO-POINT DISCRIMINATION

Experimental conditions	Distance between points in mm. applied to right middle finger	% of 5 trials correctly identified
Both eyes open, head centered	2	0
	3	60
	4	100
	5	100
Passive rotation of head to right side		
After 30 seconds	4	100
After 90 seconds	4	100
After 150 seconds	4	100
Passive rotation of head to left side		
After 30 seconds	4	80
After 90 seconds	4	40
After 150 seconds	4	20
After 210 seconds	4	0
After 270 seconds	4	0

The data given in Table 1 reflect the effect of head position on the two-point discrimination threshold in this patient. Under spontaneous conditions, 100 percent identification of two points at a distance of 4 mm from one another was obtained. Passive rotation of the head to the contralateral, right side produced no change. Passive rotation of the head to the homolateral, left side, however, led to a marked, progressive reduction in the percentage of correct identifications of the two points.

In the second patient, with a right-sided syndrome, turning of the head to the left produced a diminution of all disturbances, while turning the head to the right visibly increased them. Two-point discrimination was influenced by head posture in the same way, as seen in Table 2.

TABLE 2. THE EFFECT OF VARIATION OF HEAD POSITION ON TWO-POINT DISCRIMINATION

Experimental conditions	Distance between points in mm. applied to the left leg	% of 5 trials correctly identified
Both eyes open, head in spontaneous position	25	40
	30	60
	35	60
	40	80
	45	80
	50	60
	55	100
	60	60
	65	100
	70	100
Passive rotation of head to left side		
After 30 seconds	60	80
After 90 seconds	60	100
After 150 seconds	60	100
Passive rotation of head to right side		
After 30 seconds	120	60
After 90 seconds	120	40
After 150 seconds	120	0
After 210 seconds	120	0

The data in Table 2 illustrate the effect of head posture on two-point discrimination in the left leg. With the head in the spontaneous position, identification was 100 percent correct for a distance of 70 mm between the points. After passive rotation of the head to the contralateral, left side, identification was 100 percent correct even for 60 mm between points. When the head was rotated to the homolateral, right side, there was a distinct, rapid and progressive reduction in the percentage of correctly identified trials, even when the inter-point distance was 120 mm.

Another sensory modality whose variability under the influence of altered head posture has been investigated is that of vibratory perception. Clinical examination of these patients had already revealed a unilateral impairment of vibratory perception, manifested in an earlier extinction of sensation on the homolateral side than on the contralateral side. This impairment is also a secondary phenomenon of the basic sensory dedifferentation that results in lowered fusion thresholds for fine, closely spaced stimuli in various perceptual spheres. Vibratory stimuli are perceived by these patients on the homolateral side when, at their onset, the oscillations are widely spaced, but the perception dwindles as the spacing diminishes. Detailed examination in a series of patients revealed, moreover, that the vibratory threshold changes systematically under the influence of altered head posture. These vibratory changes will be exemplified in two patients with the features of sensorimotor induction in unilateral disequilibrium.

In one patient, with a left-sided syndrome, turning of the head to the right improved the disorders while turning it to the left increased their severity. The same effect was obtained for vibratory perception, as shown in Figure 5. The threshold values in the homolateral, left hand, under spontaneous conditions were distinctly higher than those in the contralateral, right hand. Turning the head to the contralateral, right side produced a lowering of the threshold values in the homolateral, left hand, but little if any effect on the contralateral, right hand. Turning the head to the homolateral, left side, however, led to a clear, progressive increase of the threshold in both hands, most strikingly so in the homolateral, left hand.

In the other patient, with a right-sided syndrome, turning the head to the left produced a general corrective effect, while turning the head to the right, induced a deteriorating effect. Figure 6 shows the disturbing effect on vibratory perception if the patient's head is turned to the right, homolateral side. The threshold values so obtained were markedly higher than those obtained when the head was in the spontaneous position. In fact, the threshold for vibration transcended the range of stimuli that could be supplied by our instrument. Returning the head to the normal position caused a distinct, progressive reduction of the threshold values.

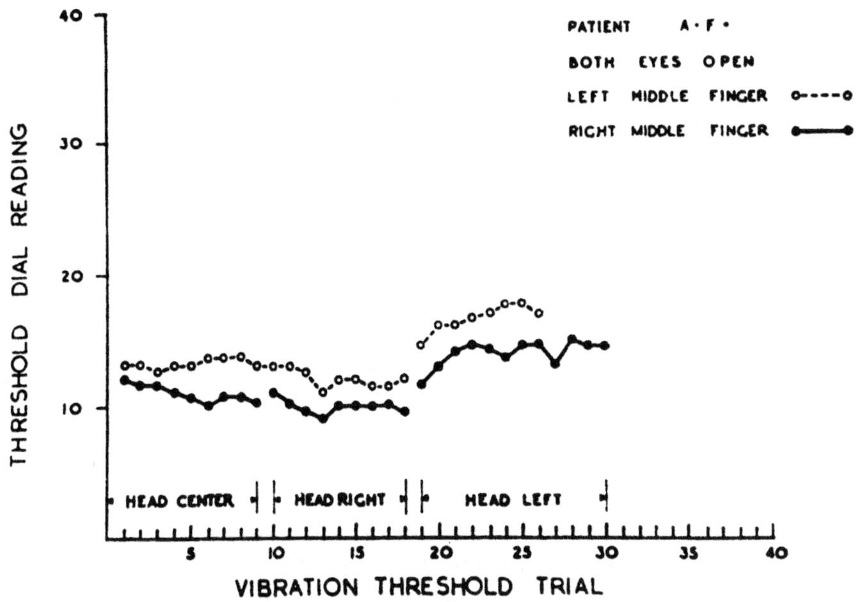

Figure 5. Influence of head position on vibratory perception in a patient with a left-sided sensorimotor induction syndrome. Turning of the head to the left produces progressive impairment of the vibration threshold.

We have also studied the influence of head posture on respiration and circulation. During routine clinical examination it had already been observed that these patients try, as far as possible, not to alter the posture of the head. When it is changed, they complain of an increasingly unpleasant sensation which is accompanied by marked pallor and acceleration of respiration and pulse rate. Actual measurement of respiratory and circulatory functions revealed indeed a systematic change of these functions under the influence of altered head posture. Displacement of the head produces the same ameliorating or disturbing effects on respiration and circulation as on the other performances (19). The data presented in Figure 7 were obtained from a patient with a right-sided syndrome, in whom turning the head to the right corrected the basic disorders while turning it to the left increased the disturbances. The figure shows that turning the head to the contralateral, left side, had an adverse effect on respiration, blood pressure and the electrocardiogram. It is worth adding that, under these conditions, the ballistocardiographic pattern also became irregular, chaotic and showed "respiratory variation," grade 2-3, even while the

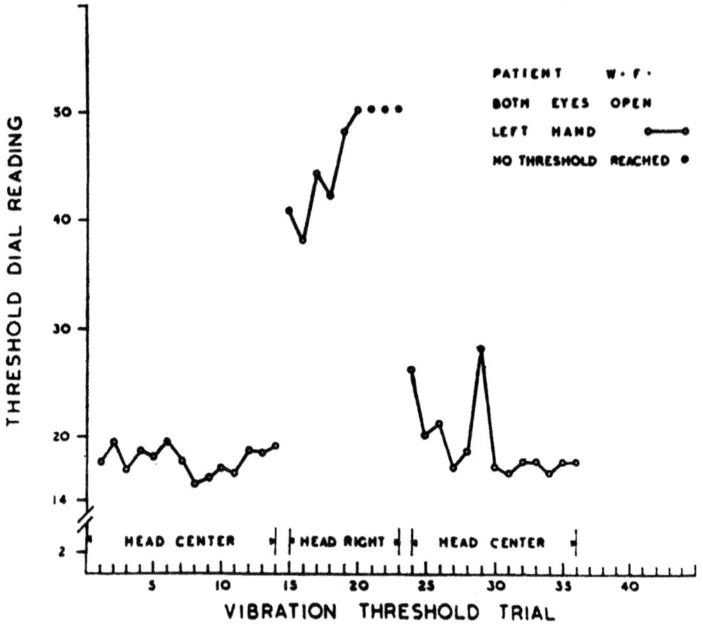

Figure 6. Influence of head position on vibratory perception in a patient with a right-sided sensorimotor induction syndrome. Turning the head to the right produces a markedly disturbing effect on vibratory perception.

patient held his breath. It is of interest that, in the same patient, turning the head to the left also had an effect on the capillaries, inducing marked capillary thinning and intracapillary red cell aggravation (20).

In considering the effect of head posture on various single functions, the question arose as to how far the general functioning of the organism is influenced by the same conditions. With this problem in mind we investigated in these patients the effect of head posture on reaction time. We obtained different reaction times as a function of the direction of head displacement. The data from a patient with a right-sided syndrome of sensorimotor induction are given in Figure 8. They illustrate this condition very clearly (16). The displacement of the head to the side which produced a disturbing effect on the other functions induced also lengthened and more variable reaction times, while shorter and more stable reaction time values were obtained with displacement of the head to the corrective side.

Thus, it is evident, from all that has gone before, that the influence of head displacement extends to many and various functions and has the same, consistent, systematic effect throughout.

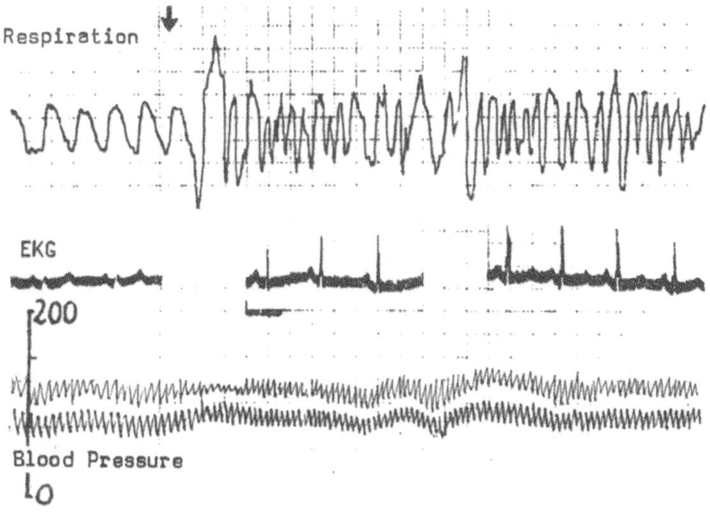

Figure 7. Influence of head position on respiration (upper record), blood pressure (lower record) and electrocardiogram (center record) in a patient with a right-sided sensorimotor induction syndrome. During the control period, the respiratory rate was 23/min. and regular; pulse rate 88/min., blood pressure 120/68 mm Hg, and the EKG normal. When the head was turned to the contra-lateral left side (at arrow), respirations became irregular at about 42/min., pulse rate rose to 115/min., blood pressure to 135/75 mm Hg, and the EKG showed flattening of the T-waves.

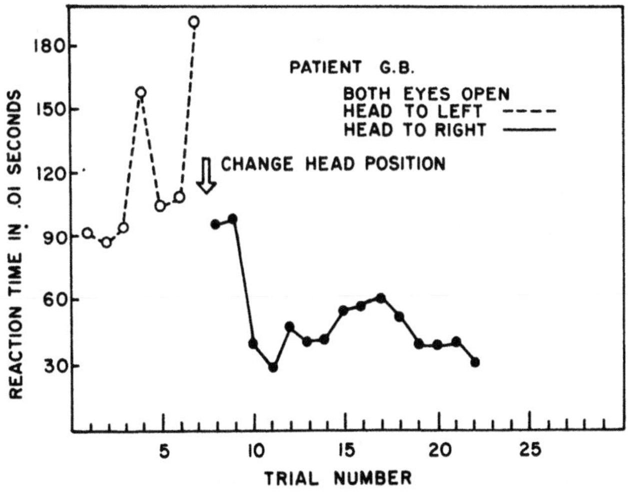

Figure 8. Reaction time values in a patient with a left-sided sensorimotor induction syndrome. Turning the head to the left has a markedly disturbing effect on reaction times, while turning to the right (corrective) side improves reaction times.

CONCLUSIONS

The posture of the head in patients with signs of sensorimotor induction in unilateral disequilibrium is an important clinical feature. The systematic, ameliorating or aggravating effect of displacement of the head on various functions is of special interest also from the neurophysiological point of view. There is no doubt that head posture in man has a significant relation to tonic neck reflexes in animals. However, while in animal experiments only the visible motor effects of head posture can be demonstrated, in human beings its influence is effective not only in the motor pattern of the limbs but also in sensory and other functions. Furthermore, it was shown that, in these patients, the spontaneous inclination of the head appears in the neurodynamics of the unilaterally disturbed equilibrium as a regulative factor; it mediates between the ameliorating and aggravating effects of extreme displacement of the head to the right or left side. The spontaneous inclination of the head represents an intermediate position and provides the organism with optimal efficiency vis-à-vis the two prevailing opposite and extreme tendencies. Along with the clarification of the principal significance of head posture, it is important to keep in mind that this phenomenon represents only a partial manifestation of the much more extensive syndrome of sensorimotor induction. This syndrome, characterized as it is by the inductive influence of unilateral disequilibrium on a variety of functions and their mutual relationships, reflects a far reaching functional disintegration. The form of this disintegration is unique; it is not seen in any other neurological disturbance. The clinical manifestations of disorders of the pyramidal, extrapyramidal or sensory systems should be recalled in this connection. Each of them pertains exclusively to its respective functional sphere. The fact that unilaterally disturbed equilibrium, in contrast to lesions of the other systems, is capable of inducing changes in a variety of functions, promotes the equilibratory system from its former obscurity to the front ranks of the important systems of the organism. The practical and theoretical aspects of sensorimotor induction in unilateral disequilibrium open up a new chapter of vestibular neurology, and they enrich our knowledge with new facts on the functioning of the organism under pathological and normal conditions.

REFERENCES

1. Goldstein, K. Über induzierte Tonusveränderungen beim Menschen. *Klin. Wochenschr.*, 1925, *4*, 294–299.

2. Goldstein, K. Zum Problem der Tendenz zum ausgezeichneten Verhalten. *Dtsch. Zeitschr. Nervenheilk.*, 1929, *109*, 1–61.
3. Goldstein, K., and Jablonski, W. Über den Einfluss des Tonus auf Refraktion und Sehleistung. *Von Graefes Arch. Ophthal.*, 1933, *130*, 395–410.
4. Goldstein, K. *The Organism.* New York: American Book Company, 1939.
5. Goldstein, K. The two ways of adjustment of the organism to cerebral defects. *J. Mt. Sinai Hosp.*, N.Y., 1942, *9*, 504–513.
6. Halpern, L. The syndrome of sensorimotor induction in disturbed equilibrium. *Arch. Neurol. Psychiat.*, 1949, *62*, 330–354.
7. Halpern, L. The syndrome of sensorimotor induction in combined cerebellar and labyrinthine injury. *J. nerv. ment. Dis.*, 1951, *114*, 137–161.
8. Halpern, L. *Le syndrome d'induction sensorimotrice dans les troubles de l'équilibre.* Paris: Masson & Cie., 1951.
9. Halpern, L., and Kidron, D. P. Sensorimotor induction syndrome in unilateral disequilibrium. *Neurology*, 1954, *4*, 233–240.
10. Halpern, L. Nouvelle contribution à l'étude du syndrome d'induction sensorimotorice dans la déséquilibration unilatérale. *Mschr. Psychiat. Neurol.*, 1955, *130*, 85–107.
11. Halpern, L. Additional contributions to the sensorimotor induction syndrome in unilateral disequilibrium with special reference to the effect of colors. *J. nerv. ment. Dis.*, 1956, *123*, 334–350.
12. Halpern, L., and Landau, J. Head posture and visual functions. *Mschr. Psychiat. Neurol.*, 1953, *125*, 148–158.
13. Halpern, L. Head posture and sensory perception. *V. International Congress of Neurology*, 1953.
14. Halpern, L., and Feinmesser, M. Head posture and acoustic perception. *Mschr. Psychiat. Neurol.*, 1954, *127*, 122–127.
15. Halpern, L. Biological significance of head posture in unilateral disequilibrium. *Arch. Neurol. Psychiat.*, 1954, *72*, 160–168.
16. Halpern, L., and Kugelmass, S. Influence of head posture on reaction time in the sensorimotor induction syndrome. *Confinia Neurologica*, 1957, *17*, 118–130.
17. Halpern, L., and Kugelmass, S. The variability of tactile two-point discrimination in the sensorimotor induction syndrome. *Acta psychologica*, 1957, *13*, 162–172.
18. Halpern, L., and Kugelmass, S. The variability of vibratory perception in the sensorimotor induction syndrome. *Acta Psychiat. Neurol. Scand.*, 1958, *33*, 181–192.
19. Halpern, L., Braun, K., and Eliakim, M. Induced respiratory and circulatory changes in unilateral disequilibrium. *Am. J. Cardiol.*, 1958, *2*, 334–341.
20. Halpern, L., and Davis, E. Capillary changes induced by motor and sensory stimuli in unilateral disequilibrium. *Amer. J. med. Sci.*, 1958, *236*, 492–495.
21. Magnus, R., *Körperstellung.* Berlin, 1924, Springer.
22. Mettler, F. A. Deviation of the head. *A.M.A. Arch. Neurol. Psychiat.*, 1959, *81*, 442–457.
23. Quadfasel, F. A. Statische Haltungsstörung und intermodale Wahrnehmungsstörungen in ihrer gegenseitigen Abhängigkeit und Beeinflussbarkeit. *Mschr. Psychiat. Neurol.*, 1937, *96*, 326–380; *97*, 90–128.

24. v. Weizsäcker, V. Über eine systematische Raumsinnstörung. *Dtsch. Z. Nervenheilk.*, 1925, *84*, 179–233.
25. v. Weizsäcker, V. Kasuistische Beiträge zur Lehre vom Funktionswandel bei stato-opto-sensiblen Syndromen. *Dtsch. Z. Nervenheilk.*, 1931, *117–119*, 716–736.

From the Department of Nervous Diseases of the Rothschild Hadassah University Hospital and Hebrew University, Hadassah Medical School.

8

The Bodily Self and Psychological Space

by DONALD M. PURDY

New York, New York

This essay is an approach to fundamental issues in the analysis of psychological space. This space is, on the one hand, something "phenomenal," and on the other, a medium for our voluntary action. Thus the topic is not restricted to the domain of perception-psychology, but is basic for behavior-psychology.

The most careful and detailed analysis of psychological space that has ever been made seems to be that of Edmund Husserl, as given in his lectures on phenomenology, and as set forth, with additions, by Husserl's student Oskar Becker in 1923 (1). This work is lengthy and full of complex detail; partial expositions of it have been given by Reiner (16) and, far more fully, by Binswanger (2); by the former in a book on volition, and by the latter in an article on the psychopathology of space.

We shall present here an analysis founded on Husserl's, but enormously abbreviated, as well as modified. Our interest will be mainly restricted to the spatiality of the visual and haptic, i.e., somesthetic, senses.

We shall begin by discussing the basic concept (not occurring in Husserl's treatment) of the psychological individual.

THE INDIVIDUAL

The psychological individual is, essentially, a living, experiencing and behaving being who is numerically one, rather than a multiplicity; although his existence, at a given moment, is highly diversified. The existent and his existence are always to be carefully distinguished.

Let us call the individual existent X. This X is not only one, at any given instant, but he preserves self-identity, i.e., he remains the same one throughout his life-course—no matter how radically the character of his existence may vary.

X is, *inter alia*, the one and only subject, or experiencer of his experience. The unity of his experience at a given moment,[1] and its unity as a single temporal stream[2] go back to the numerical singleness and identity of the experiencer.

[1] See F. C. Brentano (3), Royce (17).

[2] See Wm. James (8).

These matters have been expounded, with admirable acumen, by Alexander Pfänder (14). This author uses the term *das Ich*, which we prefer to translate not as "the ego," or "the self," but as "the individual"—a non-synonymous term, as will become clear. The individual as a "who" is radically different from any "what," or object.

THE BODILY SELF

Individual, self, and *ego* are not synonymous in common speech. One can say "That individual is angry," or "Mr. X is angry," but never "The self is angry." Even though, to be sure, anger *involves* having a self; it pertains to X as "beselved." We agree with common usage.

One can say, furthermore, that the individual called X *has* a self, but not that X *is* a self. This distinction is capital.

Mere numerical individuality and identity are, so to speak, the bare bones of selfhood. They are the purely formal, non-qualitative basis on which a self can arise. Considered as mere abstract individuals, all persons are precisely alike. But these X's have unlike selves; and a given X's self varies from one time to another. The mere individual is X taken in the narrowest sense. The individual, considered as endowed with a self, is X in a broader sense. The self is not an appendage to X; that is, X and his momentary self are not numerically two.

The entire self is a complex with many facets and sub-units; one of these is the *bodily self* (B). Schilder's term *body-image* (19, 20) is sometimes used with an essentially similar meaning.[3]

Consider voluntary, or purposive, action. When we voluntarily move, or voluntarily hold stationary, e.g., an arm, our intention is directed not toward anything physiological, but on the arm as a member of the phenomenally given *bodily self.* We do not intend a motor innervation; although our intention somehow makes it occur. Furthermore, our intention is primarily directed toward the *arm* as we experience it, and not primarily toward muscles.

When we voluntarily protrude the tongue, we do not intend a contraction of its transverse muscle—although this occurs physiologically. We simply "will" to stick out the tongue.

B is a complex unity which is experienced as "in solidarity with" the

[3] On the general topic of B, see especially Oskar Becker (1) Günther Stern (21, particularly the chapters entitled "Über die Raumindizes" and "Über das Haben."), A. Michotte (12), and J. Lhermitte (11). The literature on the phantom limb of amputees, e.g., D. Katz (9), is also instructive; as are Ponzo's remarkable experiments (15) on the experimental modifiability of the form of parts of the phenomenal B.

active and experiencing individual X, as somehow comprised in his oneness. G. Stern (21) has penetratingly analyzed the meaning of *haben* in "*Wir haben einen Leib.*"[4] It is unjust to regard B as a purely phenomenal fact. It is phenomenally given, but its essence goes beyond that. As Stern makes clear, the issue is a subtle one. Although we have no direct experience of them, our intention to move B leads to real physiological processes and to real movement of the body (as object of physics). B, far from being a pure "phenomenon," has to do with real potentialities; they "define" themselves in terms of B.

Further discussion would take us into a close consideration of the theory of voluntary action, which is beyond the scope of the present essay.

TRANSITIVE AND INTRANSITIVE AWARENESS

Pfänder (14) draws a fundamental distinction between two types of consciousness: (I) *Gegenstandsbewusstsein* and (II) *Innesein*. The terms could be translated as (I) *object-awareness*, or *objectifying awareness*, and (II) *inward awareness*.[5] We shall speak, instead, of (I) *transitive* and (II) *intransitive awareness*. Our discussion does not follow Pfänder completely.

We emphasize that the two types of consciousness are not mutually exclusive. For the "externalizing" senses of sight and hearing we have primarily the awareness of something not ourselves; and, secondarily, that of ourselves as aware of it. But note that (II) can exist without (I), as in a feeling of bodily strain or discomfort, or of general bodily euphoria.

Types (I) and (II) can exist as aspects of a single complex unity, in what may be called haptic interperception. An example of this is given when (*a*) we press against a wall, and feel its externality, and its resistance to us; or (*b*) our hand lies flat on a table, and a weight is laid on it. Here we are again aware of an external object, and also of its effect on ourselves; in this second case there is a passively experienced pressure rather than a resistance. Mere contact-experiences, as in touching or stroking an object, are still a different case.

The word *transitive* derives from *transire*, to go beyond. Intransitive awareness does not go beyond what may be called the domain of the individual. It can involve the bodily self (B), or the affective self, or, often,

[4] German has two words *Körper* and *Leib*, both translated as *body*, but often used with different shades of meaning. In a context of pure physiology *Körper* rather than *Leib* is often used. *Leib* is sometimes translatable as *bodily self* in our sense.

[5] See also Geiger (6).

both.[6] The affective and the bodily aspects of our experience often form an intimate unity.

Return to case (*a*) of "interperception": when we push against the wall, we are (intransitively) aware of ourselves as pushing; this is one "pole" of the unitary experience. The other "pole" is our transitive awareness of the wall as an external thing that resists us. And these are not two separate experiences, but a bipolar unity of experience.

When awareness is thus bipolar, it is not an object-perception in the fullest or highest sense. The latter species of perception is not an awareness of an object of interaction with us. Rather, it is the consciousness of a thing as it is in its own right, without reference to us.

The hardness of the wall is, phenomenally, an intrinsic property of the wall, which it possesses in independence of the particular push (strong or weak) that we happen to exert. However, we appreciate this hardness only by way of—through the mediation of—this push.[7]

In analogous fashion—*via* interperception—we achieve awareness of intrinsic object-properties like density, material consistency, roughness or smoothness. As Katz (10) has shown, these properties display remarkable constancy despite variation of the conditions of perception; e.g., an object retains the same properties when it is palpated through a glove, rather than with the bare hand.

Through the sense of vision we have an object-perception—a transitive awareness—which is always direct rather than mediated by *B*.[8]

B IN ITS TWO ASPECTS

G. Stern (21) says that *B* is "*ein spezifischer Bereich der Meinheit*" ("a special domain of mineness"), and at the same time "*ein Ding unter Dingen*" ("an object among objects"). In the first role, *B* is a domain of intransitive somesthetic experience, and also a motor field—a field for the definition and realization of *X*'s motor intentions.

B has a unique space of its own, which Grünbaum (7) calls the *Eigenraum* (proper space), and which is to be contrasted with the *Fremdraum* (foreign

[6] See M. Scheler (18), the section entitled *Die Schichtung des emotionalen Lebens—The Stratification of the Emotional Life.*

[7] See Conrad-Martius (4).

[8] Through hearing we appreciate sound as something that "travels over to us," and as something that issues from a place, or fills a voluminous region. The perception, though transitive, is not properly called object-perception.

The differences between the different sense-departments are penetratingly discussed by Conrad-Martius (4).

space). The two spaces meet at the surface of *B*. The boundary is capable of "artificial extension"; see below. The proper space is at once a voluminous medium for sensory "data" and a dynamic medium for action.

In the second role, *B* is, phenomenally, an "objective" thing, like a chair or a football or any other environmental object. If we are successfully to move our physical body (body as object of physics), and successfully to adjust it to the things of the outside physical world, we must have a "veridical" perception of the body—a perception that is conformable to physical reality. (The phantom limb, and other unusual phenomena, are exceptional cases of non-conformity.)

When we visually perceive one of our hands, or press it, or stroke it with the other hand, we appreciate it in its role as a mere object. We have an *intransitive* awareness which is simultaneously an *object-awareness.*

The importance of the second role for behavior is obvious. When we stoop to enter a low-ceilinged corridor, we take account of our body's "measure". Any action in which the hands, the feet or the entire frame need to be duly positioned with respect to external things is a further example; think, for example, of lifting a foot over an obstacle in one's path; or of putting a spoonful of food into the mouth, or of running after a thrown ball and catching it. Action normally conforms to veridical body-perception as well as to veridical world-perception.

SOMATIZATION

Grünbaum (7) discusses the action of reaching for an object: we reach out into "foreign space" and incorporate the object into our "proper space." The assimilation is of course not perfect. Our motor intention embraces the single unit arm-and-hand-and-object, but the object is still haptically discriminated from the enclosing hand. Even in the case of a ball we have thrown, there is a certain assimilation with the self; "our" action is not complete until the ball has attained (or missed) its destination.

The use of tools and other implements, including prostheses, offers many illustrations of what Grünbaum calls *Somatisierung* (somatization), e.g., poking with a stick, writing with a pen or pencil, hammering, and even riding a bicycle, rowing a boat, driving a car or flying a plane. As has often been pointed out, we "feel" the object at the end of the stick; we"feel" ourselves touch shore with the bow of our boat; and so on. And our clothing is so intimately included in proper space that we tend to forget our true anatomical boundary.

Goldscheider's well-known illusion (13) is especially striking. One holds in one's hand a string from which hangs a weight; on lowering the hand until the weight touches the floor, one feels a resistance—although there is actually a diminution of physical resistance. Here, as in the other cases, it is the psychological nature of our action that counts.

CENTERED AND CENTERLESS SPACE

Our visually and haptically given outer world, in "foreign space," is, phenomenally, experienced from *B* as a "center." By way of either sense, only a segment of the environment is, in the fullest way, "given" at any particular time.[9]

But, again, *B* is also *ein Ding unter Dingen*—one object among others. The "centered" space of a given moment is embedded in a centerless or, in Husserl's phrase, a "homogeneous" space, wherein one object is comparable to any other. As I walk about the room I have, to be sure, a kinematographic sequence of centered views, each phase differing from the preceding; but I also have the impression of a constant environment. And this objective environment is of primary importance for behavior.[10]

To conclude: our treatment of space has been highly condensed. We urge any interested reader not to miss the elegant and profound discussions of "being embodied" and "being in space" in Erwin Straus' writings (22 and 23)—magistral presentations fit to awaken us to the actual character of our existence in the world we daily live in.

REFERENCES

1. Becker, O. Beiträge zur phänomenologischen Begründung der Geometrie und ihrer physikalischen Anwendungen. *Jahrbuch für Philosophie und phänomenologische Forschung*, 1923, *6*, 385–560.
2. Binswanger, L. Das Raumproblem in der Psychopathologie. *Zeitschrift für die gesamte Neurologie und Psychiatrie*, 1933, *145*, 598–647.
3. Brentano, F. C. *Psychologie vom empirischen Standpunkt.* Leipzig; F. Meiner, 1924–25.
4. Conrad-Martius, H. Zur Ontologie und Erscheinungslehre der realen Aussenwelt. *Jahrbuch für Philosophie und phänomenologische Forschung*, 1916, *3*, 345–542; 1923, *6*, 159–333.
5. Duncker, K. Über induzierte Bewegung. *Psychologische Forschung*, 1929, *12*, 180–259.

---

[9] This centering in an experience-center is not to be confused with the matter of frames of reference in localization; e.g., the room wherein I stand or walk is a natural frame of reference. Phenomenally, I am in a corner of the room; it is not natural to experience the room as eccentrically oriented around me. On this topic, see Duncker (5).

[10] Woodworth and Marquis (24) review experiments on the spatial learning of rats, and emphasize that the animals ordinarily learn not specific routes but the layout of objects in space.

6. Geiger, M. Fragment über den Begriff des Unbewussten und die psychische Realität. *Jahrbuch für Philosophie und phänomenologische Forschung*, 1921, *4*, 1–137.
7. Grünbaum, A. A. Aphasie und Motorik. *Zeitschrift für die gesamte Neurologie und Psychiatrie*, 1931, *130*, 385–413.
8. James, Wm. *Principles of Psychology*. New York; Henry Holt, 1890.
9. Katz, D. *Zur Psychologie des Amputierten und seiner Prothese*. Leipzig: J. A. Barth, 1921.
10. Katz, D. *Der Aufbau der Tastwelt*. Leipzig: J. A. Barth, 1925.
11. Lhermitte, J. *L'image de notre corps*. Paris: Nouvelle Revue Critique, 1939.
12. Michotte, A. *La perception de la causalité*, 2nd ed. Louvain: Publications universitaires de Louvain, 1954.
13. Nagel, W. (Ed.) *Handbuch der Physiologie des Menschen*. Braunschweig: F. Viehweg, 1904.
14. Pfänder, A. *Einführung in die Psychologie*. Leipzig: J. A. Barth, 1904.
15. Ponzo, M. Phénomènes d'annulation perceptive avec des "stimulus" surliminaires. *Kwartalnik psychologiczny*, 1930, *1*, 7–14. Abstract in *Année Psychologique*, 1930, *31*, 707.
16. Reiner, H. *Freiheit, Wollen und Aktivität*, Halle: M. Niemeyer, 1927.
17. Royce, J. *Outlines of Psychology*. New York and London: Macmillan, 1903.
18. Scheler, M. *Der Formalismus in der Ethik und die materiale Wertethik*. Halle: M. Niemeyer, 1921.
19. Schilder, P. *Das Körperschema*. Berlin: J. Springer, 1923.
20. Schilder, P. *The Image and Appearance of the Human Body*. New York: International Universities Press, 1950.
21. Stern, G. *Über das Haben*. Bonn: F. Cohen, 1928.
22. Straus, E. *The Primary World of Senses*. New York: The Free Press, 1963.
23. Straus, E. *Phenomenological Psychology*. (Selected papers). New York: Basic Books, 1965.
24. Woodworth, R. S., and Marquis, D. C. *Psychology*, 5th ed. New York: Henry Holt, 1947.

9

Phantoms following Amputation of the Breast

by Marianne L. Simmel

Dennisport, Massachusetts

Kurt Goldstein was my teacher—a warm and generous preceptor, ever-stimulating, setting high standards, never satisfied with the easy answers or the facile pseudo-solutions of pseudo-problems. When I began to study the phantom phenomena that follow amputation or denervation he said with considerable pleasure: "That is about the only problem on which I have never published." Much of my thinking has been directed by the many discussions we had on this topic, as well as on many others. Within the last year or two I had the opportunity to tell him in preliminary fashion about the study to be presented below. He thought the problem was an important one, and the results did not come as a surprise to him.

The phantom limb which results after amputation of an extremity is a well-known phenomenon. An individual who has lost an arm or leg in an accident, or as the result of surgery, continues to feel the limb as if it were still present. The patients themselves are often puzzled by the fact that they feel they can wiggle the toes or bend the knee of the absent leg, and many report that initially they found themselves looking under the covers to verify the real state of affairs. Eventually they learn to live with the enduring enigma of their knowledge of the absence of the limb and their sensation of its continuing presence. Occasionally they forget, and try to scratch an itch on the calf of the missing leg, or reach out with the missing arm to support themselves. A small number of individuals suffer severe pain in the phantom, but this is rare and probably not germane to the present discussion.

Phantoms are a universal result after limb amputation, but their occurrence is neither limited to limbs, nor to amputation. Phantoms of amputated parts other than limbs have occasionally been reported in the literature. Of greater interest is the fact that amputation of a body part is not a necessary condition for the appearance of sensory phantoms, though it is indeed a sufficient condition. Phantoms appear just as predictably upon denervation of body parts. Denervation may be permanent, e.g., following transection of the spinal cord or lesion of the brachial plexus; or it may be transient, as with spinal anesthesia or complete brachial plexus block with local anesthetics.

In a series of earlier studies I investigated some of the conditions under which phantoms do, and do not, arise. These studies led to the conclusions that the phantom was primarily, though not solely, a kinesthetic experience; that it depends on past sensory, especially kinesthetic, experience; and that it appears whenever kinesthetic input is eliminated, and disappears when such input is re-established. In this context kinesthesis has been defined as the perception of active or passive motion through the joints and its result, i.e., the perception of the position of the limb. Furthermore, observations during recovery from spinal anesthesia have shown that kinesthesis may not be the only sensory modality involved. Recovery of some minimal degree of pressure sensitivity also plays a role in the disappearance of the phantom. While the quantitative relationships could not be specified in these observations, it seemed as if the threshold for the disappearance of phantoms consisted of some minimal "sum" of recovery of kinesthesis and pressure sensitivity, with perhaps varying contributions of the two constituents.

From a physiological point of view, kinesthesis and pressure sensitivity probably depend on the same mediating mechanism, and differ only in the site of application of the proximal stimulus: the joint capsules for kinesthesis, and the whole body surface and underlying tissues for pressure sensitivity. Yet, from the point of view of perceptual experience, the two are very different. Experienced motion through a joint does not feel like changing pressures in the joint. The question then arises: Do phantoms appear upon amputation or denervation of structures that lack joints, and thus lack kinesthesis as previously defined? Further, if such conditions do give rise to phantoms, does pressure sensitivity play any special role? The study to be reported is the first in a series specifically addresssed to this question.

The female breast differs in a number of important respects from a limb. Being without a bony joint, it obviously does not mediate kinesthesis in the above defined sense. It is, however, the site of a variety of pressure experiences in addition to those common to the whole body surface. With position changes there are pressure changes in response to gravity. As the breast enlarges during pregnancy there are accompanying sensations of engorgement which in some individuals recur regularly just prior to or during menstruation. There are the tumescent changes of the nipple in response to light touch. There are pressure sensations with lactation, and a variety of ever-changing pressure sensations in the woman who is nursing an infant.

We must note, however, an important difference between the history of sensory experiences arising from a limb and the history of sensations from the breast. Changes in kinesthetic input are a constant feature of the living individual from birth—and perhaps even before—while sensations arising from the breast can occur only after the beginning of breast development in early adolescence. Thus, if childhood sensory experience were the crucial sensory experience for the phantom, we could not expect a phantom breast to result upon amputation. Actually, such evidence as we have suggests that childhood sensory experience *per se* may be irrelevant for the phantom. It is the sensory experience during the time immediately preceding loss or denervation that determines whether or not a phantom will appear (12, 17).

Another fact which might be regarded as impeding the appearance of the breast phantom is the matter of cortical localization. It is generally assumed that only what is cortically mediated can become conscious experience, and only cortically-mediated experiences can persist and become the past experience of a later date. The breast, as far as we know, is at most minimally represented on the sensory cortex, and this might well preclude the appearance of breast phantoms.

Finally, there is the breast as the focus of special attitudes and motivations. One might expect to find an extensive discussion of this topic by Paul Schilder, but, as far as I have been able to discover, he never mentions loss of the female breast (11). On the one hand, to the extent that the breast connotes sexual attractiveness and femininity, its loss might be an especially severe blow to the patient. On the other hand, the loss of an arm or leg in a woman is noticed immediately by whomever she meets, and might thus be more traumatic than the loss of the breast which need never be evident in the ordinary social situation. In effect, the emotional impact of the loss is not relevant at this juncture. Our own previous studies of limb amputees, patients with spinal lesions or under spinal anesthesia have shown that motivational factors do not play a role in the appearance of the phantom, even though they may determine the patient's attitude towards the phantom (13).

S. Weir Mitchell is usually credited with the earliest reference to the phantom breast. The citation consists of half a sentence in a footnote and reads: "The amputated breast is often felt as present" (8, p. 350). I suspect that if Mitchell had ever examined such a patient, he would have treated us to one of his superb descriptions. In the voluminous literature on phantom limbs that has accumulated since Mitchell's treatise, breast phantoms received, until recently, only the most cursory mention. Gallinek "never observed" a phantom after amputation of the breast and concluded that the libidinous significance of the lost body part, i.e., the breast, was less important for the occurrence of the phantom than was the fact that an amputated part i.e., a limb, had been mobile (5). Riddoch stated categorically that "after amputation of the breast the nipple alone remains", and he saw this as supporting his view that only the most peripheral structures remain as phantoms because they are "anatomically most heavily endowed with sensory end organs and, physiologically, are most represented in the model of body shape" (10). In a recent publication Kolb writes as follows: "Mammary phantoms are appreciated as a percept of either the whole breast or the nipple. The perception is episodic, less realistic than that of a limb, and accentuated by menstruation or changes in the weather. The phantom may be observed as a scratching or itching of the breast or nipple" (7). Earlier he had reported his observations of a patient, a nun, with intractable pain in the mastectomy scar. "On inquiry the nun said she had not felt her breast was present after operation. However, when questioned as to when she first was aware of the loss of the breast, she declared she had not realized that the amputation had been performed until the surgeon had removed the dressing ten days after operation." And Kolb comments: "It seems plausible that a nun might deny the existence of her breast or the phantom representative of this part, in view of its unacceptable sexual or procreative significance which would offer a threat to her concept of herself as a nun" (6).

In the nineteen-fifties there appeared four separate studies of breast phantoms, with a reported incidence ranging from ten percent to sixty-five percent (1, 2, 3, 4). The lowest figure comes from Macdonald Critchley who examined thirty women after mastectomy and found that only in three of these there existed even a "soupçon de fantôme," while the remaining 27 subjects replied in the negative to his question. No other details are given (3).

Ackerly, Lhamon and Fitts interviewed 50 women who had undergone radical mastectomies for cancer from a few months to several years earlier. The patients were asked: "Have you ever felt the presence of that (amputated) breast?" Thirty-nine of the fifty patients replied in the negative, while eleven subjects replied in the affirmative; their remarks are given in the original publication. Comparison of various characteristics of those with and without phantoms yielded only one statistically significant difference, that between the mean ages of the two groups (1).

Crone-Münzebrock investigated 49 post-mastectomy clinic patients by means of a fairly detailed questionaire. Twenty-six patients reported phantoms, 23 reported no phantoms. Various comparisons between the two groups did not reveal any significant differences (4).

Finally, Bressler, Cohen and Magnussen interviewed 25 post-mastectomy clinic patients; sixteen of these described phantom sensation, the remainder did not. Only a few protocols are given in the article, and no other relevant details (2).

One striking finding is common to these four studies. The incidence of phantoms is neither zero, nor one hundred percent, but somewhere in between. To be sure, these were not very detailed investigations. Yet, even in the most rapid studies of phantom limbs following loss of an arm or leg in an adult, the incidence is usually well above 90%, and in more detailed inquiries it typically approximates one hundred percent. At the same time, we can specify conditions under which the incidence is nil, for instance, when the loss is due to gradual absorption in leprosy (12), or in amputation of a congenital malformation which had been devoid of sensitivity from birth (14, 15, 17).

The protocol material cited above, and some previous informal inquiries by the writer indicated that even those patients who did report breast phantoms did not seem to experience them as vividly as the limb amputees experience their phantom arms or legs. This observation called for more detailed questioning, and for the introduction of a situation which would allow the patient to differentiate more clearly between sensations of presence or absence of the breast. In addition, an attempt was made to obtain information on a number of conceivably relevant variables, among them also those considered previously by Crone-Münzebrock (4) and by Ackerly, Lhamon and Fitts (1).

SUBJECTS

The subjects of this study were 77 women who had undergone unilateral or bilateral radical mastectomy, in almost all cases for cancer. The majority of the patients were seen during routine clinic follow-up visits at the Massachusetts General Hospital in Boston, or The Mount Sinai Hospital in New York City, and, as far as possible, all patients attending on a particular clinic day were interviewed. A few additional patients were seen through the courtesy of Dr. Gerson Lesnick at the Central Manhattan Medical Group of New York City. Patients operated within a few days of the interview were seen as house patients at the Massachusetts General Hospital or The Mount Sinai Hospital.

Statistically the group may be described as follows: Their *ages at the time of the operation* ranged from 24 to 80 years, with a median of 49 years. *Ages at the time of the interview* ranged from 28 to 81 years, with a median of 55 years. The *interval between operation and interview* ranged from four days to 18 years. Eighteen patients were seen within a month of surgery. For the remaining 59 patients the median interval was four years and seven months. Five of the 77 patients had undergone *bilateral* mastectomies, 34 patients had had *right* unilateral operations, and 38 patients had *left unilateral* operations. Sixty-one patients claimed to be *right-handed*, seven claimed to be *left-handed* and for nine patients this information was not obtained. Sixty patients had had one or more *children*, seventeen had had none. The distribution of a variety of other characteristics will be given in the context of the results.

PROCEDURE

The patients were seen individually. They were first questioned in some detail concerning circumstances prior to surgery, especially the nature and duration of any pre-operative pain, discomfort or other sensation. They were asked about children, their ages, and whether and for how long they had nursed them; and they were asked whether they had known prior to surgery that they would lose the breast.

This preliminary information having been obtained, the conversation turned to the immediate post-operative events. The patient was asked what she had felt when she first woke from the anesthesia, whether she had been aware of the absence of the breast, and, if not, when and how she had discovered the loss. If the patient did not mention spontaneously sensations of absence or presence of the breast, the examiner tried to elicit a specific answer to a direct question.

The patient was then encouraged to talk freely about "how the breast feels now", where "now" was not restricted to the present moment, but included any sensations since the operation, both enduring and occasional ones. This conversation frequently included reports of pain or paresthesias of the scar and chest wall, along with observations of breast sensations; whenever there was any doubt to which of these the patient was referring, the examiner posed questions to clarify the distinction. Subsequently the patients were asked a series of specific questions which will be discussed in the analysis of the findings.

As previously mentioned, this interview took place either in the outpatient clinic or in the subjects' hospital room. The patients were seen while undressed, covered only with a sheet or hospital gown. This fact was used to advantage in the last part of the study, to which I shall refer as the sway exercise.

If, under ordinary conditions, a woman is not as aware of the presence of her breasts as she is, for example, of the presence of her arms and legs, it seemed important to create a situation which might heighten this awareness, and which might allow her to distinguish more clearly between sensations of presence or absence of the breast. The effect of gravity on body perception has been described by Parker and Schilder (9). While we could not replicate the condition described by these authors, i.e., acceleration and deceleration during a ride in an elevator, it seemed that the sway exercise might at least be a step in that direction. By enlisting the pull of gravity we hoped to obtain clear-cut reports even should we fail to do so during the interview.

The patient was now requested to stand up, place her hands for support on the edge of a table, bend forward, close her eyes and slowly sway back and forth. While so swaying she was asked to compare sensations on the two sides of her upper torso, and to report whether the missing breast felt absent or present.

Verbatim records were kept throughout the interview. In addition the protocols contain brief comments of the examiner's impression of the patient's intellectual and emotional characteristics, and any other striking features.

RESULTS

Since a detailed analysis of the results has been presented elsewhere (18), I shall discuss here only the major findings. The protocols contain vivid descriptions of the patients' experiences, but also a good deal of variability from one moment of the examination to another, and as a function of differently phrased questions. We had asked, for instance, on three different occasions whether the missing breast felt absent or present: in the discussion of the immediate post-operative experiences, in the context of contemporaneous sensations, and during the sway exercise. To this question we obtained between 10% and 21% "breast feels absent" answers, depending on the occasion, and between 22% and 39% "breast feels present" replies. Between 25% and 53% of the group told us that they could not really tell the difference between feelings of presence or absence of the breast, that it felt no different now from the way it had felt before operation etc. The incidence of such "no difference" responses rose strikingly when we asked patients with unilateral operations to compare sensations from the operated and the unoperated sides. Within the interview concerning the current state of affairs, 86% of the subjects replied that there was no difference; but when we asked for the same comparison during the sway exercise the incidence of "no difference" replies rose to 94%, making it all but unanimous.

It will be recalled that the "sway exercise" had been included in the examination on the assumption that, for unilaterally operated patients, the pull of gravity would facilitate the discrimination between sensations from the operated and the unoperated sides. Since we obtained almost 100% "no difference" reports, this hypothesis must now be rejected. In fact, it appears that the pull of gravity was not a crucial variable at all in this exercise. Instead, the exercise seems to have furnished the occasion for a more intense focus on breast sensations than was provided during the remainder of the inquiry. And, in view of the findings, such an intense focus produces reports of "no difference" which imply phantom sensations which, though practically universal in this group, are evidently less vivid than the usual phantom sensations reported by limb amputees. Moreover, while the limb amputee is surprised by the phantom, the patients who have lost a breast are only rarely astonished by the phantom they seem to experience. Much more typically they report that the missing breast feels "just normal"—"just like before the operation"—"no strange feelings at all." We shall return to this point in the discussion.

However, the unanimity of reports during the sway exercise was not typical of the protocols as a whole. In fact, there seemed to be rather marked individual differences among the patients' reports. It was our hypothesis that these individual differences were not a matter of chance, but were likely to be a function of variables that could be isolated, e.g. age, past sensory experience involving the breast, etc. In order to assess the impact of such factors, we grouped the protocols into six groups, according to the most striking characteristics of the reports concerning phantoms. These groups, and the criteria for classification were the following:

Group A. Phantom explicit. Patients in this group assert quite definitely that either the missing breast, or at least the nipple, feels or felt present. Twenty-six protocols were classified as belonging here.

Group B. Phantom when wearing brassiere, no phantom without brassiere. Protocols in this group are characterized primarily by the patient's assertion that she feels the breast as if it were present when she wears a brassiere, with an artificial breast or padding, and that she feels the absence of the breast when she is not wearing the brassiere. Five protocols were so classified.

Group C. "No difference." Patients whose protocols were so classified essentially assert that there is no difference in feeling of absence or presence of the breast, and/or no difference in that feeling pre- and post-operatively, and/or no difference in feeling between the two sides of the upper torso (for unilateral operations). Protocols may contain some relatively minimal comments asserting a sensation of the presence of the breast, but such comments are not prominent. If a protocol includes a statement of sensations of absence, such a statement must be contradicted somewhere within the record else the protocol does not qualify for inclusion in Class C. Thirty-two protocols were classified within this group.

Group D. No phantom. Protocols in this category assert that the breast feels absent. Such assertion need not be consistently maintained throughout— else this class would have vanished. However, a prominent contradiction within the protocol disqualified it from this class. Six protocols were classified in class D.

Group E. No information concerning phantoms. Protocols in this group provided no real information concerning the experience of presence or absence of the breast. Typically the records are very sparse and some contain grossly contradictory statements despite their brevity; some contain only descriptions of scar pain and paresthesias. Eight protocols were so classified.

Comparison of these six classes of protocols yielded the following results:

1. Patients in groups A and B, i.e., those who described phantoms explicitly, were significantly younger at the time of operation and at the time of the interview than patients in the other groups. There was, however, no significant differences between any of the groups with respect to the recency of the operation, i.e., the time between operation and interview. This finding is in agreement with a similar observation by Ackerly, Lhamon and Fitts (1).

2. On the assumption that recency of pregnancy, lactation and nursing might influence the phantom experience we had inquired about the age of the youngest child at the time of the patient's operation. Subjects in groups A and B had significantly younger "youngest" children than the other groups. As far as we can tell this is merely a function of the above indicated age difference and not an independent finding.

3. There was no significant difference between the groups with respect to the average number of children and the incidence and average duration of breast feeding. However, despite the similarity of the overall means, there are some indications of different patterns, most marked on comparison of the two large groups, A and C. Patients in Group A typically had one or two children, while patients in group C were equally likely to have no children, one or two children, or more than two children. Furthermore, patients in group C who nursed their children tended to do so for more extended periods than patients in group A.

4. Comparison of the several groups did not reveal any difference with respect to pre-operative pain and discomfort, or with respect to breast size. Thus, any notion that the experience of pain *per se*, or the loss of a large breast, are more likely to give rise to vivid phantoms than the absence of pain, or the loss of a small breast, must be discarded. Similarly, for unilaterally operated patients, loss of the right and the left breast was evenly distributed among the groups. Since only a very small number claimed to be ambidextrous or left-handed, no separate comparisons could be made for lateral dominance. Of the five patients with bilateral operations, four provided group A protocols, and the fifth fell into group C.

5. The patients in the several groups differed significantly with respect to their use of an artificial breast. Eliminating 19 patients who had been operated too recently, we find that the overwhelming majority of groups A and B wear an artificial breast, and the remainder what they describe as "padding." This is not true of the patients in groups C and D who are about equally likely to wear an artificial breast, a padding or nothing at all. In other words, explicit reports of breast phantoms are significantly related to the wearing of an artificial breast. One might be tempted to deduce from this statistical relationship that wearing of the prosthesis induces the phantom, or at least makes it more noticeable to the patient, and this is of course what the members of Group B appear to claim explicitly. However, the writer is not persuaded by this argument. As an alternative hypothesis, one might interpret the use of a prosthesis as a symptom of somewhat greater sensitivity to the reaction of one's environment and oneself, and the explicit report of phantom sensations as another sympton of greater sensitivity, or better observation of events pertaining to one's own person. This problem will be taken up again in the final discussion.

6. Information concerning the patient's emotional reaction to the surgery, and/or the diagnosis and/or the loss of the breast was culled from three sources: the patient's spontaneous remarks; the examiner's observations as noted in the protocols; and any relevant entries in the hospital chart. Essentially four types of reactions were isolated: (a) Explicit statements attesting to the presence of anxiousness and depression. (b) Remarks by the patients to the effect that the loss of the breast constituted an insult to their female pride. (c) Comments by the patients emphasizing the good adjustment they had made to the surgery, the implications of the diagnosis and/or the loss of the breast. (d) "Phobic" and "denial" reactions; the former is exemplified by the statement "I cannot bring myself to look at the scar," the latter, e.g., by reports of disbelief on being given the diagnosis, by prolonged delays of the surgery, etc.

There was no statistically significant difference in the incidence of these four types of reactions for the several groups. However, on inspection of the distributions groups A and B appear to be more likely to yield explicit reactions of anxiety and depression, while the majority of good "adjustment" comments as well as phobic and denial reactions come from group C.

DISCUSSION

The findings of this study must be evaluated against the background of the phantom experience of the amputee who has lost a limb. The first meeting between a phantom limb and its owner is, typically, a rather dramatic affair. As the patient wakes up from surgery he feels his leg present, he seems to be able to wiggle his toes quite normally—and then someone steps up to him and tells him that the operation went very well and he will be able to walk on an artificial limb in no time at all. No matter how well and how long before operation he was prepared for the loss of the leg, the patient typically cannot believe that it is really gone, until he can convince himself by looking under the covers. And though he thus verifies the true state of affairs, he continues to feel the absent limb as if it were still present. He has, as Weir Mitchell wrote, "a sense of its existence so vivid as to be more definite and intrusive than that of its truely living member." Needless to say, this is a very puzzling experience for the amputee, so much so that many have commented, "I thought I must be out of my mind."

The experience of the patient who has lost a breast is initially similar to that of the limb amputee, but then quite different. On awakening from the surgery the breast feels "no different" from before the operation; some patients report it felt present, others that they did not know whether or not it had been removed. Thereafter, when we ask the patients days or years after the operation about sensations of absence or presence of the breast, their single most typical reply is: "I have no strange feelings at all. It feels just normal, just like before the operation." If we ask about the difference of sensations between the two sides of the upper torso, almost all report "no difference." These reports imply phantom sensations. Yet, the patients are not surprised or puzzled, as are the limb amputees, by the evident contradiction between their knowledge of having lost the breast and the sensation of its continuing presence.

How can we account for the difference in the reactions of the limb amputee and the post-mastectomy patient? Specifically, are the roots of this difference to be sought in the phantom experience *per se*, or must we turn our attention to a different order of factors, for instance, questions of sampling, or "personality" differences, etc.? Though such "extraneous" factors clearly play a role in the reports we obtained, our main findings point unmistakably to a basic difference in the phantom itself.

The essential difference between the limb phantom and the breast phantom is one of vividness and articulation—in the literal and metaphorical sense. The phantom limb is a very lively and well-defined experience, with all the characteristics of the kinesthetically based experience of a normal limb, i.e., voluntary motion, position in space of the limb as a whole as well as its several parts, and thus even shape. The phantom breast is a much less vivid experience, a finding which did not come as a surprise to us, but the implications of which we had not altogether foreseen.

At the beginning of this paper several of the major differences between limb and breast were spelled out. Some of these differences led us to wonder whether a non-motile structure, such as the breast, is represented in the largely kinesthetic body scheme at all, or at least to a sufficient degree to give rise to phantom experiences upon loss. Our findings show that the breast is so represented, but more weakly than the limb, in the sense of lesser perceptual definition and clarity. Incidentally, this comparative weakness does not appear to influence the longevity of the phantom to any significant extent as far as we can tell from our data. The main effect of its relative weakness is that the phantom breast does, generally, not obtrude itself upon the individual's awareness, just as the normal breast is, under ordinary conditions, not a focus of vivid sensory experiences. It may be shapely in the eyes of the beholder, and may be a focus of emotional investment by the owner, but these facts are of a different order than sensory experience, and they evidently do not affect the breast's representation in the basic sensory scheme of the body. In that scheme the breast appears to be represented as primarily "present", without much definition or shape, and with position related only to general postural changes of the whole body. Consequently, upon loss of the breast, its continuing schematic representation expresses itself typically in but a vaguely experienced sense of "presence" which the patients formulate most easily as "no different" from the experience prior to the loss, or the experience of the remaining breast on the other side.

To the extent that the phantom breast does not obtrude itself on the individual's awareness, it does not create the hiatus between knowledge of loss and felt presence that is created by the phantom limb. This accounts for the lack of surprise and puzzlement of the mastectomy patients. And to the extent that the phantom breast lacks perceptual articulation, a variety of "extraneous" factors may influence the reports of phantoms, just as the so-called projective tests utilize ill-defined perceptual material to elicit responses the content of which is determined by factors other than the perceptual stimuli. The limb amputees, confronted with a perceptually well-articulated phantom, provide reports of their experiences which are consistent, i.e., varying very little with the examination situation, and which are practically unanimous, i.e., varying hardly from one individual to the other. In contrast to this, the poor perceptual definition of the phantom breast results in reports which vary both with the condition of inquiry and with certain individual differences among the subjects.

Fairly complex patterns of social, intellectual and personality variables seem to account for the obtained individual differences between our subjects. All these variables appear to enter into what might be described as an ability to observe events within one's own person as well as reactions of others, and to report such observations relatively accurately, and also to act on them. Intelligence in its usual definition enters into this, but so do attitudes *vis-à-vis* oneself and one's human environment. Those of our patients who gave explicit reports of phantom breast sensations received significantly fewer ratings of intellectual handicap. They seemed to be more likely to confront their own reactions of anxiety and depression in connection with the surgery, diagnosis and loss of the breast, and less likely to cling to one or the other defensive extreme of denial or phobic reactions. Their family constellations were more likely to meet present-day middle class expectations, and their practice of nursing their infants is as variable as were middle class expectations when their children were small. They respond to the present-day urban expectation when they tell us almost without exception that they wear an artificial breast. They are the "young middle-aged;" relatively more oriented to the world in which they are living than those who are approaching sixty and whose relationship to their surroundings can perhaps be characterized by the wish to avoid troublesome problems.

Given these general differences among individuals, the apparent lack of consistency of the reports from the several parts of the inquiry no longer seems incomprehensible. The direct question concerning sensations of absence or presence of the breast demands that attention be focused on a relatively unimpressive perceptual situation, and it implies a willingness to at least consider the possibility of giving a report of sensations which are contrary to the known state of affairs. To do so opens the way to problems that some people feel had better be avoided. Thus, "breast feels absent" might be viewed as an assertion of a known state of affairs rather than a report of an observation. In reply to the direct question whether the breast feels absent or present, the incidence of "breast feels absent" varies between 10% and 20%, depending on the context within which the question was asked. We also obtain between 20% and 40% of reports of sensations of the presence of the breast, and some of these come forth to the patient's own surprise, as the result of an observation not previously made at all, or only very sporadically on special occasions. A very considerable proportion of the subjects, between 25% and 65% tell us, in response to this question, that they feel no difference and/or that they could not tell whether or not the breast had been removed when they woke up from the surgery. That this report implies that the breast feels, or felt at the early time, as if it continued to be present seems not to have occurred to the majority of our subjects; though occasionally one or the other patient discovered this implication and commented on it, sometimes in surprised or even half-embarrassed fashion. This was even more striking when only the indirect question had been asked, i.e., when the patient was requested to compare the sensations between the two sides of the uppor torso, and especially when this was done during the sway exercise. Under these conditions even patients who had given the "logical" answers previously seemed to focus on sensations and joined into what turned out to be the almost unanimous reports of "no difference"—again at times to the patient's own amazement.

The lack of perceptual articulation of the breast and the breast phantom must account also, I think, for the reports of a small number of patients who tell us that the breast feels present when they wear an artificial breast and absent without the latter. At first glance this seems like a surprising report which has no equivalent among the limb amputees. On second thought, there is a precise equivalent among the leg amputees who report that while they are wearing an artificial leg the phantom leg coincides with it exactly, but as soon as they take off the prosthesis the phantom leg is experienced as telescoped. In other words, a prosthesis that rather closely replicates the everyday function of the lost limb can superimpose its own articulation and shape on the phantom, but the phantom returns to its "intrinsic" articulation upon removal of the prosthesis. The situation seems to be much the same for some of the mastectomy patients. The prosthesis supplies the normal contour and weight experience—the latter is especially mentioned by our subjects—and thus the prosthesis gives its definition to the phantom. The phantom breast without prosthesis does not have the leg's intrinsic definition. As a result, the patient contrasting the experience with and without prosthesis reports a well-defined phantom for the former situation, and an absence of that experience for the latter situation.

Finally, a brief comment on our negative findings. Despite reasonably diligent inquiry we were unable to correlate the different types of reports concerning breast phantoms to individual differences in the histories of breast sensations. We compared the several groups of protocols with respect to the incidence of pre-operative pain and discomfort, with respect to histories of pregnancy, lactation and nursing, all of which have sensory implications, with respect to differences in breast size which might well have given rise to different sensory histories. None of these showed any relationship to the kind of reports we obtained of breast phantoms.

This lack of relationship is, I think, a positive finding. It supports the notion that sensory input of the kinesthetic-pressure type primarily provides geographic information, i.e., *where* something is happening. In that sense it provides "contours" and increases perceptual articulation, and signals "presence" only incidentally. For this reason the phantom limb of the amputee assumes a long-term shape that corresponds much more closely to its representation on the Penfield-Boldrey homunculus than to the visual geometry of the limb before amputation (16). Contrast with this the relative poverty of information provided by breast sensations, especially those incident to pregnancy, lactation, nursing and breast size, which probably carry only one of two possible addresses: either they are localized in the nipple, or they are experienced as poorly localized "inside the breast." Thus they do not provide contours or articulation to the schematic representation of the breast. With the exception of the nipple, the schema of the breast remains ill-defined, and this is precisely what the ill-defined breast phantom evinces.

Presented at the Kurt Goldstein Memorial Meeting held at the 37th Annual Meeting of the Eastern Psychological Association on April 16, 1966, in New York City. The writer is indebted to several people without whose generous help this study could not have been conducted. Dr. Edward D. Churchill of The Massachusetts General Hospital, Boston, and Dr. Gerson Lesnick of The Mount Sinai Hospital and the Health Insurance Plan of New York City kindly allowed me to examine their patients. Dr. Eugenia Hanfmann and Dr. Denise Thum gave invaluable assistance in the analysis of the protocols. The study was initiated during the writer's tenure of USPHS Special Research Fellowship MF 1193 awarded by the National Institute of Mental Health. Its completion was supported by grant 61-229 of the Foundations Fund for Research in Psychiatry. The findings have been reported in detail in *Neuropsychologia*, 1966, *4*, 331–350 (18); parts of that article are reprinted here by permission.

REFERENCES

1. Ackerly, Wm., Lhamon, Wm., and Fitts, Wm. T. Phantom breasts. *J. nerv. ment. Dis.*, 1955, *121*, 177–178.
2. Bressler, B., Cohen, S. I., and Magnussen, F. The problem of phantom breast and phantom pain. *J. nerv. ment. Dis.*, 1956, *123*, 181–187.
3. Critchley, M. Quelques observations relatives à la notion de la conscience du moi corporel ("Corporeal Awareness"). *L'encéphale*, 1955, *44*, 501–531.
4. Crone-Münzebrock, A. Phantomgefühl und Phantomschmerz nach Mamma-amputation. *Langenbecks Arch. u. Dtsch. Z. Chir.*, 1950, *266*, 569–575.
5. Gallinek, A. Über die Entstehung des Phantomgliedes. *Dtsch. Z. Nervenheilk.*, 1931, *122*, 38–54.
6. Kolb, L. C. *The Painful Phantom.* Springfield, Ill.: Charles C. Thomas, 1954.
7. Kolb, L. C. Phantom Sensations, Hallucinations and the Body Image. In *Hallucinations*, New York: Grune & Stratton, 1962, pp. 239–248.
8. Mitchell, S. W. *Injuries of Nerves and their Consequences.* (First ed. 1872.) New York: Dover, 1965.
9. Parker, S., and Schilder, P. Das Körperschema im Lift. *Z. ges. Neurol. & Psychiat.*, 1930, *128*, 777–783.
10. Riddoch, G. Phantom limbs and body shape. *Brain*, 1941, *64*, 197–222.
11. Schilder, P. *The Image and Appearance of the Human Body.* (First ed. Berlin 1925). New York: International Universities Press, 1950.
12. Simmel, M. L. Phantoms in patients with leprosy and in elderly digital amputees. *Amer. J. Psychol.*, 1956, *69*, 529–545.
13. Simmel, M. L. Phantoms, phantom pain and "denial." *Amer. J. Psychother.*, 1959, *13*, 603–613.
14. Simmel, M. L. The absence of phantoms for congenitally missing limbs. *Amer. J. Psychol.*, 1961, *74*, 467–470.
15. Simmel M. L. Phantom experiences following amputation in childhood. *J. Neurol., Neurosurg. & Psychiat.*, 1962, *25*, 69–78.
16. Simmel, M. L. The reality of phantom sensations. *Social Research*, 1962, *29*, 337–356.
17. Simmel, M. L. Developmental aspects of the body schema. *Child Devel. Monog.*, 1966, *37*, 83–95.
18. Simmel, M. L. A study of phantoms after amputation of the breast. *Neuropsychologia*, 1966, *4*, 331–350.

IV

FROM APHASIA TO SCHIZOPHRENIA

10

Gelb-Goldstein's Concept of "Concrete" and "Categorical" Attitude and the Phenomenology of Ideation*

by A. Gurwitsch
New York, New York

Husserl's theory of universals as general objects and specific ideal entities has very soon acquired widespread notoriety not, however, without too often being grossly misinterpreted and misrepresented, partly on account of the not very fortunately chosen term of "intuition of essences" ("Wesenserschauung"). When Husserl established his theory of ideation for the first time in *Logische Untersuchungen*, he hardly went beyond asserting the specific nature and irreducibility of those acts through which universals in contradistinction to particular things are meant and apprehended and, correspondingly, also the specific nature and irreducibility of the objects apprehended through the acts in question. For this purpose, Husserl had to engage himself in a thoroughgoing analysis and discussion of the theories of abstraction prevailing in the tradition of classical British empiricism.

Most of the essential ideas which Husserl developed in the course of his critical discussion and refutation of the empiricistic theories of abstraction have been fully confirmed by the results to which Gelb and Goldstein have been led in their studies of brain injuries. Considering that Gelb and Goldstein carried out their investigations within a mere neurological and psychopathological setting and in complete independence of phenomenological and, quite in general, philosophical points of view and theories, their corroboration of the pertinent views of Husserl appears the more significant and conclusive. After having set forth the convergence between Husserl's and Gelb-Goldstein's theories, we shall embark upon formulating further phenomenological problems of ideation which arise on the basis of the mentioned convergence, taking also into account Husserl's later contributions towards the problem under discussion.

I. CATEGORIAL EQUALITY AND QUALITATIVE HOMOGENEITY

Empiricistic theories deny universals as ideal entities and objects *sui generis*. Ideation is reduced to, or, at least, explained by apprehension of similarity or likeness between particular things. General terms are, accordingly, held to denote classes of similar particular things. When a gen-

* This article, originally written in honor of Kurt Goldstein on the occasion of his 70th birthday, November 6, 1948, was, and is, meant not only to express the personal indebtedness of the writer to his teacher but also to show the importance of Goldstein's work for problems treated in Husserlean phenomonological philosophy. It was originally published in *Philosophy and Phenomonological Research*, 1949, *10*, pp. 172–196, and is reprinted here by permission.

eral term is predicated of a particular thing, the meaning of such predication can be but the assertion that the given thing belongs to a certain class, i.e., bears similarity or likeness to other particular things.

In his refutation of the empiricistic theories, Husserl points out that every relation of similarity or likeness between particular things presupposes a point of view from, and a respect in, which the particular things are similar or alike[1]. If two things are alike as to their color or their form, the point of view with reference to which the relation of likeness obtains is, in the former case, the εἶδος of color, in the latter case, that of form; both εἴδη have to be considered as identical ideal entities. Every object bears similarity to a great many objects; to some in one respect, to others in a different respect. To put it otherwise, every object belongs to a great many classes comprising objects which are similar to each other. Emphasizing the classes founded on similarity or likeness, but denying the identical ideal εἶδος with reference to which the relations of similarity or likeness obtain, one is confronted, as Husserl shows, with the insuperable difficulty of accounting for the constitution and unification of the very classes and also for that which separates the classes from each other and keeps them apart. A red sphere is similar to both a green sphere and a red cube; the similarities involved in either case are of a different kind. Hence similarities prove to admit of differences in kind. As the objects themselves, so similarities between objects may be compared with each other and thus turn out to be similar or alike or else to differ from each other. Similarities too may, therefore, be grouped and classified according to species. Again the problem arises as to the point of view with reference to which similarities are similar to, or different from, each other. In other words, the very problem of the εἴδη from which we started is but transferred from the objects between which similarities obtain to the similarities themselves. On the grounds of the empiricistic denial of the εἴδη as identical ideal units and entities, there remains but the resorting to similarities between similarities, and this shows that a *regressus in infinitum* is unavoidable on the mentioned grounds.

Equality or likeness with reference to an εἶδος as point of view or, as we shall likewise say, categorial equality or likeness is defined by Husserl as that relationship which obtains between objects as fall under one and the same species.[2] Since every εἶδος necessarily constitutes and defines

[1] Husserl, *Logische Untersuchungen* (referred to hereafter as *Log. Unt.*), Vol. II, II, chap. I; cf. the condensed but faithful rendering by M. Farber, *The Foundation of phenomenology* (Cambridge, Mass., 1943), chap. IX A.

[2] Husserl, *Log. Unt.*, Vol. II, 1, p. 113, "Gleichheit ist das Verhältnis der Gegenstände, welche einer und derselben Species unterstehen"; cf. also *Erfahrung und Urteil*, p. 393 "*. . . Gleichheit nur ein Korrelat der Identität eines Allgemeinen. . . .*"

a class, namely the class of objects which fall under it,[3] the relation of categorial equality may be said to obtain between objects by virtue of the latter's belonging to one and the same class. For any objects to state that they belong to the same class or that they stand in the relation of categorial equality are but two expressions of the same state of affairs. Objects between which the relation of categorial equality is ascertained, to obtain, are not taken in themselves in all their individualities and particularities, but are rather considered with reference to a certain species as particularizations of the latter, or as representatives of the class to which they belong by virtue of their actualizing the εἶδος in question.

From equality in the categorial sense there is to be distinguished the sensuous factor of equality (*"das sinnliche Gleichheitsmoment"*), the latter being to the former what "figurale Momente" by means of which pluralities are perceptually recognized are to pluralities as apprehended through genuine representation.[4] For the apprehension of a plurality in the latter mode, there are required as many acts as the plurality contains elements, each element being apprehended through one of these acts; in addition to these acts of individual apprehension, there is furthermore required an act of synthesis through which the individually apprehended elements are colligated and united.[5] Such genuine apprehension of a plurality by means of explicit colligation cannot be assumed to occur when, e. g., looking at the sky we instantaneously see "many" stars or entering a hall perceive at a glance "a lot" of people.[6] To account for the apprehension of pluralities under circumstances which preclude explicit colligation, Husserl refers to "quasi-qualitative Momente" or "figurale Momente" as perceptual features exhibited by certain groups.[7] In speaking of the perception of a "row of trees," a "column of soldiers," a "swarm of birds," etc., we render by the terms "row," "column," "swarm" a certain aspect, a certain characteristic property or organizational form with which the group in question presents itself in very sense-experience. Geometrical configurations, all kinds of

[3] *Id., Erfahrung und Urteil,* p. 423.

[4] *Id., Log. Unt.,* Vol. II, 1 p. 282 note.

[5] *Id., Philosophie der Arithmetik,* pp. 79 f.

[6] *Id., ibid.,* pp. 219 ff.

[7] *Id. ibid.*; pp. 228 ff.; cf. also Farber, *loc. cit.,* pp. 46 ff. In the present context we cannot dwell at some length on Husserl's concept of "figurale Momente"; we wish, however, to point out that the phenomena referred to by Husserl are the same which Chr. v. Ehrenfels studied in his consequential article "Ueber Gestaltqualittäten" in *Vierteljahrsschrift für wissenschaftliche Philosophie,* Vol. XIV (1890). Concerning the complete agreement between Husserl and v. Ehrenfels as to the theoretical interpretation of the phenomena in question, cf. A. Gurwitsch, "Quelques aspects et quelques développements de la Psychologie de la Forme" pp. 415 ff. in *Journal de Psychologie Normale et Pathologique,* Vol. XXXIII (1936).

arrangements of points and lines belong here as well as the characteristic aspect of the chess-board pattern, the specific nature of a rhythm, a melody, etc. *"Figurale Momente" denote characters, properties, aspects of groups, and are no more and no less a matter of mere sense-experience than the groups themselves and the "elements" of which the groups consist.* Among such group-aspects there must also be reckoned, and it deserves special attention in the present context, the perceptual feature of qualitative homogeneity. We see at a glance "a heap of apples" or "a heap of nuts," without resorting to, and, in most cases, without even being able to resort to $\frac{n(n-1)}{2}$ comparisons, *n* being the number of elements involved.[8] The group in question displays the perceptual feature of qualitative homogeneity of a specific kind, by virtue of which the "heap of apples" presents a group-aspect different from that of a "heap of nuts." Qualitative homogeneity is involved in both cases, but is differently specified in either.

There is then a mere perceptual apprehension of equality in the sense of qualitative homogeneity which neither requires nor implies any reference to an εἶδος. Sensuous equality between the members of a perceived group is exhibited by the group as a specific perceptual character of its own, as a "figurales Moment" of a special kind. By the same token, the group-character in question, as every "figurales Moment," is confined and restricted to the very group as experienced in actual perception. Suppose the perception of a certain number of red objects, all of identical chromatic properties (as to hue, brightness, etc.). For the perception of such a group, the perceptual apprehension of qualitative homogeneity specified in a certain determinate manner, is characteristic. Still the *perception of the group* in question *with its characteristic group-aspect is not only entirely different from, but does not even convey or found the idea of the class of red objects,* no more than that of the class of red objects of a certain completely particularized chromatic determination. Such a class, understood as the extension of a concept or εἶδος, which is a necessary correlate of the εἶδος is essentially an infinitely open class, comprising whatever objects have the properties in question, whether or not they happen to be given in actual experience.[9] Considered as that perceptual phenomenon as which it presents itself in experience, qualitative homogeneity, on account of its sensuous nature and the ensuing restriction to actual sense-experience, contains no motivation leading beyond actual perception, in particular toward the idea of a class in the conceptual sense. On the other hand, a genuinely conceptual class, e.g., that of red objects, which, as shown before, cannot be

[8] Husserl, *Philosophie der Arithmetik*, p. 233.

[9] *Id.*, *Erfahrung und Urteil*, §82 and pp. 422 f.

constituted and unified except with reference to an εἶδος does obviously not present itself as an experiential or perceptual whole.[10] Its unity is not of a sensuous nature, but is derived from the unity of a categorial intention, the class itself being the correlate of that intention. It follows that in contradistinction to sensuous equality or qualitative homogeneity, categorial equality, defined as the relationship between objects which belong to a certain class or, what amounts to the same, fall under the corresponding εἶδος, proves a mere conceptual relationship established by categorial thought, and not a relationship of sensuous or perceptual nature.

As the result of Husserl's discussions and distinctions, we may state the unaccountability of ideation in terms of equality, insofar as categorial equality presupposes, and is rendered possible by the apprehension of an εἶδος, whereas qualitative homogeneity does not found the presentation of a class in the conceptual sense, at least not without the intervention of specific mental activities and operations.

II. GELB-GOLDSTEIN'S ANALYSIS OF A CASE OF AMNESIA OF COLOR-NAMES

Husserl's views have found hitherto unnoticed corroboration by Gelb-Goldstein's concepts of "categorial" and "concrete" attitude, concepts which the mentioned authors have laid down on the basis of their studies of numerous psychopathological cases presenting most various symptoms. For the sake of conciseness and brevity, we shall essentially limit ourselves to their analysis of a case of amnesia of color-names;[11] the symptoms involved being closely related to the phenomena dealt with by Husserl.

a. The symptoms and the perceptual experience of the patient

Gelb-Goldstein's patient, Th., manifested the familiar difficulty in naming a color shown to him; even the suggestion of the correct name was of little, if any, avail. Presented with color-samples and requested to choose a sample fitting to a color-name, Th. repeatedly uttered the name, but it seemed that the word had no meaning for him. He could no more indicate the name of the color of an object which was mentioned to him than he was able to point out a color corresponding to a color-name. If, however, instead of being asked to *name* the color of an object, the patient was requested to choose a sample fitting to the object in question, he succeeded very well due to his excellent visualization, provided a fitting specimen was there. He never chose a wrong color. If the specimen did not match perfectly the color of the mentioned object, Th. was not satisfied and continued looking for better fitting ones.

[10] *Id. Log. Unt.*, Vol. II, 1, pp. 282 f.

[11] A Gelb and K. Goldstein, "Ueber Farbennamenamnesie . . ." in *Psychologische Forschung*, Vol. VI (1924).

Particularly interesting and revealing was the behavior of the patient, when he was given a color-specimen (e.g., a red one) and was requested to sort out all those specimina as agreed with the former in hue, though they might differ as to brightness, warmth, etc.[12] Th. proceeded with much uneasiness and hesitation. Sometimes he tried to assort specimina of equal or very similar hue, sometimes specimina of different hue which, however, agreed as to brightness. It happened not infrequently that, having already chosen a correct specimen (a red one), he laid it aside or that he paid no attention at all to the red specimina. Some of his choices appeared quite incomprehensible. There arose the impression, rejected, as we shall see, by Gelb and Goldstein, that the patient was unable to abide by his principle of coordination and shifted from one principle to any other; assorting sometimes according to hue, sometimes according to brightness. The patient himself was far from satisfied by his own procedure. Having made a first selection of specimina, he again and again compared each one of the selected specimina with the sample of reference until he finally accepted a few, but very few only, as fitting, not without expressing doubts as to whether he might not find still better fitting ones. The meticulosity with which the patient proceeded in choosing a color-specimen corresponding to the color of an object either presented or merely mentioned, reappeared in his assorting. For Th. to be satisfied with his choice, the color-specimina had to agree in both color and brightness, i.e., to be identical. In fact, when his task was to match identical nuances, the patient succeeded perfectly.

Starting from the procedure of their patient in assorting color-specimina, Gelb and Goldstein explain all the symptoms presented by Th. as well as by other patients who had been studied by various authors, as effects of a general reduction from the level of "categorial" behavior and attitude to that of "concrete" attitude. Confronted with a color-specimen, the patient has of the latter a characteristic perceptual experience in which, according to the objective qualities of the specimen, the factor of hue, that of brightness, or some other factor may prevail.[13] *It is by that characteristic experience with its individuality and particularity that the patient abides and cannot help abiding.* When, e.g., in the experience of the specimen of reference the factor of hue is predominant, whereas in that of another sample which Th. compares with the former, the factor of brightness prevails, the patient cannot persuade himself to group the two specimina, on account of the difference in brightness, though both are of the same hue, say red. Conversely when the factor of brightness prevails in the experience of either specimen and when the latter are of the same, or nearly the same, brightness, the patient considers them as fitting together, the eventual

[12] *Id.*, *ibid.*, I, §3.

[13] *Id.*, *ibid.*, pp. 148 f.

difference in hue notwithstanding. It goes without saying that Th. sometimes grouped specimina agreeing in hue. Whether or not two color-specimina appear to him as fitting together depends entirely and exclusively upon whether or not he has the experience of *concrete agreement, accordance,* and *coherence* ("konkretes Kohärenzerlebnis") on account of the particular, characteristic individual aspects which the specimina present to him. In the case of identical specimina, the patient obviously experiences concrete agreement to the highest possible degree; hence he is prompt and unhesitating in assorting such specimina. On the other hand, when the samples selected by the patient are not identical, but merely very close to each other, he still assorts them on account of his experience of concrete accordance. The latter, however, appears to him as not quite perfect and somehow increasable; therefore he does not feel completely satisfied with his choice. If in the case of Th., the experience of concrete accordance depended upon factors like hue or brightness, it could, and did in other cases,[14] also be attached to esthetic effects, suitability for practical purposes, etc.

Confronted with the same task as the patient, *viz.*, the task of grouping color-specimina according to hue, the normal person unhesitatingly assorts two, say, red specimina, though the one may be very dark, the other rather bright. In so doing, the normal person is not unaware of the difference between the specimina. Carrying out the assignment given to him, however, the normal person does not take the specimina in their particularity and individuality, but rather sees in either a special case of redness. To express it in Husserl's terminology, the normal person does not depend for his assorting upon sensuous equality or likeness, but may, and does, group specimina according to the relation of equality in the categorial sense, which obtains between the specimina in question insofar and *only* insofar as the latter are considered as particularizations and actualizations of the εἶδος of redness. In his grouping, the normal person is not confined to abiding by the immediately given experiential features of perception, including among the latter the experience of concrete agreement and accordance. He may impose a principle of classification upon the data of perception, he may consider these data from a certain point of view, in the case under discussion from the point of view of hue.

It is just this attitude, the "categorial" attitude, that brain-injured patients are utterly unable to adopt, an inability which, according to Gelb and Goldstein, defines the essential difference between normal persons and patients. Confined to the content of perception as actually experienced, the patients abide by that content in all its singularity and particularity; they are unable to see in it the representative of a color-species or of a cate-

[14] Cf. K. Goldstein, "L'analyse de l'aphasie et l'étude de l'essence du langage," *Psychologie du Langage* (Paris 1933), pp. 480 f.

gory or class of colors.[15] To the patient's mind, the given color-specimen stands out as that as which, and exactly as it, presents itself in perceptual experience without any reference whatsoever to any thing beyond itself. Especially, the patients cannot regard their perceptual experience in the light or under the perspective of a principle extraneous to that perceptual experience in the sense that it is not embedded in, but somehow imposed upon the latter. Hence the patients prove unable to refer their actual experience to any ideal or conceptual order; they cannot take a stand or a view with regard to their perceptual experience, not to speak of varying views so that, according to the view taken, sometimes these, sometimes other features of the perceptual content appear as particularly relevant or essential.[16]

Every brain-injury entails, according to Goldstein,[17] a regression to the level of merely concrete behavior and attitude. Only that exists for the patient which offers itself in perceptual experience. Within the content of actual experience, there is no differentiation between the experiential features as to their relevancy and significance. All features of the perceptual content are of equal importance for the patient; each of these features is of paramount importance for the mere reason that it is encountered in actual perception. The patients are somehow overwhelmed and overpowered by actual experience imposing itself upon them by a force of constraint from which they cannot emancipate themselves. Thus the patients are unable to conceive of eventual changes or modifications in the experiential content, i.e., to conceive of the latter as possibly being different from what it actually is. This goes so far that brain-injured patients cannot make or even repeat statements which are at variance with actual experience as, e.g., repeating the sentence "Today the weather is bad and it is raining," when in fact the sun is shining.[18] All that these patients can do is act (in the broadest sense of the word) under the suggestions and imperatives as arise from the given concrete situation. To the extent to which problems can be solved in this direct and immediate way, the patients succeed, for their actions, oriented with regard to and dictated by the experienced concrete situation, prove adequate to the latter. When, however, the patients are confronted with problems that cannot be solved by actions directly and

[15] Gelb and Goldstein, *loc. cit.*, pp. 152 f.; Goldstein, *loc. cit.*, pp. 453 ff. and 473 ff.; cf. also E. Cassirer, *Philosophie der symbolischen Formen*, Vol. III, pp. 258 ff., (Berlin, 1929).

[16] Cassirer, *loc. cit.*, pp. 261 ff.

[17] Goldstein, *loc. cit.*, pp. 453 f. and 470; *Der Aufbau des Organismus* (Haag, 1934), pp. 18 ff.

[18] Cassirer, *loc. cit.*, pp. 295 f. and 314; cf. also W. Hochheimer, "Analyse eines Seelenblinden von der Sprache aus," *Psychologische Forschung*, Vol. XVI (1932), pp. 30 f.

immediately induced by the very experiential situation, they always fail. One might say, the patients are at the mercy of actualities so as not to be able to conceive of possibilities or to look at the given situation from a distance.[19] The latter attitude requires and implies a certain detachment from the experienced concrete situation which, without losing its character of actuality and reality, yet loosens its grasp upon the experiencing subject's mind so as to permit him to consider the given situation under varying angles, from different points of view, and to display some initiative in its respect. Since it has become impossible for the patients to detach themselves from the given situation and to look at the latter from a distance, they prove deprived of any initiative whatever.

b. Theoretical interpretations

Considered in the light of Gelb and Goldstein's general characterization of the "concrete" and "categorial" attitudes, the behavior of their patient Th. in assorting color-samples becomes understandable. Already holding in his hand a sample agreeing with the specimen of reference as to hue, the patient, as mentioned above,[20] not infrequently put the "correct" sample aside to choose another one of different hue, but of equal or nearly equal brightness as the specimen of reference. It must not be concluded herefrom that the patient inconsistently shifted from one principle of classification to another. To assort color-specimina with reference to a principle of classification requires adoption of the "categorial" attitude, whether the principle of classification is adhered to consistently, i.e., for a certain length of time or is adopted for a brief moment only. Maintaining that their patient is utterly unable to adopt the "categorial" attitude, Gelb and Goldstein conclude that he has no principle of classification at all.[21] Hence Th.'s behavior has to be explained by an alternation and succession upon each other of different experiences of concrete agreement. Suppose the specimen of reference to be experienced in concrete agreement as to hue with a specimen *a*, and the patient to notice at this moment another sample *b* which, though of different hue, is highly similar to the specimen of reference as to brightness, even more similar in the mentioned respect than *a* is as to hue. While the factor of hue had thus far prevailed in the experience of the specimen of reference, that of brightness now becomes predominant. An experience of concrete coherence based on brightness supersedes the previous experience of concrete coherence based on hue. Guided exclusively

---

[19] Goldstein, *Der Aufbau des Organismus*, p. 19; Gelb, "Remarques générales sur l'utilisation des données pathologiques pour la psychologie et la philosophie du langage," *Psychologie du Langage* (Paris, 1933), pp. 415 f.

[20] *Supra*, pp. 123ff.

[21] Gelb and Goldstein, *loc. cit.*, pp. 149 ff.; Gelb, *loc. cit.*, pp. 409 f.

by that experience of concrete accordance which proves stronger and more imperative, the patient is thus led to prefer *b* to *a*.

This interpretation is borne out by Gelb and Goldstein's observations of their patient Hac.[22] Requested to sort out those color-samples which seemed to him to fit with a given specimen of reference, Hac., differently from Th., selected a rather great number. A closer examination of Hac.'s choices revealed that any two specimina selected in immediate succession were highly similar to each other as to certain optical qualities (e.g., hue, brightness, warmth, and other properties hard to describe and to formulate), so that they may well have been experienced to be in concrete accordance. Such, however, was not the case when all the selected specimina were compared with the given specimen of reference. In the course of assorting samples, Hac., in contradistinction to Th., did not abide by the given specimen of reference. His specimen of reference varied from moment to moment in that at any moment the sample which he had last chosen became the specimen of reference for the subsequent selection. Th. performed *one single process of selection* in that he persistently referred his choices to the given specimen of reference and thus, after many vacillations and hesitations, he came to assemble only very few samples, since only these few were experienced in concrete accordance with specimen of reference. When Hac. selected a great many specimina and established a series in which two neighbors, but only neighbors, stand to each other in the relation of concrete accordance, it is because, instead of one single process of selection, he performed a *set of partial choices* with varying specimina of reference, looking out at each choice for a sample as agreed with that which he had selected just before. Whatever the difference in the procedure of the two patients, both of them were determined in their choosing entirely and exclusively by the experience of concrete agreement and coherence.

To gain more insight into the procedure of assorting color-samples on the basis of the experience of concrete accordance, let us describe the phenomenal aspect of that experience. Gelb and Goldstein point out[23] that the experience of concrete coherence must not be misconstrued as a secondary experience supervenient to those of the specimina themselves and their chromatic qualities. In other words, it is not that the specimina in question are first experienced independently of each other, each one determined by definite chromatic properties of its own and are then, subsequently, related by concrete accordance. Rather the specimina in question are experienced but *within the relation of concrete coherence*. This is to say, the specimina—for the sake of simplicity let us assume there are but two—present themselves as members or "parts" of a *contexture of which, on account of its*

[22] Gelb and Goldstein, *loc. cit.*, pp. 171 f.
[23] *Id.*, *ibid.*, p. 153, note 2.

uniformity, the phenomenon of concrete agreement is the specific and distinctive feature. From the point of view of the specimina, the uniformity of the contexture of which they are "parts" appears as qualitative homogeneity. The two specimina present themselves as platforms on the same plane, with no rise or fall from the one to the other, with no tension between them. Obviously this characterization holds for the specimina but as members of the contexture in question which offers the typical aspect of a level-phenomenon.[24] Within this contexture, either specimen occupies a definite place and plays a specific role which, to be sure, is the same for both specimina in a contexture of the kind as here considered. It is from the contexture with the properties which the latter has of its own and with reference to all the other members of the contexture that each one of the members derives its functional significance and that qualification which defines its phenomenal status in a given concrete case. All the examples to which Husserl refers for "figurale Momente" and v. Ehrenfels for "Gestaltqualitäten" are contextures with characters and properties of their own, though, of course, not all of them are of the type of the "level-phenomenon," as this is easily seen in the case of a melody, a rythm, an ascending scale, etc. Accordingly, all the component members of a contexture have not always the same functional significance. However, what holds for the members of any contexture, of whatever type and kind, is that each member is experienced with, and as defined by, a specific functional significance which, in turn, is determined by the role which the member plays within the contexture in question. The structure of such contextures has to be accounted for in gestalttheoretical terms of the kind of those which we have used. A further clarification of these terms is not within the scope of the present discussion.

Assorting color-specimina on the basis of concrete agreement, the subject looks for samples as lend themselves best to forming a contexture of the mentioned kind together with the specimen of reference. All he has to do is to select such specimina which are experienced as belonging together with the specimen of reference in the sense of concrete agreement to the highest possible degree. For that purpose, the subject does not need to go beyond the very experience of concrete agreement. In particular, it is not necessary for him to analyze the latter experience and to recognize the agreement as agreement by equality of, say, brightness.[25] It may well happen that the agreement is in fact based upon the factor of brightness which thus actually determines the perceptual experience. Still the factor

[24] As to level-phenomenon in contradistinction to step-phenomenon cf. K. Koffka, "Perception: An Introduction to the Gestalt-Theorie," *The Psychological Bulletin*, Vol. XIX (1922), pp. 540 ff. Koffka has introduced these concepts in discussing quite different problems.

[25] Cf. Gelb, *loc. cit.*, p. 411.

of brightness, is, so to speak, but silently effective. The subject acts under the imperatives of its silent effectiveness, without disengaging and apprehending the factor of the brightness as to the role which it actually plays for the experience of concrete coherence. When, on the other hand, specimina *are* assorted with reference to brightness as point of view and principle of classification, there may again occur, at the outset, an experience of concrete agreement. Here, however, the subject does not merely experience concrete coherence, but proceeds from that experience toward disengaging the factor which is constitutive for that very experience. Apprehending the concrete agreement as founded upon equality of brightness, the subject discloses the factor of brightness in its effectiveness and may then choose the factor thus thematized as principle of classification. The difference is between concrete coherence founded in fact on brightness and concrete coherence explicitly recognized and apprehended as thus founded, between the factor of brightness actually effective and the thematization of that factor in its determinant role. Previously[26] we mentioned a certain detachment from experienced situations as prerequisite to the adoption of the "categorial" attitude. Such detachment permits the normal person not merely to experience the actual situation and to undergo the effectiveness of operating factors, but also to explicate the given situation, to apprehend and thematize effective factors, and, eventually, to orient his actions with respect to factors thus rendered explicit. Reduced as the patients are to passively accepting experiential situations in their actuality and to acting only under their direct inducements, explication and thematization have become operations impossible for them to perform.

If Gelb and Goldstein's patient Th., who had an excellent capacity of visualization, found no difficulty at all in choosing a specimen whose color matched that of an object pointed out or mentioned to him, it is because the "categorial attitude is not required for that purpose. Evoking a mental image of the object in question, all the patient had to do and did in fact was to select a specimen whose color was experienced by him to be in concrete accordance with that of the object.[27] Normal persons do not act differently when they are confronted with the same task.

Required to sort out specimina of the same color as that of a certain object, we select, like the patient, very few shades only, *viz.*, those as exactly fit and concretely cohere with the color of the object. Asked, e.g., to point out the color of blood, we do not accept a pink specimen, not any more than a green one. Actual mental visualization of the object in question is not even indispensable for the accomplishment of the task under discussion.[28] The selection may and, more often than not, does take place on the basis of

[26] *Supra*, pp. 125f.
[27] Cf. Gelb and Goldstein, *loc. cit.*, I §2.
[28] *Id.*, *ibid.*, pp. 135 f.

mere recognition of a specimen as fitting with the color of the object, no mental image of the latter being evoked. What is important, and is alone important, is the occurrence of the immediately "intuitive experience of fittingness" ("das anschauliche Erlebnis des Passens"), whether on the basis of visualization or mere recognition. It is obviously with respect to only very few specimina that the mentioned experience takes place, whereas other specimina of the same hue, but of brightness, saturation, and other chromatic properties different from those of the object in question appear inappropriate and incongruous. Under certain circumstances, in the face of certain tasks, normal persons also adopt the "concrete" attitude. When, however, we are given the assignment to assort samples of the same hue as a certain specimen of reference, we select all specimina as fall under the class represented by the specimen of reference. Prevented from adopting the "categorial" attitude, Th. resorts to the same procedure with respect to either task. Herein reappears the difference between the behavior of the patient and that of normal persons.[29]

Finally we have to mention the interpretation which Gelb and Goldstein give of the affections of speech proper. Since these affections are the most conspicuous symptoms in amnestic aphasia, older theoreticians had explained the latter by a deficiency of words, at least by a considerable difficulty on the part of the patients to find certain words. Against this explanation, Goldstein points out that the very same words which the patients are unable to find under *certain circumstances* are spontaneously and easily uttered under *different circumstances*.[30] Whether or not a certain word is found by a patient does not depend upon the word itself, but upon the meaning with which the word is to be used in a concrete situation of speech.[31] Color-names like "red," "blue," etc., do not designate individual and particular chromatic phenomena in all their singularity; they rather denote classes or categories of colors. It is with this categorial meaning that the subject has to use the terms in question when he is asked to name a color shown to him or to point out a color to which a given name applies. Since patients suffering from amnesia of color-names are not able to consider a given color as representative of a class of colors, words whose significations are of an as predominantly conceptual nature as is the case of color-names, have lost all meaning for them.[32] The inability of the patients to

[29] Gelb and Goldstein, *loc. cit.*, p. 150.

[30] Goldstein, *loc. cit.*, pp. 471 ff.; cf. also pp. 449 f.

[31] As to this view, first advocated by H. Jackson, cf. Cassirer, *loc. cit.*, pp. 245 ff.

[32] Gelb and Goldstein, *loc. cit.*, I §5; Gelb, *loc. cit.*, pp. 411 f.; Goldstein, *loc. cit.*, pp. 475 ff. The preeminently eidetic signification of color-names also appears in that mentioning the correct color-name, even its utterance by the patient himself, hardly produces any effect in contradistinction to cases of amnesia of names of objects (Gelb and Goldstein *loc. cit.*, pp. 184 ff.; Goldstein, *loc. cit.*, pp. 487 ff.). This not only

use words which have an essentially eidetic signification and their characteristic behavior in assorting color-specimina thus appear, according to Gelb and Goldstein, as two manifestations of the same fundamental modification, *viz.*, regression from the "categorial" to the "concrete" level. Neither manifestation, however, must be considered as the cause of, or in any sense primary with respect to, the other. Both must be regarded as coordinate to each other and must equally directly be referred to the fundamental modification of attitude.

When Th. speaks of colors, he often uses expressions as "grassy" (grassartig"), "like a cherry" ("kirschartig"), "like a violet" ("veilchenartig"), etc.[33] Of another patient Goldstein reports that she consistently used color-names like "red," "green," etc., with reference to only a few determinate shades, mostly highly saturated ones. As to other shades, the mentioned terms did not apply; in their stead, the patient had expressions like "dark yellow" ("jaune foncé"), "bright blue" ("bleu clair"), "leaf-green" ("vert feuille"), or "fashion color" ("couleur mode"), "spring color" ("couleur printanière"), etc.[34] If inferences from the verbal formulations of the patients to their chromatic experiences are warranted, one might presume that colors do not appear to the patients as "pure qualities" but as attributes and properties of objects, in attachment to and adherence in objects. Tendencies to designate colors after objects have also been observed among primitive peoples.[35] We furthermore refer to the thesis of Pradines who asserts the priority, from the genetic, especially the phylogenetic point of view, of colors as well as sounds as essentially related to agents and objects over colors and sounds divested of objective significance and thus given the status of "pure qualities."[36] According to Pradines, "pure qualities" are no primary data, not even data at all, but rather products of mental operations by means of which the realm of sensibility is surpassed. It thus seems that their reduction to the "concrete" level of behavior and

leads to the question, discussed by Gelb and Goldstein, as to whether all terms which are of general applicability have by this very token a genuine eidetic signification; it also gives rise to the problem as to whether there are εἴδη with reference to all objects, of whatever kind and description, and to all properties, attributes, characters, etc., of any objects. In the present context, we must confine ourselves to noting that a problem debated in Platonism as well as in platonizing philosophies (e.g., that of Malebranche) also arises out of a mere psychopathological discussion.

[33] Gelb and Goldstein, *loc. cit.*, pp. 133 f.; Goldstein, *loc. cit.*, p. 476.

[34] Goldstein, *loc. cit.*, pp. 480 f. and 483 f. As to both denominating and assorting colors, the patient exhibited the symptoms of amnestic aphasia.

[35] Cf. D. Katz, *Der Aufbau der Farbwelt* (Leipzig, 1930), pp. 4 f.; Cassirer, *loc. cit.*, pp. 265 ff.; and also the remarks by Gelb and Goldstein, *loc. cit.*, p. 134.

[36] M. Pradines, *Philosophie de la Sensation*, Vol. I (Paris, 1928), Livre I, chap. IV; cf. also M. Merleau-Ponty, *Phénoménologie de la Perception* (Paris, 1945), p. 352, who distinguishes between "couleur-fonction" and "couleur-qualité."

attitude purports for the patients the inability not only to consider a given color as member of a class, i.e., to perceive the color with reference to a species, but also to sever the relatedness of the color to some object whose property and attribute it is. Such severance is necessary for the conception of a purely qualitative order, i.e., an order in which colors figure as mere chromatic phenomena, as "pure qualities," detached from objects to which they adhere. We thus venture the hypothesis that if patients, reduced to the "concrete" attitude, speak of colors in terms implying essential reference to objects, it is because their confinement to accepting actual experience in all its concreteness prevents them from performing mental operations upon the data of experience, in the case under discussion, divorcing colors from the objects whose attributes they are and thus experiencing the colors as pure chromatic phenomena, with the exception, perhaps, of the limiting case of identity of shades or similarity to such high degree as borders upon identity. The propounded conception of colors as originally and primarily attributes of objects also makes understandable the fact previously[37] pointed out that even normal persons do not adopt the "categorial" attitude when they are required to assort specimina whose color matches that of some object mentioned to them. Under the conditions of the assignment, the color reassumes its primary function; it is perceived with reference to some object; it is experienced, so to speak, as an envelope of the latter which in a certain specific manner announces itself in the very chromatic experience. A closer examination of the phenomenal impliedness and involvement of objects in colors or, for that matter, in sounds, cannot be attempted here. It has its place within the broader frame of the phenomenology of perception.

III. PHENOMENOLOGICAL PROBLEMS OF IDEATION

a. Convergence of Husserl's and Gelb-Goldstein's views

Husserl's distinction between equality in the categorial sense and sensuous equality appears, in the light of Gelb-Goldstein's theory, as a special case of the distinction between acts which are performed in the "categorial" attitude and those which belong to the "concrete" attitude. We cannot here discuss the question as to whether and, if so, in which sense, the same holds for Husserl's distinction between multiplicities apprehended through acts of genuine explicit colligation and multiplicities which in very sense-experience are perceived as such by means of "figurale Momente." Sensuous equality, as previously mentioned,[38] is counted by Husserl among "figurale Momente." When we speak of the distinction between sensuous and categorial equality as of a *special* case of that between "concrete"

[37] Pp. 130f.

[38] P. 122.

and "categorial" acts, it is because the latter two concepts comprise much more than the phenomena which, for the sake of the discussion, had to be emphasized in the present context.

Guided in his assorting of color-specimina by the experience of concrete agreement, coherence, and accordance, i.e., in Husserl's terminology, by the experience of sensuous equality to the highest possible degree, Gelb and Goldstein's patients prove utterly unable to conceive of the relationship of equality in the categorial sense. This observation of Gelb and Goldstein's bears out our previous conclusion as to the impossibility to account for ideation by apprehension of equality.[39] *Both Husserl's and Gelb-Goldstein's theories converge towards recognizing ideation as an act sui generis with a specific nature of its own.* Patients of the kind here considered have become unable to perform acts of ideation, an inability which also appears in that color-names, when used in an eidetic sense, have no longer any meaning for them. It is the specific act of ideation that renders possible the apprehension of a particular thing or of a plurality of particular things with reference to, or under the perspective of an εἶδος.[40] Among the latter acts, there are to be included those through which a particular thing is conceived of as belonging to a class which, in turn, is constituted with respect to an εἶδος. Husserl's distinctions and theoretical ideas further clarify and complement Gelb and Goldstein's concepts.

Expounding Th.'s procedure in assorting color-specimina and emphasizing the difference between the patient's procedure and that of a normal person, Gelb writes: "Rapprocher . . . les teintes également claires, parce qu'elles s'accordent en fait,-et que momentanément c'est ce rapprochement et non tel autre qui s'impose—est toute autre chose que de connaître ces teintes *en tant qu'analogues* par la clarté, puis de choisir cette propriété comme principe de classement."[41] This argument of Gelb's is reminiscent of Husserl's discussion of the logical presentation "*all A*." For the latter presentation to be conceived it is not sufficient to survey in fact all A, even if the number of the individuals in question is finite. "Wie viele Einzelheiten wir . . . durchlaufen, und wie eifrig wir sie kolligieren mögen, bestenfalls wären, wenn die Erschöpfung des Begriffsumfanges wirklich gelänge, all A vorgestellt, und doch wären nicht *alle A* vorgestellt, die logische Vorstellung wäre nicht vollzogen."[42] In both Gelb's and Husserl's arguments, reference is made to an operation of consciousness which we propose to term *thematization*, meaning hereby disengagement and disclosure of factors which previously to the operation in question are present to consciousness

[39] Pp. 122f.
[40] Cf. Husserl, *Log. Unt.*, Vol. II, II, §1; cf. also Farber, *loc. cit.*, pp. 246 f.
[41] Gelb, *loc. cit.*, p. 411.
[42] Husserl, *Log. Unt.*, Vol. II, 1, p. 173; cf. also Farber, *loc. cit.* p. 268.

in a rather implicit form. In Gelb's example, the nature of thematization is quite obvious. It denotes the afore-mentioned[43] transition of the factor of equality by brightness from the state of silent effectiveness in determining the phenomenal aspect of perception to the state of explicit apprehension. It is just this transition which cannot be performed in the case of amnesia of color-names. As to the example referred to by Husserl, it is conceivable that in proceeding from one A to another and thus actually exhausting the extension of the concept, the experiencing subject is not aware at all of his covering all A. Under these conditions, there is no thematization, not any more than a motivation to form the logical presentation *all A*. We therefore consider the case in which at the end of his survey the subject is aware of all A having been covered. Still the logical presentation *all A* cannot be conceived, the totality of the A cannot be explicityly apprehended and stated, unless the mentioned awareness is rendered explicit and thematized, rather than accompanying, in an implied and involved form, the act of consciousness experienced in the final phase of the survey. To both the apprehension of logical forms and the process of ideation, the operation of thematization proves essential.[44] Concerned with ideation, we have to assign to the operation of thematization its systematic place within the whole of the process of ideation.

b. The problem of the perceptual basis of ideation

To obtain an idea of the phenomenal aspect which the heap of color-specimina presents to their patient, Gelb and Goldstein had a few normal persons move the specimen of reference forth and back over the heap.[45] These observers were instructed to look at the heap as passively as possible and especially to refrain from placing themselves at a point of view or adopting a principle of classification. Specimina identical with, or extremely similar to the specimen of reference appear in concrete accordance and coherence with the latter. When there are no identical or highly similar specimina, the heap sometimes presents an aspect of instability, fluctuation, unrest and agitation. Incipient contextures between color-samples are formed and dissolved almost at once. Different groupings of color-specimina conflict with each other. Experiences of concrete agreement and accordance of various descriptions compete with, and supersede upon each

---

[43] Cf. *supra*, pp. 129ff.

[44] As to the apprehension of logical forms, cf. Husserl, *Formale und Transzendentale Logik*, pp. 69 f. Husserl's operation of "nominalization" (*Log. Unt.*, Vol. II, V, §§35 f. and *Ideen zu einer reinen Phänomenologie und phänomenologischen Philosophie* (referred to hereafter as *Ideen*) §§119 ff., 134, 148) seems to us a special case of that of thematization.

[45] Gelb and Goldstein, *ibid.*, pp. 151 ff.

other. It is more or less under this phenomenal aspect that Gelb and Goldstein presume the heap of color-specimina to appear to their patient. When, however, under the influence of a given assignment, e.g., that to assort all red specimina, the normal person abandons his heretofore passive attitude, the instability and agitation of the heap of color-specimina, the vacillation of conflicting contextures, the alternation between and fluctuation of inchoate groupings, dissolved almost as soon as formed, etc., all at once give way to a reorganized perceptual field. All red specimina acquire predominance and emerge from the rest which in turn forms a more or less irrelevant background. Since the organization and grouping of colors is not immaterial to the phenomenal appearance of the latter, Gelb and Goldstein conclude that their patient's experience of colors differs from the chromatic experience which the normal person has, when he adopts the "categorial" attitude.[46] In Gelb and Goldstein's theory, the behavior of the patient is not interpreted as a mere intellectual deficiency, *viz.*, the loss of the ability to subsume perceived colors under categories, while the very perceptual experience of colors remains unaltered, i.e., is with the patient the same as with normal persons. Merleau-Ponty[47] sees herein the "existentialist" rather than "intellectualist" character of their theory: "... l'activité catégoriale, avant d'être une pensée ou une connaissance, est une certaine manière de se rapporter au monde, et corrélativement un style ou une configuration de l'expérience." Accordingly, "... le trouble de la pensée que l'on découvre au fond de l'amnésie ... concerne moins le jugement que le milieu d'expérience où le jugement prend naissance, moins la spontanéité que les prises de cette spontanéité sur le monde sensible et notre pouvoir de figurer en lui une intention quelconque."

Emphasizing the difference between the chromatic experience of their patient and that of a normal person adopting the "categorial" attitude, Gelb and Goldstein still seem to admit, at least in their article on "Farbennamenamnesie," that there is hardly any difference between the chromatic experience of the patient and that of a normal person, provided the latter adopts the "concrete" attitude. This is borne out by Gelb and Goldstein's explanation of the failure to detect anomalies in the chromatic perception of their patient by means of certain ophthalmological methods.[48] What is examined by the methods in question is but the experience of homogeneity and inhomogeneity between colors. For that experience, the adoption of the "categorial" attitude is not required. To the extent to which the normal person perceives colors in a mere intuitive, i.e., "concrete," attitude, his chromatic experience is not assumed by Gelb and Goldstein to differ sub-

---

[46] Gelb and Goldstein, *loc. cit.*, p. 162.

[47] Merleau-Ponty, *loc. cit.*, pp. 222 ff.

[48] Gelb and Goldstein, *loc. cit.*, pp. 161 f.

stantially from that of their patient. Yet in an article written subsequently to that on "Farbennamenamnesie," Gelb cautions against assimilating the perception of the patient to that which the normal person has when he adopts the "concrete" attitude.[49] From the fact that the normal person may, and with respect to certain tasks, does adopt the "concrete" attitude, the conclusion must not be drawn that the patient experiences and acts like the normal person does in the "concrete" attitude. Whereas the patient is reduced and confined to the "concrete" attitude, the latter is with the normal person but *one phase* of a more comprehensive process, it is integrated into a total process of experience which also comprises phases of "categorial" attitude, of detachment and contemplation from a distance. In the life of the normal person, the "categorial" and "concrete" attitudes —the latter more immediate and direct, more "manual"—fecundate each other and it is from this integration into the total process of experience that either derives its full meaning and significance.

Gelb's remarks, it seems to us, must not be construed to mean that the integration in question is but a fact ascertainable by an onlooking observer, and not by the experiencing subject himself. On the contrary, we submit that a perception experienced in the "concrete" attitude appears in itself as integrable into a wider context, is descriptively characterized as a phase of a more comprehensive process. For a perception thus to present itself, it must include a specific phenomenal tinge or feature by means of which a more encompassing context is referred to, through which the possibility of the "categorial" attitude is somehow preannounced and anticipated in the very perception experienced in the "concrete" attitude.

To formulate more precisely what we mean by the inclusion in an act pertaining to the "concrete" attitude of a possible "categorial" attitude, let us proceed by way of contrast. Confined to abiding by perceptual data as they actually present themselves, the patient cannot experience such data except in that organizational form in which they impose themselves upon him. If, as in the case of a heap of color-samples which contains no identical or highly similar shades, the perceptual field exhibits no unambiguously determined organization, the field appears unstable and fluctuating with conflicting groupings superseding each other. The normal person, on the contrary, may adopt the "categorial" attitude, and impose upon the perceptual field an organizational form which that field does not possess in its own right. He may even impose upon the field varying forms of organization according to different points of view. As we have seen,[50] the perceptual field accepts organizational forms determined by the point of view at which the subject chooses to place himself.

[49] Gelb, *loc. cit.*, pp. 413 ff.

[50] Pp. 135f.

In the perception of the normal person, there is then a certain readiness to receive forms of organization imposed from without, a certain *ambiguity* and *plasticity* which are in marked contrast to the rigidity characteristic of the perception of the patient. To the normal person's mind, the things perceived do not appear as *mere* actual data and facts, as they do to the patient, but rather, without in the least being divested of their character of real things given in actual experience, as *eventual examples*, as *potential varieties of an invariant*. Even when the normal person does not adopt the "categorial" attitude, his perception is not mere perception in a "pure" state, but, we tentatively submit, is pervaded and permeated by some consciousness or awareness of possibilities, of possible reference to a non-perceptual order. Such consciousness of possibilities does not necessarily exist in an entirely explicit and distinct state; more often than not it assumes the form of greater or lesser inarticulation, latency, and implicitness. The reference is, especially in the latter case, to the realm of possibilities as such rather than to any specified possibility. To a greater or lesser degree of implicitness, the perceptual experience of the normal person is oriented with respect to non-perceptual orders and possibilities so that, even when a thing is perceived in itself and for its own sake, without actual reference to a conceptual order, it still is experienced as *referable* to such an order; even when it is not perceived as an example, it still appears as thus *perceivable*. All perceptual experience is encompassed by the horizon of an at least potential consciousness of possible non-perceptual perspectives. In every perception experienced in the "concrete" attitude, there is implied a more or less vague, indistinct, and inarticulate consciousness of and reference to a possible transition to the "categorial" attitude. It is by the plasticity in the sense as just sketched that experiences which the normal person has, when he happens to adopt the "concrete" attitude, seem to us to differ substantially from those of the patient who by virtue of the profound modification which he has undergone is confined to the "concrete" attitude.

c. The operation of "free variation"

Already in *Logische Untersuchungen* Husserl mentions the operation of "free variation." To be sure, in *Logische Untersuchungen*, the operation in question is not introduced in order to account for the apprehension and phenomenological constitution of εἴδη, but rather as a method for establishing *a priori* laws between εἴδη, as, e.g., between the εἶδος of color and that of extension.[51] In the very performance of "free variation," certain limitations become apparent which the operation under discussion is bound to respect. Eidetic laws *a priori* are formulations of such limitations. Start-

[51] Husserl, *Log. Unt.*, Vol. II, III, chap. I; cf. Farber, *loc. cit.*, chap. xA.

ing, e.g., from a colored surface, we may imagine the surface to vary arbitrarily as to size and shape, and still the color remains unaltered. When, however, we go as far as imagining the size of the surface to decrease until the extension vanishes altogether, we see that the color vanishes as well.[52] Color and extension do not coexist merely accidentally. It appears from the mental experiment by way of "free variation" that no instance of color can exist except in connection with an instance of extension. By virtue of an eidetic law *a priori* there is an essential and necessary relationship between color and extension. Because this relationship is founded on the very εἴδη of extension and color, it extends to every instance of either εἶδος.

Even when it starts from some actual experience, the operation of "free variation" leads—of necessity, as we shall presently see—to forms which are not and have not been given in actual experience, which for empirical reasons will, perhaps, never be actually experienced. Since eidetic science in not interested in matters of fact, but in possibilities, the eventual existence or inexistence of forms arrived at in the process of "free variation" is of no relevancy whatsoever.[53] Geometry, which is an eidetic science itself, sets the example. Arbitrarily modifying his figures, passing from form to form by way of continuous transformations, the mathematician is not in the least concerned with the question as to whether or not the products of his geometrical imagination correspond to something in empirical reality. To assure the geometrical validity of these forms it is both necessary and sufficient that they may be contrived in the process of "free variation" oriented in a certain direction. In other eidetic fields, the situation is not different. Setting out to disclose the εἶδος "material thing," we may be led to consider golden mountains and winged horses. As far as their function as exemplifications of the εἶδος in question is concerned, the mentioned products of the fancy are no more and no less valid possibilities than are stones and trees given in actual experience.[54] Since εἴδη are exemplified in facts of actual experience as well as in creations of the imagination, the operation of "free variation" is not bound to start from real existents. Products of the imagination may serve as starting-points as well.[55] At any event, whatever its starting-point, the operation of "free variation"

---

[52] This argument has been advanced by C. Stumpf, *Ueber den psychologischen Ursprung der Raumvorstellung* (Leipzig, 1873), pp. 112 ff. Taking over the argument, Husserl (*Log. Unt.*, Vol. II, III, §§4 ff.), presents it in an ontological rather than psychological setting.

[53] Cf. Husserl, *Ideen*, §§4, 7, 70; *Méditations Cartésiennes*, sect. 34.

[54] *Id.*, *Ideen*, §149.

[55] *Id.*, *ibid.*, p. 12, (Wir) "können . . ., ein Wesen selbst und *originär* zu erfassen, von entsprechenden erfahrenden Anschauungen ausgehen, *ebensowohl aber auch von nicht-erfahrenden, nicht-daseinserfassenden, vielmehr 'bloss einbildenden' Anschauungen.*"

must lead to, and pass through, merely imaginary forms. Otherwise the process would be confined to actualities which form but a subclass of possibilities, whereas it is the very purpose of the process of "free variation" to yield a survey of what is possible in a certain domain, regardless of its actualization in empirical reality. Imagination thus proves the "organ" of eidetic knowledge.[56] The process of "free variation" by means of which not only eidetic laws and relations between εἴδη are established, but εἴδη themselves are apprehended and constituted, is carried out in imagination.

If the process of "free variation" leads to the constitution of εἴδη, it is because certain features and structures prove to remain unaltered throughout the process in question. Starting from a musical sound, whether actually experienced or merely imagined, we engender a series of auditory phenomena which originate from each other by way of variation and transformation. All members of the series prove congruent in a certain respect by which the members of the mentioned series differ from the members of that series which would have been engendered, if we had started from a color and applied to it the process of variation and transformation. Throughout all varieties which are encountered in the very process of "free variation," there appears an *invariant general form, an invariant structure* exhibited by every member of the series. Different as the members in question are from each other and must be on account of their orgination, they all exhibit congruity as to an *invariant identical content.*[57] Congruity with other members of the series as to the invariant is the condition for any member to belong to the series in question, the latter being conceived as generated by "free variation" and transformation of a certain exemplar, e.g., a musical sound. *Ideation reaches final completion with the disengagement, disclosure, explicit apprehension, briefly, thematization of the invariant in question.* This invariant is the εἶδος in the Platonic sense, to be conceived without any metaphysical connotation.

Constituted as an invariant which manifests itself in the very process of "free variation," the εἶδος presents itself in genuine apprehension as ἓν επὶ πολλῶν, i.e., in opposition and therefore, in *necessary* relatedness to a multiplicity of varieties which, however differing from each other, are all actualizations of the same invariant form.[58] The εἶδος is apprehended as an identical ideal entity in contradistinction, and with reference to an infinite multiplicity of possible varieties, since the significance of the εἶδος

[56] Cf. Fr. Kaufmann, "On Imagination," pp. 372 f. in *Philosophy and Phenomenological Research,* Vol. VII (1947).

[57] Husserl, *Erfahrung und Urteil,* §87 a and e.

[58] *Id., ibid.,* §87 c; *Log. Unt.,* Vol. II, 2, p. 162 ". . . gegenüber der Mannigfaltigkeit von einzelnen Momenten einer und derselben Art, diese Art *selbst,* und *zwar als eine und dieselbe vor Augen* stehen kann . . . wir werden uns . . . auf Grund mehrerer individueller Anschauungen der Identität des Allgemeinen bewusst. . . ."

lies in that it is an invariant with regard to all possible varieties of a certain domain, e.g., that of musical sound, the reference can obviously not be to those varieties only as have actually been considered in a given process of "free variation" which, like any process actually performed, is by necessity finite. Though the process is in fact broken up after a certain number of steps, it is, however, carried out with the consciousness that it can be continued *ad libitum*.[59] It is this consciousness of a possible continuation that renders possible the reference of the εἶδος not only to the varieties which have actually been taken into account, but also to more varieties to be contrived *ad libitum*. The very phenomenological constitution of the εἶδος, which here we can but roughly sketch, accounts for the above-mentioned[60] essential correlation between the εἶδος and its extension as an infinitely open class. It also appears that the extension in question does not comprise real objects and their real properties, but rather pure possibilities, i.e., possible varieties.[61] If it is justified to speak of an empirical extension of an εἶδος, and if eidetic relationships hold, and hold even necessarily and *a priori*, for matters of fact, it is because every real occurrence may, and must, be considered as a possible variety which happens to be actualized. By the same token, the distinction, upon which we previously[62] insisted, between a class in the conceptual sense and a perceptual grouping which exhibits the "figurales Moment" of, e.g. qualitative homogeneity, finds here its ultimate validation.

As already mentioned, the process of "free variation" is carried out in imagination. All the forms which originate from each other by way of transformation and variation, play their roles as, and *only* as, possible varieties, i.e., as possibly contrivable in imagination. This holds without exception for every member of the series generated in the process under discussion. It also holds for the member from which the process starts, even when the member in question happens to be a real occurrence. For the process of ideation to apply to an object given in actual experience, the latter object must be subjected to what Husserl occasionally calls "eidetic reduction."[63] By eidetic reduction, the real existent is divested of its actuality, of its existential character, its spatio-temporal determinations from which it derives its individualization, and also of all those characters as accrue to it on account of its integration into the real world.[64] Every real existent can be regarded as an actualized possibility. Under the eidetic reduction, the

[59] *Id.*, *Erfahrung und Urteil*, §87 b, "Es kommt . . . darauf an, dass die Variation als Prozess der Variantenbildung selbst eine *Beliebigkeitsgestalt* habe, dass der Prozess im Bewusstsein beliebiger Fortbildung von Varianten vollzogen sei."

[60] Cf. *supra*, p. 122.

[61] Husserl, *Erfahrung und Urteil*, §§90 f. [62] *Supra*, pp. 122ff.

[63] Husserl, *Ideen*, p. 4. "Eidetic reduction," it must be stressed emphatically, ought not to be confounded with phenomenological or transcendental reduction.

fact of its actualization is considered as immaterial and, hence, is disregarded. What is encountered as a matter of fact, is "irrealized"; i.e., considered as to its imaginableness, and not as to its actuality; it is transformed into a "pure possibility" among other possibilities.[65] From the status of a real existent, it is transferred to that of an example or exemplar lending itself to "free variations" and thus becoming apt to function as starting point for an infinitely open series of possible, i.e. imaginable, varieties.[66] Eidetic reduction is obviously a necessary condition for a real existent to play a role in ideation. Only possibilities can find insertion into a process whose very purpose is to yield a survey of what is possible in a certain domain.

Recalling Goldstein's characterization of the modification undergone by brain-injured persons,[67] we can, in the light of the results which we have now attained, understand the incapacity of the mentioned patients to perform any operation which involves ideation. Overwhelmed by the actuality of factual experience, the patients in question are unable to conceive of possibilities; they cannot imagine any actual experience to be possibly different from what is actually is.[68] In the case of the patients, the very precondition of ideation, which we found to be conception of facts as actualized possibilities and free variability of the latter in and by imagination, is not realized. Expressing it in Kantian terms, Merleau-Ponty[69] speaks of an affection of productive imagination rather than understanding ("entendement"). By its very structure, the perceptual experience of the patients resists being subjected to imaginational operations, processes, and transformations. Thus we are brought back before the rigidity in the perception of the patients in contrast with what we tentatively described as plasticity in the perceptual experience of normal persons.[70] When we refer to psychopathological findings, it is because, by way of contrast, these findings permit us to disclose conditions which, just on account of their realization in the case of normal persons, are likely to be taken for granted and, hence, to be overlooked. The structure of perceptual experience, proves, we submit, a necessary condition of ideation and, therefore, an important problem for the phenomenology of ideation. It is to this problem that we wish to call attention.

[64] Cf. Husserl, *Ideen*, §2; *Erfahrung und Urteil*, §89.

[65] *Id.*, *Méditations Cartésiennes*, pp. 59 f.

[66] *Id.*, *Erfahrung und Urteil*, pp. 410 f. [67] Cf. *supra*, pp. 178 ff.

[68] We wish to stress that the modification in question is not peculiar to amnesia of color-names alone. Impairment of imagination in the mentioned sense has been observed by Gelb and Goldstein on numerous patients exhibiting the most diversified symptoms.

[69] Merleau-Ponty, *loc. cit.*, p. 224. [70] Cf. *supra*, pp. 190 f.

11

On the Problem of Cortical Syndromes: Experimental Studies

by Egon Weigl
Berlin, G. D. R.

As one of Kurt Goldstein's oldest students and collaborators, I consider it an honor as well as my duty to make a modest contribution to this volume published in his memory. I welcome the opportunity to express my deep gratitude to this outstanding man at whose home—first in Frankfurt, and later in Berlin—I had the privilege of being warmly received whenever I called.

The seminars for the study of the after-effects of brain lesions, which were held in the nineteen-twenties at the University of Frankfurt by Kurt Goldstein and Adhémar Gelb were an experience never to be forgotten by those privileged to attend them. Here we witnessed the classical investigations of aphasia, agnosia and apraxia in patients who were to become famous; and we were encouraged to conduct our own experiments under the guidance of these two unique teachers.

The ideal cooperation and severe, mutual criticism practiced in Frankfurt in those days by the eminent experimental psychologist Gelb, and the internationally known neurologist and brain expert, Goldstein, continues to serve as a model for neuro-psychological research.

Hitler's disastrous seizure of power put a sudden end to this personally and professionally so stimulating contact with Kurt Goldstein, the great friend and teacher. Physician and university lecturer of Jewish origin, known to be a Democrat, he managed to escape Hitler's bloodthirsty hangmen, almost as if by a miracle, at the very last moment.

While writing these lines, I have in front of me Kurt Goldstein's last letter to me. In this letter he expressed his great satisfaction that his former pupil and collaborator had remained loyal to aphasia research, the field he himself had loved so much. In this letter, written in 1962, he told me that, despite his advanced age, he was incessantly at work, getting "immer mehr in das Fahrwasser der Philosophie"; and he added, "... man hat das Gefühl, es hat alles nicht mehr so sehr viel Sinn in dieser Welt," a remark that sounded somehow like a sigh. Its interpretation must be left to those who had the privilege of being among his close friends during his last years. But of those who know the true value of his contribution to science, none will share his doubts as to the "use" of his own life.

Kurt Goldstein is a classic in the field of brain pathology. His work, his deep insight into the intricate mechanisms of the normal and impaired human brain, will remain an inexhaustible source of knowledge for many a generation of scientists to come.

Many decades ago, Goldstein made profound contributions to the problem dealt with in this paper, i.e., the problem of higher cortical syndromes. He expressed his far-reaching ideas mainly in his papers *Zur Theorie der Funktion des Nervensystems* (1), *Das Symptom, seine Entstehung und Bedeutung für unsere Auffassung vom Bau und der Funktion des Nervensystems* (2), *Über Aphasie* (3), and finally in his comprehensive work *Language and Language Disturbances* (4). The method of psychological case analysis which he elaborated jointly with A. Gelb, and his attempt to regard cortical syndromes not as "ein zufälliges Nebeneinander" of single disturbances due to local injury (3, p. 27), but as the result of *disturbances of a system*, in the sense of impairment of certain "basic functions" (4, p. 3), justify his being regarded as the founder of modern neuro-psychology (*cf.* 8, 10, *et al.*).

I have tried to find a new approach to the problem of cortical syndromes, following my own way of studying the disturbances of higher cortical functions, to be described in this paper. Proceeding from the examination of patients with different cortical syndromes, we pursue questions concerning the reciprocal structural and dynamic relations between the various disturbances of single functions, their hierarchy, the extent of their impairment, and potential avenues of relief.

The experimental study of syndromes is carried through with the help of the *deblocking method* (14, 18). In order to facilitate the understanding of this paper, a brief description of this method follows.

The deblocking method makes use of the fact that the capacity for decoding, coding and recoding verbal information (6) is not completely obliterated in most aphasic patients. Though examination of these processes via certain "channels" may show them to be more or less severely disturbed, an examination utilizing other "channels" might indicate that the processes are completely—or almost completely—intact; the specific findings depend on the localization of the lesion, i.e., on the "type" of aphasia. The alexic patient, for instance, understands without difficulty the meaning of a certain word when hearing it, yet he fails to do so when reading it, i.e., verbo-visually; conversely, the patient with sensory aphasia remains "deaf" to the meaning of a word spoken to him, while he is able to understand the same word as soon as it is shown to him in writing.

The conditions underlying disturbances of decoding, illustrated in the foregoing examples, are similar to those that underlie disturbances of coding and recoding. A patient suffering from disturbances in naming of objects may well be able to read a certain word aloud, whereas he fails, when asked, to name the respective object, i.e., in the expressive use of the same word. Patients with expressive-alexic disturbances can react quite normally when requested to name objects, while reading aloud the very same words proves to be an insurmountable difficulty.

In the elaboration of our deblocking method, we proceeded from these relations between intact and disturbed functions of speech which are well known in aphasia research and rehabilitation work. The deblocking effect is attained through use of the intact channel leading to a certain "meaning," in order to eliminate the "blocking" when the same meaning cannot be decoded, coded or recoded via other channels. This is achieved through prompting of the intact speech performance just before we test the disturbed verbo-receptive or verbo-expressive function. If, for example, a patient with word-deafness is requested first to read a given word, he will subsequently be able to understand its meaning upon hearing it. The same applies to patients with disturbances of repetition who can repeat a word which they have previously copied in writing.

The phenomenon of deblocking in aphasic patients consists in removing, for longer or shorter periods, total or partial disturbances of various speech and other performances. The deblocking effect (D-effect) is attained through linking two semantically related performances of a preserved and a "blocked" function, evoking the unimpaired *prior* to the disturbed performance.

"SIMPLE" DEBLOCKING

Example # 1. Deblocking of impairment of auditory word understanding through intact picture naming in a case with predominantly sensory aphasia.

Control experiments. a) A list of words is drawn up, the meaning of which the patient does not understand when they are spoken to him.[1] b) It is ascertained that the patient is capable of naming correctly all pictures used for deblocking later on.

Main experiment. In order to deblock one of the words not understood by the patient, e.g., "slipper," the patient is first shown a number of

[1] In order to avoid "pseudo-deblocking," one must take into consideration the possible fluctuations of performances. In the control experiments we make sure that disturbances of naming certain pictures do not appear and disappear from one experiment to the next. Thus we carry through quantitative controls in order to assess the extent of the disturbance that is being studied.

pictures, among them one of a slipper (1st input). The pictures are then removed, and the examiner pronounces a number of words, among them the word "slipper" (2nd input). The D-effect consists in the patient's remaining "deaf" to all these words, with the exception of the word "slipper."

Example # 2. Deblocking of disturbances of anomia through preserved auditory word understanding in a case with amnesic aphasia.

Control experiments. a) A record is made of pictures which the patient cannot name, even though he is able to recognize them. b) Auditory word understanding is checked, mainly of the "critical" words to be used later.

Main experiment. In order to deblock the naming of those pictures that the patient failed to name in the control experiment, e.g., one showing a slipper, the examiner pronounces several words, among them the critical word "slipper" (1st input). Following this, the patient is shown several pictures (2nd input), and he is able to name only the one showing the slipper.

In a similar way, we succeeded in eliminating experimentally disturbances of oral repetition, of reading, of writing, etc., in various types of aphasia. It is possible, for example, to deblock disturbances of repetition by means of intact word reading, or, conversely, disturbed word reading by means of intact repetition. We have also obtained the D-effect in disturbances of written naming by means of intact copying; in agraphia on dictation by means of intact reading, etc.; finally, we have been able to deblock non-verbal, gnostic disturbances, such as disturbances of picture recognition, by having the patient read the names of the objects before presenting the pictures of the objects to be named.

As we have shown in detail elsewhere (14, 18), the main difference between the deblocking method described above and the usual facilitation methods (e.g., in cases of word-deafness, the patient is asked to select pictures named by the examiner; or, in cases of alexia, the patient is asked to match words offered in writing with simultaneously presented pictures) consists in the patient's complete lack of insight into the procedure. In our experiments, the patient cannot possibly know which of the items (pictures, words) offered in the control experiments (1st input) will prove to be the "critical" one in the test that follows. Deliberate memorization of all items (five as a rule) is either exceedingly difficult or completely impossible for patients with brain lesions which ordinarily impair short-term memory to some degree. In order to prevent the patient right from the beginning from "discovering" the principle underlying our method, we usually include "neutral" series among the actual deblocking series. For example, when deblocking disturbances of anomia through intact oral repetition, we include in the first input some series that contain not one single word corresponding to the pictures to be named later; correct picture naming can, of course, not be expected in these instances. In this way, the majority of our patients do not become aware at all of how we evoke their correct response. When asked how it is that all at once they can understand, write or read a certain word, the patients usually express their conviction that they "suddenly remembered it." Typically they cannot even remember having spoken, heard, read, or copied the very word beforehand, and they reject the idea when it is suggested by the examiner.

It must be stressed that the D-effect is by no means limited, e.g., to deblocking word-understanding in cases of word deafness by means of naming the picture corresponding to the critical noun; or, in cases of anomia, to deblocking the naming of a certain picture by means of hearing the critical noun beforehand. Modifications in our experimental technique made us realize that the critical word need not necessarily be contained in the series offered for the first input. For example, we were able to deblock the auditory understanding of verbs, such as "to close," when we offered the antonym "to open" within the first input series. Similarly, we could deblock the name of an onion through having the patient repeat aloud in the first input series "hot, tears, sharp, frying," etc. This means that the D-effect need not be restricted to the identical object or word, as we had presumed in the beginning (14, p. 355). Instead, the D-effect is the result of *prestimulation* of a certain "semantic field"[2] within which certain related concepts, e.g., synonyms, antonyms, generic nouns, are ontogenetically connected. These may lead to deblocking the "blocked" stimulus—or at least, facilitate its deblocking—much as do the identical concepts.

The above-mentioned fact, that the patients are neither directly nor consciously engaged in this process of deblocking, indicates the automatic, stereotype character of these processes, during which stored connections can be reactivated, connections which the patient, due to his cerebral lesion, is not capable of reactivating on his own.

From the neurophysiological point of view, which we cannot enlarge upon within the scope of this paper, these effects probably must be ascribed

[2] Only vaguely similar to the use of this term in linguistics, e.g., by Trier, we define "semantic fields" as ontogenetically developed systems of meaning, comprising not only logical and linguistic but also psychological and social relations, and, therefore, differing from individual to individual (see also 9, p. 89).

to a process of *summation* between a pathologically subliminal and a supraliminal stimulus (*cf.* 20, p. 317ff.).

"CHAIN" DEBLOCKING

The investigations described heretofore pertain to certain discrete symptoms of various aphasic or agnostic syndromes. I have previously reported (14) on a method that could serve a more direct study of syndromatic connections. This method consists in having a given deblocker successively deblock a "chain" of single performances of various impaired functions, instead of deblocking only one particular impaired performance, provided all intact or disturbed performances involve one and the same semantic field. The following examples will illustrate our method.

Example #3.[3] Patient M. M., age 57, retired, formerly employed in the textile trade; first admitted on 11th May 1953. Speech difficulties had appeared suddenly two weeks before admission. Slight signs of right hemiparesis. Diagnosis: hypertensive disease and cerebral arteriosclerosis; sensory aphasia. The patient was hospitalized on repeated occasions in 1957, 1959 and 1960.

Aphasia examination. Spontaneous speech and dialogue: frequent verbal stereotypy, polite formulae, etc.; telegraphic style with long intermittent pauses, literal and verbal paraphasia, perseveration, small vocabulary. Automatic speech and repetition as well as naming, completely or almost completely abolished. Total word deafness for abstract and unusual words, as well as for sentences (obeys only simple orders), only partial word deafness for concrete words and simple sentences. Total receptive alexia for abstract words and simple sentences, much less marked for letters and common words; total expressive alexia for sentences, only partial alexia for single words, no literal alexia. Total agraphia for words and sentences on dictation, in contrast to intact writing when copying. Almost complete acalculia. It must be noted that word deafness as well as verbal receptive alexia are considerably diminished by means of visual stimuli (pictures) or auditory ones (words uttered by the examiner). *Conclusion: mixed aphasia.*

Control experiment (see Figure 1). The patient can neither name correctly the picture of a boy (he tries to circumscribe what he sees), nor write the word "boy" correctly on dictation (he scribbles some meaningless word

[3] The reports of the Roumanian patients M.M. and T.J., including Fig. 1 and Fig. 2, are taken from the above mentioned paper (14, pp. 342, 344 and 354–355). These investigations were carried out at the Neurological Institute of the Academy of Science of the Socialist Republic of Roumania (Professor A. Kreindler, Director).

Image Word	before deblocking			after deblocking		
	naming	writing on dictation	repetition	repetition	writing on dictation	naming
tînăr (youngman)	"tovarăsul mic este" (the comrade small is)	Vie	"crii... pro" (paraphasic)	correct	tiner	correct
vultur (eagle)	"nu pot" (I can't)	[illegible]	"proc" (paraphasic)	correct	vultur	correct
tobă (drum)	"nu pot, nu stiu" (I can't, I don't know)	[illegible]	"proc" (paraphasic)	correct	tobă	correct
covor (carpet)	"nu pot să vorbesc" (I can't speak)	[illegible]	"vro... plo" (paraphasic)	correct	Covor.	correct

Figure 1. *Patient M.M.* Successive deblocking of naming, writing on dictation, and repetition through reading aloud

consisting of three letters), nor repeat the word "boy" (he merely articulates in a totally paraphasic manner meaningless sequences of sounds).

Main experiment. Some days later the patient is offered the written word "boy" which he can read promptly. Silent reading—at least of concrete words—is still intact. This intact performance now effects the deblocking of the following: He is able to repeat correctly the word spoken to him, to write it correctly on dictation, and to name correctly the corresponding picture when it is shown to him.

The three other control experiments also showed the patient to be completely anomic when requested to name pictures ("I can't," "I don't know"); to be capable only of producing brief sequences of letters without meaning, when requested to write on dictation (frequent perseverations); and to utter totally paraphasic sequences of sounds (*pro, plo, vro,* etc.) when he was asked to repeat. In the main experiments, however, the earlier reading aloud of the critical word deblocked the whole chain of verbal performances consisting of repetition, writing on dictation and naming.

Example #4. Patient T. J., age 64, retired laborer; admitted to the hospital on May 12, 1960. Apoplexy five days before admission, followed by speech disturbances. High arterial blood pressure with left ventricular hypertrophy. Marked tendon reflexes in upper limbs, especially on the right side. Right homonymous hemianopsia; bilateral hypoacusia. EEG, December 15, 1960: bilateral temporal foci. Diagnosis: left posterior temporal cerebral thrombosis; aphasia.

Aphasia examination: Appreciably disturbed spontaneous speech and dialogue, literal and verbal paraphasia, frequent perseveration, diminished vocabulary. Partially preserved automatic speech. Appreciably deteriorated sentence reading and auditory receptive verbal functions (does not obey spoken or written words). Word repetition also completely abolished (paraphasia), as is naming of real and pictured objects; partial disturbance of color naming. Relatively well preserved are reading aloud of letters and of common concrete words, as well as copied writing. Total agraphia on dictation. Total acalculia. Difficulties of silent reading can be temporarily removed by means of auditory adjuvant stimuli (the written word is spoken aloud by the examiner) or visual ones (exhibiting a picture corresponding to the written word). *Conclusion: mixed aphasia.*

In this case too (Figure 2), we applied the chain deblocking method to impaired picture naming, repetition and writing on dictation. Here, however, we used a *combined deblocker:* reading aloud and copying. This combination had proved necessary in the control experiments primarily in view of picture naming, which could be deblocked neither through copying alone nor through reading aloud by itself, but only when both these performances were combined. Comparison between the single performances during the control experiments and in the main experiment shows the chain-like effect of deblocking of several discrete performances.

We thus succeeded in both patients in deblocking "in a chain" the three impaired functions in aphasic syndromes with anomia, agraphia-on-dictation and disturbances of repetition.

Thanks to the chain deblocking experiments carried on subsequently, in collaboration with Erika Metze and Renate Böttcher, we have gathered additional information concerning the significance of this method for aphasic syndrome research.

Example #5. Patient M. J., age 55, retired employee of a trade enterprise, was first admitted to the municipal hospital ("Oskar-Ziethen-Krankenhaus," Berlin) on January 27, 1965, and then to the University Neurological Clinic, Charité, Berlin (Prof. K. Leonhard, Director) on

Image Word	before deblocking			Deblocking by copying and reading	after deblocking		
	naming	repetition	writing on dictation		naming	repetition	writing on dictation
pălării (hats)	"par...plu...part" (paraphasic)	"pălăride" (paraphasic)	Palăngk	Pălărei	correct	correct	Pălărie
divan	"ratoite" (paraphasic)	"vecer" (paraphasic)	C	Divan	correct	correct	Divan
scurtă (coat)	"nu pot" (I can't)	"curte" (paraphasic)	Corte	Scurtă	correct	correct	Scurtă
pădure (wood)	"schela" (scaffold)	"nu pot" (I can't)	Pode	Pădure	correct	correct	Părdure Pădure

Figure 2. *Patient T.J.* Successive deblocking of naming, repetition, and writing on dictation by combined stimuli (copying and reading).

March 31, 1965. A myocardial infarction was followed three weeks later by a cortical embolism and diabetes mellitus with aphasic, apraxic and visual agnosic disturbances. No other findings on neurological examination. EEG: Irregular, with minor general changes; left temporal-basal focus extending into occipital region, predominantly subcortical in character.

Aphasia examination: Spontaneous speech and dialogue are much better, i.e., more fluent, than reactive speech, yet they show many paraphasic failures, perseveration, and word finding disturbances; other verbal-expressive functions, such as automatic speech, repetition, oral naming and reading aloud, are severely impaired or even abolished. Among the verbal-receptive functions, auditory understanding of concrete words and simple sentences is relatively intact, but there is word deafness for abstract and unusual words and for more complicated sentences; silent reading is intact. Total agraphia for spontaneous writing, writing on dictation and written naming. When tested a year later, copying and drawing were found to be intact. Color perception intact, but color naming and understanding of names of colors are disturbed. Visual, auditory and tactile gnosis intact. Slight facial and pantomimical apraxia. Acalculia: only simple written arithmetical operations can be executed. "Abstract" thinking as tested by sorting tests is reduced. *Conclusion: mixed aphasia (primarily sensory aphasia).*

The peculiarity of this case lies above all in the fact that "simple" deblocking, i.e., deblocking of the performances of a particular impaired function through one (or several) preserved functions, was not possible. With patients M. M. and T. J. we had succeeded in deblocking disturbances of repetition and naming by means of reading aloud, either alone or in conjunction with copying. In the case of patient M. J. such "simple" deblocking accomplished but little for repetition and writing on dictation, and failed altogether for oral and written naming and for reading aloud. These performances could only be deblocked within "a chain."

Furthermore, we found with this patient, as with others, that the greatest possible D-effects could be guaranteed only if the links of the chain had *a certain sequence.* The sequence is shown in our protocol (Figure 3) and consists of the following order: repetition—writing on dictation—oral naming—written naming—reading aloud. This sequence is based on our observations during several preliminary experiments. We had found that if, for instance, reading aloud was removed from the 6th position in the chain to an earlier position, the D-effect could not be obtained; the same applies to oral naming, which could only be deblocked after writing on dictation. Comparison with other patients shows that this succession

	copying	repetition	writing on dictation	oral naming	written naming	reading aloud
I	Wange Gürtel Papagei	"Krieg ich nicht"	Par Pagen	legaex	Pagel	nicht möglich
II	Stirn Ampel Klammer	nicht möglich	a S Klapper	fange	nicht möglict	Kanne
III	Matrosen Tulpe Palme	"saleweinger"	Mali Mali	lege	nicht möglich	trase
IV	Pinsel Uhr Sahne	nicht möglich	nicht möglich	lame schekin	S Malter malen Pipe Pinsel	Pinsel
V	h Axt Kekse Amsel	Keks	Ax Kekor Kekse	Kekse	Kekse	Kense
VI	Rose hase Decke	Decke	Decke	'ne Decke	Decke	Decke
VII	Sand Nadeln Maus	Nadel	-hadel	Feder.....Stege	Nadel	Ladel
VIII	Dackel Bank Falte	'ne Dacke	Dacket	Deckel, Dackel, Deckel	Dackel	Deckel..Dacker
IX	Lilie Regal Blitz	Dicks	Biltz Blitz	liks	Blitz	Bix
X	globus Rose Buch	Globus	globus globus	der lege..legök	Globus	ein lebes
XI	Stein Schlauch Raupe	'n Strauch..... Strauss	l Schlauch	'n Stauch...... Schlauch	Schlauch	Schlauch
XII	Wolf Fuss Nest	Nest	Nest	Nest	Nest	Nest
XIII	Krebs Seide gas	Krebs	Krebs Krebs Krebs	'n Krebs	Krebs	Krebs
XIV	Kiste Fuchs Linde	Füchs	Fuchs	Füchs	Fuchs	Füchs
XV	motte Bier Kragen	streiger	Kragen Krachen	Krägen	Kragen	Krägen

Figure 3. *Patient M.J.* "Chain" deblocking.

varies from case to case, which means that it must be ascertained empirically for each new patient.

In contrast to our procedure with patients M. M. and T. J., we could forego control experiments to check the impaired functions in the case of patient M. J., as he showed complete absence of repetition, agraphia-on-dictation, anomia (orally as well as in writing), and expressive alexia.

One complete protocol of the deblocking experiments carried out with patient M. J. is given in Figure 3.[4] The mistakes can be divided into three main groups: 1) total failures, i.e., the patient is completely unable to repeat, name, write on dictation, etc. (see Figure 3, Papagei, Klammer, Matrosen, Pinsel); 2) in other instances the patient's responses are totally paraphasic ("saleweiniger" instead of "Matrosen" on repetition), totally

[4] These experiments were carried out by my collaborator Erika Metze.

paralexic ("ein lebes" instead of "Globus" when reading aloud), or partially paragraphic ("Pagen" instead of "Papagei" when writing on dictation); 3) yet, most mistakes are, in fact, true deblocking effects, as they are merely literal-paraphasic or literal-alexic reactions ("Kense" instead of "Kekse," "Ladel" instead of "Nadel," "Dacke" or "Dacker" instead of "Dackel," "Füchs" instead of "Fuchs," "Krägen" instead of "Kragen," etc.); literal-paragraphic deviations did not occur.

RESULTS

1. Chain deblocking can be evoked through performances of a variety of preserved receptive or expressive functions.
2. Performances of a single function or, should this be insufficient, of combined functions (e.g., reading and copying) can serve as deblockers.
3. The succession of the performances of impaired functions to be deblocked is not important, as long as the discrete performances can be restored by means of "simple" deblocking, i.e., not within a "chain."
4. In a number of cases, performances of certain impaired functions could not be deblocked except within a "chain" (for example: oral naming and reading aloud in the case of patient M. J.).
5. In the latter cases the sequence of the links of the chain cannot be interchanged arbitrarily. The D-effect is obtained only if the performance to be deblocked follows several performances of other functions. The succession of the performances is to be ascertained in each case through preliminary experiments.

DISCUSSION

The study of the deblocking phenomenon appears to be highly suitable for the investigation of the problem of aphasic syndromes. A number of problems concerning the reciprocal relationships between preserved and disturbed speech functions, on the one hand, and relationships between various symptoms of aphasia, on the other hand, can thus be investigated experimentally.

The method of "simple" deblocking makes use of the fact that verbal decoding, coding and recoding of the meaning of a given word or sentence may be possible for the aphasic via some "channels," even though other "channels" may be "blocked." Certain aphasic disturbances can be eliminated for shorter or longer periods through successive experimental linking of intact and impaired functions.

We have shown in detail in earlier papers (14, 18) that the means by which D-effects can be obtained are manifold indeed. It is possible to deblock not only expressive but also receptive impairments via visual as well as via auditory, tactile or verbo-motor analyzers. It was further shown that preserved understanding of words or sentences, naming of objects, repetition, reading or writing can all serve equally well as deblockers. On the one hand, D-effects can be evoked on the level of receptive functions, (e.g., preserved silent reading can deblock impaired auditory word understanding), while, on the other hand, it is possible to eliminate expressive disturbances through the utilization of preserved performances, e.g., disturbances of repetition through reading aloud. Finally, expressive aphasic disturbances can be deblocked receptively,[5] and vice versa, e.g., the inability to read aloud can be deblocked through hearing the words spoken; word deafness may be deblocked through repetition.

Although we carried through our deblocking experiments primarily with verbal performances in the widest meaning of this term, deblockers—as well as disturbances to be deblocked—may be non-verbal. It is possible, for example, to deblock disturbances of object naming through perception of corresponding noises (e.g., naming of an animal after having heard the relevant typical animal sounds), or picture-agnosia through hearing the words to be deblocked (15, 16).

These facts comprise a number of important aspects which allow us to draw conclusions regarding the nature of syndromatic disturbances. The numerous interrelations between various discrete functions, functional levels and analyzers, indicate above all—as Goldstein has pointed out repeatedly—that after-effects of brain lesions are disturbances of *systems*.

The qualitative and statistical analysis of data collected from a sufficiently large number of different syndromes would seem a promising approach to the comparative study of the structure of these syndromes.

Going beyond the results that can be attained with the method of "simple" deblocking, the method of "chain deblocking" is an instrument for a more comprehensive analysis of the dynamic structure of syndromes. The main feature of the phenomenon of chain deblocking is the fact that single or combined deblocking stimuli can eliminate not only the performance disturbance of one impaired function, as in the case of "simple" deblocking, but that, in certain cases, the disturbances of several component parts of a given syndrome can be eliminated simultaneously.

---

[5] In a separate paper (17) we have dealt with the problem of expressive disturbances being deblocked by purely receptive means through the exclusion of even latent speech movements.

Examples of some of our chain deblocking experiments are summarized in Table 1; they illustrate clearly the polyfunctional effect of the deblocking stimuli. In all the cases listed in this table, earlier reading, be it aloud or silent, or hearing the spoken word, in some cases combined with copying, was sufficient to deblock simultaneously the performances of several component parts (up to five) of the respective aphasic syndromes. This is due to the fact that, under certain conditions, the effect of semantic information radiates over the language-functional system as a whole. This means, for example, that through hearing a word (decoding) all other forms of decoding, coding and recoding of this word—such as receptive understanding, repetition, reading aloud, writing—are simultaneously put into a state of readiness. This process of radiation is to be regarded as a form of simultaneous pre-stimulation of the "blocked" channels which favors the deblocking of the impaired speech performances.

TABLE 1. EXAMPLES OF DIFFERENT FORMS OF CHAIN-DEBLOCKING.

Patient	Deblocking functions	Functions to be deblocked →	→	→	→	→
Schw. W.	silent reading and copying	oral naming	written naming			
G. P.	word-hearing and copying	silent reading	reading aloud	oral naming		
M. M.	reading aloud	repetition	writing on dictation	oral naming		
T. J.	reading aloud and copying	oral naming	repetition	writing on dictation		
D. E.	silent reading and copying	repetition	writing on dictation	oral naming		
T. B.	silent reading and copying	writing on dictation	reading aloud	oral naming	written naming	
M. J.	silent reading and copying	repetition	writing on dictation	oral naming	written naming	reading aloud

The assumption of polyfunctional effects of this kind cannot be restricted to the pathological sphere, but must be regarded as a characteristic feature of the language-functional system.

In order to understand fully the specificity of this radiation, its *selective* character must be stressed. As indicated above, the verbal deblocking stimuli that we use do not lead to a general functional readiness of the impaired component parts of the language system. The functional readiness is, in fact, specifically related to the *semantic field* to which the particular verbal deblocking stimulus belongs. The selective character of deblocking or radiating is, therefore, primarily determined by the factor of meaning. These findings seem to confirm Goldstein's thesis of the importance of the problem of meaning in the interpretation of disturbances of higher cortical functions. He writes: "Thus, the problem of meaning assumed *central importance* in the interpretation of aphasic symptoms" (4, p. 23). Using Lotmar's term, Goldstein speaks of a "sphere of meaning," referring to observations made on patients with amnesic aphasia[6] who produce "other words that belong to the sphere of meaning of the demanded words" (5, p. 47).

In this connection, we must point out that receptive and expressive reactivation of meaning connections by our deblocking method takes place on a level of language behavior that does not permit the use of Goldstein's dichotomy "concrete-abstract." Although deblocking enables patients to code, decode and recode correctly both "concrete" and "abstract" meanings, the reactivation of these verbal reactions takes place quasi-automatically, without active and conscious participation of the patient. The verbal behavior of aphasic individuals during the successful deblocking process is similar to that of normal subjects when given the task to understand, repeat, read, or write familiar words or sentences, or to name well-known objects. Goldstein referred to this form of behavior in connection with the "automatisms" of thinking when he wrote, "Thereby, not only present events play a role, but also the remnants of previous thinking that were fixed as thoughts in the form of automatisms. They become more or less effective, facilitating the active process of thinking. Thus we have also in thinking to distinguish an active and a passive part. The fixated thoughts often appear in words. That form occurs particularly when the concern is not so much with creation of new concepts but with reproduction of old ones for special purposes . . ." (5, p. 44).

In the case of our deblocking, we are dealing just with this "reproduction of old ones," i.e., of words or sentences "in the form of fixed automatisms."[7]

[6] Nevertheless, it must be stressed that our statements concerning "semantic fields" are not limited to amnesic aphasia, but apply to all types of aphasia.

[7] For the sake of avoiding misunderstandings, it should be pointed out that the abovementioned "automatisms" are not identical with those showing a complete absence of all meaningful language behavior, e.g., the mere mechanical reproduction of sequences of letters, words or figures, etc., or, as Goldstein calls it, "reproductions of simple associations of sound complexes to a particular object" (5, p. 41).

We think we are not mistaken in the assumption that a more profound study of the level of the stored thought and language patterns would lead to a clarification and revision of the problem of so-called concrete and abstract behavior. In such a study the deblocking method might be utilized, along with other methods.[8]

The polyfunctional effects of the language system also help to explain other phenomena of chain deblocking. In our experiments, we found that the *sequence* of the links of the "chain" plays an important part. Through variation of the sequence of these links we could show that, in certain cases, such as patient M. J., these links cannot be interchanged at will. Only if performances of certain functions are deblocked first can failure in subsequent performances be eliminated. This proves that a positive induction radiates from the disturbed performances as soon as they are deblocked, affects the links that follow, and intensifies the effect of the actual deblocker. It is this *summation* of deblocking effects which is ultimately responsible for the elimination of the impairment of performances of certain severely disturbed functions. At times it is necessary for several pre-deblocked performances to participate in this intensification of the D-effect. In the case of patient M. J., the inability to read a certain word aloud could only be eliminated through his reading the same word first silently, and then copying it (the actual deblocking process), before his inability to write the word on dictation, or to use it as the name of an object orally and in writing could be deblocked.

The variety of these phenomena raises a number of questions concerning the structure and dynamics of the language-functional system, its disturbances and the possibilities of removing them (deblocking). The interrelations existing within the "chain" seem to indicate a certain *hierarchy* among the functions involved, a hierarchy which determines for any given disturbance the possibility of its being deblocked and, once deblocked, the likelihood that the regained performance will induce additional positive effects. Without doubt, the final analysis of these interrelations will lead to more definite conclusions concerning relationships within and among syndromes. Statistically significant evidence has yet to be collected and analyzed before the ideas outlined here can be said to contribute comprehensively towards the systematic analysis of the structure and dynamics of these syndromes.

In concluding this paper, written in memory of Kurt Goldstein, I wish

[8] The author in no way excludes his own views of "concrete" and "abstract" behavior, published as early as 1927 and 1933 (see 11 and 12) from this necessity of revision.

to stress once more the sincerity of my feelings for this great man, for whom I cherish a deep feeling of love, respect, and gratefulness—the sincerity of which remains unaltered, even though my path in research may deviate from the direction he had shown me many years ago.

REFERENCES

1. Goldstein, K. Zur Theorie der Funktion des Nervensystems. *Arch. Psychiat. & Nervenkr.*, 1925, *74*, 370–405.
2. Goldstein, K. Das Symptom, seine Entstehung und Bedeutung für unsere Auffassung vom Bau und der Funktion des Nervensystems. *Arch. Psychiat. & Nervenkr.*, 1925, *76*, 84–108.
3. Goldstein, K. Über Aphasie. *Schweiz. Arch. Neurol. Psychiat.*, 1926, *19*, 3–39; 292–322.
4. Goldstein, K. *Language and Language Disturbances*. New York: Grune & Stratton, 1948.
5. Goldstein, K. Thinking and speaking. *Ann. N.Y. Acad. Sci.*, 1960, *91*, 38–51.
6. Jakobson. R. Towards a linguistic typology of aphasic impairments. In: A CIBA Foundation Symposium, London, 1964, Churchill Ltd., p. 21–46.
7. Lotmar, F. Zur Pathopsychologie der erschwerten Wortfindung bei Aphasischen. *Schweiz. Arch. Neurol. Psychiat.*, 1933, *30*, 86–158; 322–379.
8. Luria, A. R. Kurt Goldstein and neuropsychology. *Neuropsychologia*, 1966, *4*, 311–313.
9. Luria, A. R. and Vinogradova, O. S. An objective investigation of the dynamics of semantic systems. *Brit. J. Psychol.*, 1959, *50*, 89–105.
10. Teuber, H.-L. Kurt Goldstein's role in the development of neuropsychology. *Neuropsychologia*, 1966, *4*, 299–309.
11. Weigl, E. Zur Psychologie sogenannter Abstraktionsprozesse. *Z. Psychol.*, 1927, *103*, 2–45.
12. Weigl, E. Sprache und Ordnen. Kritisches und Prinzipielles zu den von Kuenburgschen Zuordnungsversuchen bei Gesunden und Sprachgestörten. *Z. ges. Neurol. Psychiat.*, 1933, *144*, 507–561.
13. Weigl, E. On the psychology of so-called processes of abstraction. *J. abn. soc. Psychol.*, 1941, *36*, 3–33.
14. Weigl, E. The phenomenon of temporary deblocking in aphasia. *Zeitschr. Phonetic, Sprachwiss. Komm.*, 1961, *14*, 337–364.
15. Weigl, E. Deblockierungen akustisch und optisch agnostischer Störungen. In: *Ber. Tag. Oto-Neuro-Ophth.* Dresden, 1962. Leipzig, 1963, Thieme-Verlag, p. 264–266.
16. Weigl, E. Deblockierung bildagnostischer Störungen bei einem Aphatiker. *Neuropsychologia*, 1963, *1*, 91–107.
17. Weigl, E. Die Bedeutung der afferenten, verbo-kinästhetischen Erregungen des Sprechapparates für die expressiven und rezeptiven Sprachvorgänge bei Normalen and Sprachgestörten. *Cortex*, 1964, *1*, 77–90.
18. Weigl, E. The experimental deblocking of aphasic verbal defects, a method of

investigation of processes of cerebral dynamics. *Vopr. Psychol.*, 1964, *149–159* (Russian).
19. Weigl, E. Neuro-psychological studies of structure and dynamics of semantic fields with the deblocking-method. In: *18th Internat. Congr. Psychol. Abstr. II*, Moscow, 1966, p. 424.
20. Weigl, E. and Kreindler, A. Beiträge zur Auffassung gewisser aphasischer Störungen als Blockierungserscheinungen. Temporäre Deblockierungen sprachmotorischer Reaktionen durch Wortlesen bei motorischer Aphasie. *Arch. Psychiat. Zig. Neurol.*, 1960, *200*, 306–323.
21. Weigl, E. and Metze, E. Gesteuerte verbale Kettenreaktionen bei Aphatikern. (In press).

From the Laboratory of Language Pathology, German Academy of Sciences, Berlin, G.D.R.

12

Goldstein and Vygotsky

by EUGENIA HANFMANN

Watertown, Massachusetts

At the time I was asked to contribute to this volume, I was preparing a brief essay on the Russian psychologist L. S. Vygotsky, whose chief work I had translated a few years earlier. This essay seemed to me to be an appropriate contribution to a volume dedicated to Kurt Goldstein, since the two men had had a central area of interest in common: the "higher psychic functions" as described by Vygotsky, coincide, or greatly overlap, with Goldstein's categorial or abstract attitude. Although Vygotsky's interest in this specifically human level of functioning arose originally within the framework of developmental psychology, not of psychopathology, he knew of Goldstein's work and must have been influenced by it. In the outline of Vygotsky's work, which forms the first part of the present communication, similarities with Goldstein's theories will be obvious to the reader.

There was also another phase in the interchange of ideas between the two men, one in which I was involved personally more than thirty years ago. It so happened that one segment of the younger man's work did in turn stimulate Goldstein's thinking. I believe that this stimulation was directly responsible for strengthening Goldstein's interest in schizophrenia and causing him to place this topic among his active research interests. In this interaction I myself functioned as a link between the two scholars, by conveying to Goldstein some of the Russian's findings and conclusions a few years after the latter's premature death. A report of this episode forms the second part of this essay; I did not attempt to integrate it with the first part since, being based on my own memories, the second part has a more personal tone than the first.

I. VYGOTSKY'S WORK[1]

Before trying to characterize Vygotsky's work, I want to comment briefly on the man himself—the most outstanding representative of humanistic psychology in Russia. As a student, Vygotsky read widely in liguistics, philosophy, the social sciences, and the arts; he focused his work on psychology only in 1924, ten years before his death. In these ten

[1] A paper delivered at the 74th annual meeting of the American Psychological Association, New York City, September 1966, under the title: "Vygotsky's 'Thought and Language.' "

years he launched a series of experimental investigations in developmental, educational and abnormal psychology, published close to one hundred articles and books and wrote many that were not published during his life. I learned from one of Vygotsky's personal friends that he was also a serious student of classical languages, a poet, a theater critic whose opinion and advice were highly valued by some of the innovators of the stage; his circle of friends included actors, writers, philosophers, and rabbinical scholars. His wide erudition, his originality, and his effortless grasp of various disciplines make him appear to have been a near genius, a true renaissance man. Vygotsky seems not to have been interested in politics, and he succeeded in avoiding it as much as was possible; in his psychological writings he makes no strenuous efforts to bring his theories in line with the prevailing political doctrines. Yet he applied some of the tenets of Hegelian dialectics to the consideration of psychological issues in a very productive, imaginative way.

For about twenty years following Vygotsky's death his works were not republished, and his approach to psychological issues received no official support, though it continued to be influential, particularly among workers in the field of educational psychology. Since 1956 three volumes of Vygotsky's works have been published—or republished—in Russia. The first, *Selected Psychological Studies*, included the monograph on thought and language, together with various studies pertaining largely to child development: an experimental investigation of the development of the higher forms of attention, a discussion of the relationship of instruction and maturation during the preschool and school ages, an approach to a theory of mental retardation, and a study of conceptual disturbance in schizophrenia. This volume was followed in 1960 by one entitled *The Development of Higher Psychic Functions* which contained some of Vygotsky's works never published before: an unfinished treatise on the development of higher mental functions; a lecture series dealing with perception, memory, thinking, emotion, imagination and volition, particularly in their genetic aspects; a popular presentation comparing animal and human behavior; a discussion of his views on the localization of mental functions. A book on the psychology of (literary) art forms had been completed by Vygotsky quite early, in the 'twenties, but for some reason it had not been published at the time. In this book, after reviewing and criticizing various approaches to aesthetics (including that of literary formalism), he formulates a theory of his own, a psychological theory of the nature of a work of art, and illustrates it by analyzing various literary forms. This book, *Psychology of Art*, was published for the first time in 1965. There is a good chance that it will be translated eventually into English: like *Thought and Language*, this work is of interest to more than one discipline.

Valuable as the contents of all these volumes are, *Thought and Language*, completed by Vygotsky shortly before his death, represents the culmination of his work, the most mature formulation of many converging lines of exploration he had been pursuing. I shall not try to discuss this work in detail: I could not do justice to it in a brief review, and the book is available in English, even as a paperback (12). I shall merely recapitulate some of the main theses of *Thought and Language*, pointing out their relationships to Vygotsky's general theories of mental development and to some of his other empirical studies.

In reviewing the literature on child and animal intelligence, Vygotsky notes that there is a pre-linguistic stage of thinking—manifested, for instance, in the use of tools—and a pre-intellectual, social-emotional stage of language. As the child begins to acquire representational language in the second year of life, these two lines of development start converging and, through their convergence, the foundation is laid for *verbal thought*, the specifically human achievement. In time, child language, which is globally social at first, becomes differentiated into communicative language proper and language for oneself—the so-called inner speech. This description of the child's linguistic development differs in some important points from that given by Piaget. According to Piaget, the younger child's autism gradually yields to socialized thought and speech, the children's egocentric language being the transitional stage between the former and the latter. Vygotsky conducted several studies of the factors that promote or hinder egocentric speech; the evidence he collected indicated that this type of speech often served problem solving, arising, for example, when the child's pursuits met with difficulties. Vygotsky concluded that egocentric speech should be viewed not as a residue of autism, but rather as speech on the way towards internalization, the beginning of a dialogue with oneself in which we excel as adults and which becomes the main vehicle of our intellectual achievements.

These formulations of a specific developmental trend exemplify some of the main theses of Vygotsky. The structure of the psyche, the interrelationship of the various psychological functions—in this case, of language and thought—is not constant: it changes as these functions develop. Consequently, all psychology must be developmental, not static. It is also, by necessity, social, since the development of the specifically human functions is mediated by socio-cultural factors. But Vygotsky does not stop with this thesis, which is too general to be useful. He goes on to explore the specific processes through which cultural factors help modify the very structure of individual consciousness.

The experimental study of the development of concept formation in children has a bearing on this issue. Vygotsky describes three stages, corresponding to changes that meanings of words undergo as children grow older. The early syncretistic stage is followed by the stage of thinking in complexes: the common name of a group of objects means to the child that these objects are related to each other in some concrete factual way, as are members of a family; but the basis of similarity can differ from one pair to another. Even if it happens to be the same, as in a group of *red* blocks, this property is not seen by the child as the common characteristic defining the group; if he describes the group as red, this word must be viewed as a pseudo-concept. Words come to stand for generalized concepts only later, in adolescence, and this raises verbal thought to a radically new level.

It should be pointed out here that the method used in the study of concept formation is an example of the method Vygotsky advocated for the study of all higher mental functions: he calls it the method of double stimulation. The child is given some task, e.g., that of memorization; he is provided, first, with the material to be memorized, second, with a different group of items, or stimuli, which may be used to facilitate this task. In the concept formation test, the nonsense words written on the blocks serve as these additional stimuli: If the subject understands that they refer to some common properties of the blocks, he can use these words as guidelines to the "correct" ordering of blocks. In Vygotsky's study of the development of voluntary attention, the pointing finger of the examiner serves as an additional stimulus which often creates a shift useful for the solution of the problem. Another method is patterned after a familiar game; the child must answer questions, for instance, about the colors of different objects, but must remember to refrain from using certain words, such as "yes" and "no," or "black" and "white." Later on he is provided with some bits of colored paper which he can use to make this task easier. While a young child is unable to do this effectively, the school-age child's performance improves greatly through a planned use of these visual reminders; the adult no longer needs this external help for controlling his attention and memory.

Vygotsky maintains that every mental function undergoes a development similar to the one observed in the experimental studies described above. Spontaneous and unmediated at first, responsive to a wide range of stimuli, each mental function of the child is gradually brought under the control of the social environment with the help of some recurring additional stimuli which come to function as signs; later on the child internalizes these signs and thus gains a conscious control over the given mental function. In order to further this process maximally, instruction, both formal and informal, must keep a few steps ahead of maturation, introducing tasks likely to result in some strain and, consequently, in some movement, in the growth of the child's capabilities. Accordingly, the child's developmental level is to be measured not so much by the kind of problems he can solve through his own unaided efforts, but by the extent of his ability to utilize help effectively in the performance of a mental task he can not yet perform by himself. Throughout his discussion of maturation and instruction, Vygotsky shows how they determine each other, and how their interplay determines development; in his polemics he turns equally against excessive "biologizing" of the conception of the human being and against considering culture either as an all-powerful factor, or as a higher existential level, without solid roots in biological foundations. It should be noted that Vygotsky's genetic analyses never remain on these levels of generality: he ably uncovers the minute steps through which the interaction of the two factors proceeds from a given developmental level to the next higher one.

Let me add a few words on Vygotsky's ideas concerning the psychological essence of art, specifically of the art forms that use words as their material. He maintains that the formal elements of a literary work—for example, the sequence in which events are presented, as different from their true chronological sequence—are aimed at creating an emotional response in the reader, a response that is radically different from the one inherent in the material as such. Catharsis is the essence of art; in Vygotsky's conception, catharsis is the resolution of the tension created by the divergent directions in which our emotions are led to develop by the content and structure of a work of art. In this resolution the recalcitrant material is mastered and subdued; it is, as it were, de-materialized by the form, much as in a statue of winged victory the weight and inertia of marble are transformed into weightless flight. This idea is elucidated by Vygotsky in a series of sensitive analyses of the structure of various literary forms—fables, short stories, Shakespearean tragedies—and of the emotional effects of these various structural moments. The concrete sources of these effects are not obvious at a glance—art consists in concealing art—but these formal elements—sequences, arrangements, rhythms—are of utmost importance in the emergence and functioning of a work of art. Content alone does not explain art's psychological effects. Elements of emotional contagion, conscious or unconscious feelings aroused by the content of a story, may be part of the material the author works with, but they are not what makes a work of art. A verbal composition attains the artistic level of cultural endeavor only when it succeeds in resolving emotional tension, the dialectic which has been created and maintained through the interaction of content and form. This process of resolution or catharsis occurs in a similar way in different people, even if the emotional response to the specific content of a literary work varies to some extent from person to person. In promoting this common experience, the effects of a work of art transcend the sphere of individual psychology, and art becomes part of a culture, a shared possession of a social group.

II. VYGOTSKY AND GOLDSTEIN ON SCHIZOPHRENIA[2]

My first contact with Goldstein took place a few months after he arrived in the United States in 1935, when I was a member of the research staff at Worcester State Hospital. At that particular time I was engaged, together with Maria Rickers-Ovsiankina, in studying a puzzling patient, Lanuti, who, after having sustained an apparently slight head injury some months earlier, continued to appear dazed and to behave strangely. The medical staff was divided between the diagnoses of traumatic neurosis and of malingering—there was some insurance money involved—but the Rorschach test administered by Rickers-Ovsiankina yielded a clear-cut picture of an organic condition. We then embarked on a series of tests, including those for agnosia, aphasia, and apraxia, and in this context I read or reread many of Goldstein's writings. I had been familiar with his basic theoretical formulations, but reading them in conjunction with the rich data we had collected on our patient's behavior and performance was a novel and an eye-opening experience. Those psychological theories of which I had detailed knowledge—like those of K. Koffka whose research assistant I had been earlier—had to be fitted to the experimental observations in a careful elaborate fashion; many of the facts serving as supports of these theories were "minute," difficult to elicit and observe. Now I saw Goldstein's theories meet the observed clinical facts halfway, as it were, with no strenuous efforts on my or anyone's part, as if the two had been fitted for size. In the light of his formulations the previously discrete data

[2] This report is not intended as a systematic review of the two authors' contributions to the study of schizophrenia: I have used it largely as a vehicle for some reminiscences about Goldstein, and about the effect of the encounter with him and his work on me personally.

suddenly acquired meaning and coherence, things clicked and fell into place in a most plausible, if not always the most simple way.

Hand in hand with this demonstration of the effects of a "concordant," material-congruent theory, went the discovery of how much can be learned from a well-understood single patient with whom the examiner has come to empathize. For me this discovery was a very personal matter, as it must have been for many others. During this period, when any aspect of the "concrete attitude" was being discussed, I found myself reproducing those of Lanuti's expressions, actions, or words that embodied this aspect; for instance, at any mention of the numbers one, two or three, I would automatically raise a corresponding number of fingers. There was no psychological issue which I did not find possible to illuminate and to clarify by reference to some of the patient's productions; friends accused me of believing that "the world has been generated by Lanuti." But at least an important part of my personal world, the collaboration and friendship with Goldstein, was generated by Lanuti, though not without the help of a mutual friend, Fritz Heider. After the patient had been demonstrated to him, Heider encouraged me to get in touch with Goldstein who, he felt, would enjoy hearing about a case that confirmed his theories in such a dramatic and striking fashion. In following this suggestion I visited Goldstein in New York; he was enthusiastic about my report, and I was exhilarated by his response to it. Soon after my visit to him, Goldstein came to Worcester to meet the patient in person and to give him a few more tests; he agreed to be a co-author of *Case Lanuti* (9).

A few years later, when the study was completed and I was writing the first version of the monograph, I spent a few weeks in New York, working on the manuscript and discussing it with Goldstein for a few hours every second or third day. The discussions were lively, at times heated, and some of our disagreements remained unresolved, but Goldstein's high spirits and contagious enthusiasm made the sessions exhilarating throughout. After a coffee break he would get up, exclaiming: "And now back to work—that is what we are here for!" ("Denn dazu sind wir ja da.") This sounded less as a reminder of a job to be done than as an invitation to a joyous feast, and it was indeed a feast and a delight to watch Goldstein's mind at work.

Soon after I first met Goldstein I moved from Worcester to Howard State Hospital to start work on a schizophrenia project sponsored by Jacob Kasanin, a Russian-born psychiatrist with strong research interests; he had recently visited his native country where he had met Vygotsky. Kasanin was greatly impressed by Vygotsky's work on the development of concepts and charmed by the elegance of the "Concept Formation Test" which the

Russian had adapted from an experimental procedure used by N. Ach (7). Vygotsky was mainly interested in the performance of children of different ages, but he had also given the test to some schizophrenic patients. In 1932 he had communicated his conclusions in a short article without much information on the patients' test performance. He stated that the onset of schizophrenia brings with it a loss of the capacity for strictly conceptual thinking, the highest level of thinking which is acquired in adolescence; consequently the patients resort to more primitive, "complex" thinking, specifically to its later forms typical of pre-adolescence. This communication had fired Kasanin's imagination. On returning to the States he started the manufacture of the test blocks which Vygotsky had given him, translated and published Vygotsky's article (11), obtained a research grant from the Masonic Foundation for Research in Dementia Praecox, and charged me with the task of replicating Vygotsky's study in a controlled, systematic fashion. The results of this research were published in monograph form only much later, in 1942 (8), but almost from the start of the study it became increasingly evident that, for some patients at least, Vygotsky's conclusions held. I felt certain of this long before the experiments were completed, particularly after some supplementary studies had shown that the patients experienced similar difficulties in a variety of tasks, some of them much less exacting than the Concept Formation Test. The credit for this extension of the findings to a wider area of performance goes primarily to one schizophrenic young woman, who, after having taken the test, started frequenting my office with requests for more work to do; she thus made herself the subject of a comprehensive study. Josephine was given a variety of tasks, some of them selected for a specific reason, others at random. In analyzing her performance I benefited from having been sensitized, through the study of Lanuti, to a great variety of "concrete" approaches to different tasks. Though Josephine showed no circumscribed disturbances of perception, action or speech, her inability to select and organize perceptual material, the "literalness" of her thinking and her use of language suggested a drastic impairment of the "categorial attitude," a disturbance which Goldstein had discovered in cases of brain injuries. Josephine's performance met all criteria of the "concrete attitude" exhibited by Goldstein's brain-injured patients (5).

Startled by this finding, I reread Vygotsky's article on schizophrenia and found, in a previously unnoticed paragraph, that I was not the first one to be startled (11). In talking about the changes which meanings of words may undergo in pathology, Vygotsky tells of having first seen one type of this change in patients with amnestic aphasia for whom, he says, the disturbance of thinking in categories or in concepts, as described by Gelb and Goldstein, is in the foreground; in these cases he found a drastic disturbance of the ability to understand and to use words in a figurative, non-literal sense, as demonstrated, for instance, within the context of proverbs. He then tells of having been "deeply astonished" to find a similar disturbance in schizophrenic patients, even though their speech was wholly intact and there were no striking surface indications of the dissolution of conceptual structures. In the same text I also found a statement confirming another conclusion suggested by the case of Josephine and of some other patients, namely, that in some schizophrenics the loss of conceptual thinking is a basic disturbance accounting for a large part, if not the whole, of the patient's symptomatology. Kasanin later designated such cases as those of "primary thought disorder" (10).

Armed with these quotations, with the group results of the Concept Formation Test and with a record of Josephine's performances, sayings and doings, I went to see Goldstein. I was not entirely at ease in preparing to deliver my message. Vygotsky's brief reference to amnestic aphasia did not seem to me to express an adequate recognition of the role Goldstein's work has played in opening up this new perspective on the schizophrenic disturbance of thinking. The thesis of Vygotsky seemed to me to represent essentially an extension of Goldstein's findings to schizophrenia, and I was afraid that the absence of an explicit acknowledgment of this situation by the Russian might annoy him or hurt his feelings; I was ready with plausible explanations of this omission as due to the fact that Vygotsky had arrived at his conclusions by a different route, using methods different from Goldstein's. But my misgivings proved unfounded: no explanations were necessary. Goldstein was both greatly intrigued and greatly pleased with Vygotsky's findings and my confirmation of them. As I read the records, he repeatedly expressed his amazement at their strong similarity to the performance of organic patients.

At that time Goldstein was engaged, together with Scheerer, in preparing an analytic description of a series of tests he had found useful for the differentiation between abstract and concrete behavior (4). He included some schizophrenics in the group of subjects who were given these tests, and, to his great satisfaction, found the results of his procedures to be consistent with Vygotsky's findings (1). When Kasanin, in 1939, arranged a symposium on language and thought in schizophrenia, Goldstein spoke of Vygotsky as "the pioneer who adopted our general concept and methodological procedures in his attempt to determine the fundamental mental change in schizophrenia" (3). He cited several findings from my studies, especially from the *Analysis of the thinking disorder in a case of schizophrenia*, as exemplifying the schizophrenic's abnormal concreteness (5, 6). In the same talk Goldstein also pointed out that the concrete performance of the schizophrenics, though similar to that of the brain injured, was not identical with theirs, and that the similarity did not necessarily indicate the presence of an organic factor in schizophrenia: the concreteness of schizophrenics might be considered as a way out of an unbearable conflict, a protection against the danger of a severe catastrophe. Gradually this latter interpretation became dominant in Goldstein's view of schizophrenia. He learned through clinical observation that the abnormally concrete behavior does not occur under all conditions, but seems to depend on the demands confronting the patient. He concluded that the schizophrenic's concreteness is a protective mechanism against anxiety, a mechanism which originates in early youth and which functions selectively (2). During the period of Goldstein's association with Brandeis University he occasionally discussed with me the possibility of studying this selectivity in a systematic fashion, working with those patients who manifest clear shifts from one type of behavior to the other. To my regret I was unable to make time for this project; I would have greatly enjoyed exploring this problematical area in collaboration with Kurt Goldstein.

REFERENCES

1. Bolles, M. and Goldstein, K. A study of the impairment of "abstract behavior" in schizophrenic patients. *Psychiat. Quart.*, 1938, *12*, 42–65.
2. Goldstein, K. Concerning the concreteness in schizophrenia. *J. abn. soc. Psychol.*, 1959, *59*, 146–148.
3. Goldstein, K. Methodological approach to the study of schizophrenic thought disorder. In: *Language and Thought in Schizophrenia*, ed., J. S. Kasanin, New York: Norton, 1964, pp. 17–39.
4. Goldstein, K. and Scheerer, M. Abstract and concrete behavior, an experimental study with special tests. *Psychol. Monogr.*, 1941, *53*, No. 2, pp. 151.
5. Hanfmann, E. Analysis of the thinking disorder in a case of schizophrenia. *Arch. Neurol. Psychiat.*, 1939, *41*, 568–579.
6. Hanfmann, E. Thought disturbance in schizophrenia as revealed by performance in a picture completion test. *J. abn. soc. Psychol.*, 1939, *34*, 249–264.
7. Hanfmann, E. and Kasanin, J. A method for the study of concept formation. *J. Psychol.*, 1937, *3*, 521–540.
8. Hanfmann, E. and Kasanin, J. Conceptual thinking in schizophrenia. *Nerv. ment. Dis. Monogr.*, 1942, No. 67, pp. viii & 115.
9. Hanfmann, E., Rickers-Ovsiankina, M. and Goldstein, K. Case Lanuti: extreme concretization of behavior due to damage of the brain cortex. *Psychol. Monogr.*, 1944, *57*, No. 4, pp. 72.

10. Kasanin, J. S. The disturbance of conceptual thinking in schizophrenia. In: *Language and Thought in Schizophrenia,* ed. J. S. Kasanin, New York: Norton, 1964, pp. 41–49.
11. Vygotsky, L. S. Thought in schizophrenia. *Arch. Neurol. Psychiat.,* 1934, *31,* 1063–1077.
12. Vygotsky, L. S. *Thought and language.* Translated and edited by E. Hanfmann and G. Vakar. Cambridge, Mass.; M.I.T. Press (Paperback), 1965, pp. xxi & 168.

13

Contributions from Schizophrenia to the Understanding of Normal Psychological Function

by David Shakow
Bethesda, Maryland

INTRODUCTION

It seems particularly appropriate in a memorial volume for Kurt Goldstein to introduce this essay with a consideration of the importance of the psychopathological for the understanding of normal behavior. Goldstein consistently argued from this point of view. It is especially evident in his two theoretical volumes, both of which make direct reference to pathology in their titles: *The Organism: A Holistic Approach to Biology Derived from Pathological Data in Man* (16), and his William James Lectures, *Human Nature in the Light of Psychopathology* (18).

This, however, is not necessarily a point of view that is generally accepted. So many of us regard this approach, in addition to the direct one, so essential, that to find others rejecting it comes as a great surprise. An understanding of this neglect may come from an examination of the three possible factors involved.

The first originates in the psychologist's dual identity as both human being and scientist which provides the inherent dichotomous base of his discipline. Considering the current relatively primitive stage of both man's and psychology's evolution, the psychologist has undertaken the difficult task of differentiating himself as objective observer from himself as subject, in an attempt to deal with the "fallacy" which William James long ago assigned to the psychologist and which is so peculiarly his own. An understandable lack of security and ease in this dual role makes us sensitive to the implications of abnormality. We defend ourselves against these implications by transposing Thomas à Kempis' observation of "out of sight, out of mind" to "out of mind, out of sight." But one naturally asks: What about the converse—the *over*preoccupation with the abnormal which is characteristic of some of our clinically-oriented colleagues? This would appear to be compensatory and only the other side of the same coin. I do not say this unambivalently for I recognize that any field, science included, often advances because of the productive clashes between extreme positions.

The second source of the psychologist's frequent rejection of the interrelationship of the abnormal with the normal originates in the attitude of those of us who are concerned with scientific purism. It is characteristic of the purist in psychology, as in other fields, to insist on a narrow and rigid definition of the discipline, limiting it to only the most immediate areas and to the most direct approaches.

But another facet of purity appears to be involved as well: I refer to the fear of contamination by the applied. Study of the abnormal seems in its very essence to demand that something ameliorative be done—illness naturally calls for help. As a result, those concerned with a psychology that they wish to keep uncontaminated tend to look on even the *investigation* of the phenomena of the abnormal as contact with the "non-kosher," a contact which their deeply ingrained orthodox attitudes find abhorrent.

For such reasons, we have been obliged to rely mainly on the paradigm-breakers, in psychology and related fields, to emphasize the importance of the abnormal. Among these, William James repeatedly stressed the significance of the borderline areas of mental functioning. Writing to Stumpf in 1894, he claimed that Janet's book on hysteria was "worth more than all 'exact' laboratory measurements put together" (35, p. 121). Again in his Presidential Address to the American Psychological Association (32) in 1895, he asserted that the phenomena of dissociation such as hypnosis, hysteria and the trance cast more light on human nature than did the products of the psychophysical laboratories. The sentiments James expressed in "The Energies of Men" (31), his welcome of psychoanalysis as a movement (35, p. 122), and his Lowell Lectures on "Exceptional Mental Phenomena" (35, p. 123) provide further examples of this continuing interest in the study of extreme states.

It was Freud's emphasis on the primacy of the irrational that clearly revealed the close affinity between the normal and abnormal (13). With the gradual permeation of Freud's thinking into the substance of psychology, the principle of the normality/abnormality continuum became widely accepted. Indeed, the emphasis on abnormality became so great that Bernard Hart's important little volume devoted largely to conflict and defense could be misnamed "The Psychology of Insanity" (20) without provoking vehement objections. Although Freud emphasized the principle of the continuum repeatedly throughout his life, it is stated most strongly in his later writings: *Fetishism* (12), *Splitting of the Ego* (15), and Chapter VIII of the *Outline* (14).

Goldstein has already been mentioned in this connection.

Prominent biologists have also recognized the interrelations of the normal and abnormal. Almost a century ago, Darwin made repeated references to the phenomena of insanity and idiocy in his *Expression of the Emotions* (1872). Today, analogous principles are found in Paul Weiss' systematic investigations of deformations and deformities that have contributed so significantly to the understanding of developmental processes. Weiss states the case for the interrelationship of the abnormal and normal so clearly that I feel compelled to present a few quotes from the Lowell Lecture (65) in which he summarizes his views.

> "While there is thus no doubt that understanding of development has been furthered by the study of abnormalities . . . the preoccupation with the grossly abnormal has also had the unfortunate side effect of grooving the mental habit of separating the 'abnormal' from the 'normal' as a distinct and disparate phenomenon, as if the processes themselves were less sound in one case than in the other. It is important, therefore, to restore perspective by emphasizing that even the grossest deformity is produced by the same rigorously lawful molecular and cellular interactions that govern normal development. All that has happened is that the proportions among the component processes, whose harmony is predicated on proper dosing and timing, have become grossly distorted during the course of development because of either some major initial flaws in the . . . endowment or some disruptive variations in the environment. . . . The point to keep in mind is that these major deviations, though being more spectacular, are no different in kind from the more minor and less conspicuous variations. . . .
>
> "Pathology and developmental biology must be reintegrated so that our understanding of the 'abnormal' will become but an extension of our insight into the 'normal,' while, *pari passu*, the study of the 'abnormal' will contribute to the deepening of that very insight. Their common problems should provide foci for common orientation so that, as they advance in joint directions, their efforts may supplement and reinforce each other to mutual benefit. . . . "

The case could not be stated more forcefully.

In recent psychology, however, the principle of considering the normal and the abnormal conjunctively has been bypassed because of a trend to "accentuate the positive" and to disregard the negative. This new emphasis on the "positive" is even reflected in psychoanalysis in connection with the development of ego psychology. As Rapaport once argued, and as we see more clearly with time, Freud himself made a definite contribution to the "positive." This facet of his work was originally neglected because there are times when we require only one aspect of a particular person's message. On these occasions, we select from his total contribution just the material which meets our needs, and neglect the rest. In the earlier days of the period of receptivity to Freudian notions, psychologists were ripe for an emphasis on the id. We were starved for motivational concepts, and we found these in Freud. Later, when "there shall ego be" became the prevailing cry, our attention focused instead on this aspect of Freudian theory.

This latest movement follows what at times appears to be an historical dictum that calls for advance only through extremes. It may reflect as well a radical reaction to the extravagant stand taken by some who have argued that, since a normality/abnormality continuum exists, normality is not distinguishable from pathology.

Is not the current counterswing toward the affirmative, however, equally exaggerated? "Mental disease" has been replaced by "mental health," a change which is understandable and reasonable. But for some this shift in emphasis does not appear to go far enough. We are now told about *positive* mental health, as if there were a negative mental health! This slogan has caught the public eye to such an extent that conferences have actually been organized on the topic. A concurrently related development appears to be an excessive concern with the important principle of the uniqueness of the individual. This involves, at least in the existentialist interpretation, an exaggerated emphasis on unpredictability.

Do we not need to achieve a balance? Is it necessary to advance faddishly—to move with the swinging pendulum from one extreme to the other? To achieve such a balance we need a variety of approaches. We need not only studies centered on normal subjects, but also studies of normal subjects contrasted with particular pathological groups, and comparative and differential studies of abnormal groups themselves—among them the various psychoses and neuroses, the brain-damaged, the senile and the retarded.

I must emphasize that I am actually much encouraged by today's broadening trends. Increasingly we see a tendency toward a breaking down of barriers between traditional areas of concern and an overlapping into adjacent fields. Thus sociologists have become interested in psychology, psychiatrists in normal process, and psychologists in abnormal process. The special backgrounds and approaches that these disciplines bring to extensions of their customary areas can result in nothing but gain for behavioral science as a whole.

THE PHENOMENA OF SCHIZOPHRENIA

My presentation will necessarily be limited, since I shall devote myself almost entirely to investigations of schizophrenic patients that have implications for normal functioning. These investigations, with rare exceptions, were carried out in the context of studies of the normal. Additionally, in many studies we collected data from other pathological groups for comparison with the normal.

Moreover, my comments are based primarily on the results of studies with chronic patients. Although research carried out on this limited population does present some disadvantages, it also has many advantages. The defensive processes in the acute patient, especially those of restitution and regression, are exceedingly complex and require careful teasing out. Although such processes also occur in the chronic patient, they have become less complex and more stabilized by this stage; they are, therefore, simpler to theorize about as well as to observe.

A discussion of the implications of research on schizophrenia for the understanding of normal functioning can most satisfactorily be presented, I believe, in two sets of successive steps—four steps concerned with schizophrenia and three with normal performance. For schizophrenia these are: 1) The phenomena actually found by objective studies of schizophrenic patients; 2) the direct inferences from these findings and their categorization; 3) an effort to theorize about the variety of specific inferences; and 4) further theorizing to account for the etiology of the disturbances found.

For normal subjects, the following steps are called for: 1) A discussion of the implications from schizophrenia for normal characteristics; 2) an attempt to place these implications into a broader theoretical framework; and 3) a theory which provides reasons why schizophrenic disturbances do not occur in normal mental functioning.

For our present purposes I shall, however, limit myself to the first three steps for the schizophrenic and the first two for the normal, interlacing to some extent the consideration of these two contrasting groups. I shall not speculate about the etiology of schizophrenia or the nonoccurrence of schizophrenic-like behavior in the normal since such a discussion would take us too far afield.

I shall try to distill, from the results of the numerous studies carried out by my colleagues and myself, the implications of our work on schizophrenia for normal functioning. These investigations were executed over several decades at the Worcester State Hospital, the University of Illinois and most recently at the National Institute of Mental Health.[1]

Our data are derived from the application of experimental techniques and objective test methods to the investigation of questions of the *what* and *how*, rather than the *why* and *about what*, of the psychological functioning of schizophrenic patients. These projects were undertaken as part of an effort to understand the nature of schizophrenia—something about its psychological structure and function. We attempted to study the effects of pathology both on the personality itself and on the schizophrenics' adaptations to the pathological state, as represented in their restitutive and regressive efforts. Ego function was emphasized in the selection of areas for study, particularly single ego functions such as psychomotility and learning. In some ways, this approach to psychopathology is not so intriguing as research focused on the *why*, because it does not, on the one hand, immediately relate to the florid aspects of the psychosis, or, on the other, contribute to understanding the developmental aspects of normality. Studies of etiology, however, are more likely to receive their most plausible answers from complex longitudinal studies which necessarily lend themselves less readily to experimental control. Nevertheless, taken in the context of clinical and organic studies which I shall at least touch upon, our essentially descriptive studies may give us some hints as to the *why* as well.

The schizophrenic patients we studied most intensively were chronic, male, with a mean age of approximately 30 years, a mean schooling of 9 to 10 years and a mean hospitalization age[2] of approximately 7 years. As I have already suggested, the relative stability characteristically achieved by chronic patients reduces the intra-individual and, indirectly, the inter-individual variability. Such stability obviously facilitates research. Even in research with chronic patients, however, the problem of variability remains sufficiently great to warrant continued attention, indeed caution.

The controlled approaches to schizophrenia that we utilized ranged widely. They included quite simple physiological functions, such as patellar tendon reflex latent time; simple motor functions, such as steadiness, tapping and reaction time; studies of sensory threshold, perception and apperception; and studies of memory, learning, intelligence, association and thinking. They encompassed, as well, experiments involving such

[1] I have summarized some or other of these findings in different ways in four previous publications (49, 50, 53, 54).

[2] Hospitalization age is defined as the time elapsed since first hospitalization for mental disorder.

behavior as accessibility, interruption, substitution and aspiration. Among the more complex studies we carried out were some involving learning under social conditions of cooperation and competition.

Instead of presenting an extensive discussion of quantitative findings, I shall, as a background for a discussion of the implications of these findings for normal functioning, draw a composite word picture of the chronic schizophrenic's characteristic modes of response. This is based on those of our studies in which we found statistically significant differences between patient and normal groups.[3]

The psychological disturbance in schizophrenia does not appear at the relatively simple level of psychophysical organization represented by the patellar tendon reflex (25) or even at the sensory level (24). The schizophrenic does not seem to be affected either in reflex latent time or, after the initial period of testing, in a sensory function such as direct current threshold. The disturbance appears to begin at the level of response where voluntary behavior is involved. It is particularly evidenced in voluntary behavior demanded by the environment such as reaction time, behavior that is experimenter-controlled and programmed (29).

In practically all new experimental situations, the schizophrenic patient shows an immediate adaptive difficulty, one which might be thought of as a kind of neophobia—a disturbance that occurs when dealing with the new. This is strikingly reflected in learning situations (27, 28) where he is particularly affected in the earlier trials. The difficulty prevents the schizophrenic from initially achieving anywhere near his capability level. By this I mean that there is a marked discrepancy between the level of performance at which he ordinarily works and his capability level. Under certain conditions, however, the schizophrenics' capability level becomes more manifest. This may occur when one or several of these following situations prevail: when he is permitted to work repetitively for a long period on a task (28), when the experiment involves stronger than ordinary social motivation (59), when he is put under stress (47), when his organism is shocked (40, 48), when considerable time between sessions is permitted to elapse (27), when he has time to prepare himself (57), or when he gets fully involved in a task (26, 57).

It seems desirable to repeat, at this point, what I have already said elsewhere (49) about the specific way in which I use the terms *capability* and *capacity*. In ordinary, and even in psychological, discourse, these words are too often used interchangeably with the word "ability." Per-

[3] The reference to the original study is provided in the context of its discussion, for those who are interested in the details of the particular experiment.

sonally, I prefer to use these more rigorous psychological definitions: *capacity* indicates the level of performance that a subject can potentially reach under optimal conditions, *viz.*, the region of the physiological limit; *capability* indicates the upper limit of functioning that a subject can reach under ordinary day-by-day conditions when he is not hampered by deep-rooted disturbances of relatively long duration, such as special physical disabilities, depression, or inaccessibility; *ability* refers to the level of performance that a subject can reach in daily activity when he is not hampered by such temporary interfering factors as fatigue, emotional upset, passing physical illness or inadequacy, or poor external conditions for examination.

The schizophrenic's poor adaptiveness is evidenced not only in situations calling for voluntary overt response (as in learning), but it also appears in situations that call forth cryptic autonomic reactions (as in those involved in response to physical pain or to noise). Thus, one of our studies (8) indicated that the heart rate of schizophrenic subjects, when measured during the middle of the inter-stimulus period in response to ten successive pain stimulations given five minutes apart, does not diminish as it does in the normal person. Further, in a series of studies over many years, the most recent and detailed ones carried out at NIMH (67), we have found that the galvanic skin response, heart rate and finger pulse volume to a repeated noise stimulus—a situation of low demand where the subject does not have to respond voluntarily—tended to be greater in schizophrenic than in normal subjects and remained at approximately the same higher general "arousal" level over the experimental period. In situations of high demand, such as the reaction time, where the subject has to respond voluntarily, the reverse is true: they are significantly lower in the autonomic responsivity measured simultaneously. And within the schizophrenic group the slower reactors have the higher autonomic nonspecific responsivity (66).

Although the schizophrenic is generally accessible to the environment, he is so only in a partial and superficial way; he does not really become involved with it in a full sense (36). Apperceptive devices such as the Word Association (56, 58) and the Rorschach (38) Tests reflect, in the frequency of unusual and individual responses, the degree of this isolation.

The schizophrenic subject's lack of adaptiveness and inadequate manipulation of environmental situations are also brought out in the relatively superficial nature of the tasks which he chooses when given a free opportunity to occupy himself in any way he wishes (36), in his nonresumption of impersonal tasks when these are interrupted (37), and in his apparent inability to use substitute modes of activity for interrupted impersonal tasks (39). His responsiveness seems more directed to intrinsically personal situations or to impersonal situations that he apparently endows with personal significance. Thus, in contrast to his behavior on impersonal tasks, the schizophrenic *will* resume interrupted ego-involving tasks (3). The schizophrenic's tendency to subjectivity is also supported, to some extent, by the frequency of his idiosyncratic responses on the Kent-Rosanoff Word Association Test and by his tendency to introduce subjective interpretations spontaneously into play constructions (46).

Even though the composite of intellectual functioning represented in mental age scores does not seem to reveal any very marked disturbance, the psychosis apparently does interfere with the balanced distribution of intellectual functions, as evidenced by the lesser impairment of vocabulary scores when compared with measures of other psychological functions (1). Schizophrenia also seems to affect the ability to conceptualize (41,64); this may, however, be merely the secondary effect of another trend.

Findings from our reaction time investigations are particularly relevant to the picture I have just drawn. (Huston, Rodnick, Rosenthal, Zahn and I have been the main investigators in these studies.) Reaction time is important because it deals with a basic adaptive process; it utilizes two basic functions, speed and psychomotility, which are parts of all response. Since, in addition, it lends itself to rigorous and quantitative experimental procedure, we have concentrated a fair proportion of our research on this approach.

In schizophrenic subjects, reaction time appears to be related to mental health status, as confirmed by a correlation of .89 between a reaction time index and ratings of mental health (43). Schizophrenics are consistently slow in their reaction time, even when the situation is deliberately simplified as much as possible (29). In this situation, the patient "knows" not only what the stimulus and response are to be, but also the exact length of time before the stimulus will appear; that is, he can determine from repeated exposure the length of the "preparatory interval," the time between the warning signal and the stimulus. When this situation, where the length of the preparatory interval is constant, is compared with one in which the interval is inconstant, the schizophrenic, even at his own lower level of performance, is able to take advantage of this knowledge only for the shorter intervals. (The actual length of these shorter intervals varies between two and six seconds, depending upon the context.) The schizophrenic is, further, inordinately disturbed by the immediately preceding interval (68) and similarly affected by the preceding extended context (69). Thus when a series of longer preparatory intervals, which characteristically yield longer reaction times, precedes a series of shorter ones, the reaction times of schizophrenics for this shorter series are lengthened markedly (69). In a more complicated reaction time situation, one that involves a discrimination response, the schizophrenic subject's reaction times are lengthened significantly when interpolated not-to-be-reacted-to stimuli are introduced. When given an opportunity to work under circumstances in which he does not know or control the warning interval (an experimenter-controlled condition) or under circumstances in which he himself has control of both (an autonomy condition), he performs best in the experimenter-controlled situation. When asked to state his preference for the setting in which he would like to work, the schizophrenic patient chooses the experimenter-controlled condition (9).

I stated earlier that the schizophrenic disturbance begins to show up when voluntary behavior is involved. But, within this category, it is clear that there are varying degrees of autonomy for the subject. For instance, although the schizophrenic had no control over the situation in the tapping task we used, in the sense of actually patterning the task himself, our procedure allowed him, without his knowledge, to set his own pace at least in part. His performance then was relatively high. In our ordinary reaction time situations, however, the procedure did not favor the schizophrenic, for here the demands came exclusively from the environment in the form of experimenter controls and programming. If, in contrast, he was given almost complete control of the reaction time situation so that he programmed the entire experiment, the schizophrenic's performance, in keeping with his own stated preferences, was poorest. Thus, there seems to be a negative relationship for the schizophrenic between the degree of autonomy he is *openly* given and the level of his performance; but, if the experiment is so arranged that it takes advantage of his own pacesetting *without attention being called to it*, he performs relatively well.

This composite sketch of the psychosis has obviously neglected the striking variation that is actually found among schizophrenic patients—a problem that I have discussed at length elsewhere (55). To provide a somewhat more accurate picture of the syndrome I shall attempt to define the range of variation. This might be accomplished most simply by depicting the differences between some aspects of the personality patterns of the two major subtypes of schizophrenia—the paranoid and the hebephrenic. Members of these diagnostic groups consistently seem to handle situations in distinctive ways. The paranoid subject usually resembles the normal far more than does the hebephrenic, but in many instances the paranoid and hebephrenic behavior fall on *either* side of the normal. This consistent observation emphasizes the striking differences which may exist between these subtypes. The paranoid organizes his environment in a limited but relatively effective manner (2, 46). Although he is quite rigid in his response, he is sufficiently preserved intellectually (41) and has sufficient "ego strength" to protect his personality against the inroads of the environment (45, 46). The hebephrenic subject, on the other hand, is quite disturbed intellectually. This extends even to a considerable reduction in vocabulary performance, a function which is surprisingly stable in other schizophrenic groups as well as in many other pathological states. Actual tests indicate that his vocabulary level is not different from one of the lowest of the disordered groups we have studied, the general paretic (41). He seems to be at the mercy of the environment, constantly being buffeted about by it (45, 46), and he consistently takes the "easy way" out. He thus prefers to repeat a task that he has completed (44); or, in contrast with the normal and the paranoid who maintain the same level, he lowers his aspiration level after failure (59); or, again, he vacillates in a free situation, shifting his attention from one aspect of the environment to another without apparent plan (36). The distinctive behavior styles of each of these subtypes may be interpreted as being alternative methods of responding to the same basic difficulty. The paranoid appears to be overreacting to the underlying trend towards disorganization which exists in the psychosis by organizing his resources to fight the disruption; the hebephrenic, on the other hand, appears to give way to the trend.

INFERENCES FROM THE PHENOMENA FOR SCHIZOPHRENIA

In my attempts to organize the inferences from such data on schizophrenics, I have often found a five-stage model useful in dealing with the transactional (stimulus-response) process as represented in the response to both internal and external stimulation. I have employed this model in the context of the underlying motivational one of need/tension/gratification/tension reduction, which I have adapted and modified from Rapaport's model of primary tension maintenance (51). I consider this model primarily psychological, but it is also translatable into neurological terms. Although the stages tend to follow one another in time, it is important to recognize the reverberating feedback processes that take place during the several stages leading to consummatory response. By this I mean that while there is a general forward-going process in the successive appearance of these stages, there is, at the same time, both a simultaneous and backward-testing process of spontaneous examination of what has been happening in these advancing stages. What results is a "halting" kind of progress; as it were, something like three steps forward and one step backward. We must therefore be careful not to overemphasize the apparent sequential nature of the reaction. Because of their importance, these simultaneous forward and backward processes call for detailed examination.

The five stages I have made reference to are: 1) a generalized preparation for a wide range of responses represented in curiosity, general anticipation, and readiness for novel situations. When the need object is available, as it was in the studies I have described, the other four stages follow; 2) a stage of preparation for specific input—a specialized preparation for response, a readiness to respond to an expected specific stimulus or class of stimuli; 3) a stage involving the stimulus input itself, consisting of both a sensory substage and a perceptual-cognitive-discriminative substage; 4) a central stage, involving both integrating and inhibiting aspects; 5) an output stage—a motor stage which may consist of a body movement, speech, thought, or other kind of consummatory act. With the completion of the transactional cycle, the organism achieves gratification and reduction of tension. At this point, however, the organism automatically re-enters the first stage of generalized preparation and is readied for the cycle again. This regenerative aspect seems to be an integral part of the transactional chain (19).

A few general comments are in order before I go on to the inferences to be drawn from our studies on schizophrenia in the context of the transactional model I have just proposed. The model, at the first level of consideration, is a cross-sectional one covering a single transaction. Although the stages follow in sequence, they overlap temporally; they also have their distinct feedback aspects. It is, therefore, often difficult to assign a particular defect in function to one stage of the transactional process. Sometimes one stage is involved, frequently several. For simplicity's sake I have tended to assign the defects to the particular stage in which they appear most strikingly. While I recognize that this is quite arbitrary, it seems acceptable to do so for expository purposes. To repeat, it is important to recognize that the five stages, under which I consider the inferences from our studies, exist in the framework of the need/tension/gratification/tension reduction paradigm that I have mentioned. After I have dealt with the characteristics of individual transactions in which there are deficits (and it must be recognized that there are many transactions in schizophrenia that do not show deficits), I shall then consider the persisting pattern of transactions as reflected in structure. This is a second level of discussion—the consideration of the underlying permanent structure from which individual transactions derive.

The *first* stage, *the generalized preparation for input*, is characterized by curiosity, search for stimulation, general anticipation and preparedness for stimulation. Certain broad inferences about schizophrenia can be drawn from studies focused on this initial interval in the cycle.

Curiosity and search for stimulation seem particularly weak in the schizophrenic. He appears to suffer from the kind of neophobia I have alluded to, that is, the disturbance that results from entry into new settings, from contact with the uncertain. He seems to prefer old, already-experienced situations. His lack of involvement with his environment, seen for example in his poor cooperation, is another aspect of this deficit. When given the choice he prefers superficial to demanding tasks; he neither resumes tasks after interruption nor utilizes substitute tasks to deal with the tensions presumably created by incompletion.

Another common characteristic of the schizophrenic is the lack of spontaneity in his behavior. A superficial glance at a hebephrenic patient leaves the naive observer with the impression that the patient is functioning at the acme of spontaneity. The patient appears *so* responsive to his environment, both the outer and the inner. Careful observation, however, would soon convince this same observer that the responsivity does not have the goal-directed curiosity and search for stimulation characterizing true spontaneity. It consists rather of a superficial flightiness, a succession of sporadic responses which is intermittent in character and which has no persistent structure.

I have been considering the case of the chronic patient in relation to this basic quality of generalized preparation for input. In the acute patient the curiosity, the search for stimulation that we have found missing in the chronic patient, appears especially prominent. But here again, if we examine the patient carefully, we find our first surmise to be misleading. In acute schizophrenics this curiosity and search for stimulation, instead of being focused on the external environment, is actually directed inwardly. The patient finds his internal world so rich in stimuli, so full of new and constantly changing experiences, that he seems to have little interest in contact with the outside environment.

Let us now turn to the *second* stage of the transactional process, the one that I have characterized as *preparation for specific input.* At this stage the organism is in a state of readiness to respond to a particular stimulus or class of stimuli. Here one major defect is predominant in the schizophrenic—an extreme sensitivity to irrelevancies. This defect, I believe, helps to explain many of his peculiar responses. His signal-to-noise ratio is low; he appears to react to stimulus situations under the influence of what

I have for a long time called "remorating"[4] factors. He displays a tendency to focus on irrelevant aspects of the ground, rather than to concentrate on the figure itself. The schizophrenic seems to violate Freud's principle of *Reizschutz* (11)—that protection against stimuli which is so important in the economy of personality functioning. He is vulnerable not only to nonfocal aspects of the external stimulus situation itself, but also to both external irrelevant distracting factors and internal irrelevant preoccupations.

In the *third* stage, that of *actual input*, schizophrenic disturbance is not evident at the sensory substage but is at the other, the perceptual/cognitive/discriminative substage. I recognize that the isolation of the sensory from the other aspects of the perceptual is a somewhat arbitrary division. I believe, however, that it is important on theoretical grounds to stress the differences between the two. The schizophrenic seems to be plagued with unrealistic perception, reflected in extremes of behavior with regard to scanning and articulation (62). He either over- or underscans, and over- or underarticulates. This extreme reaction appears related to his responsiveness to the irrelevant which we have already mentioned.

It is in the *fourth, central* stage that I concentrate a considerable number of the defects characteristic of schizophrenia. Variability, individuality, approximateness, inappropriateness, poor thinking, slow habituation, weak goal behavior, poorly controlled, quite pervasive affect, and inappropriate personalness can all, in one way or another, be assigned to the central process. But it is equally clear that many of these may in part be placed elsewhere in the response cycle, particularly in the output stage.

Since performance is ordinarily measured at the *fifth*, or *output stage*, it is not surprising that the bulk of the inferences about schizophrenic inadequacy is based on data from this part of the sequence. Although we have already mentioned some of these characteristics, it may be desirable to summarize them at this point. Schizophrenic behavior may be characterized as perseverative, slow, subjective, variable, inordinately affected by context, inadequately guided by the information that is available, and anomalous. The schizophrenic habituates slowly and his goal behavior is inadequate.

We have thus far, of course, been discussing only isolated transactions. The schizophrenic deficit *is* a deficit, however, because the inadequate responses are not single or casual; it is a deficit because these responses reflect a persistent pattern of aberrant reaction; they indicate some

[4] "Remorating" factors are named after the remorae, the fish which attach themselves to sharks by their sucking discs and thereby impede the shark's progress.

underlying abnormal psychological structure. This structure is characterized in its most general aspects by performance considerably below capacity level, a slowness in adaptation to a situation, a difficulty with "time-binding," and a weak ego and mechanism of control. These deficiencies manifest themselves in the complex of disorganization we think of as so characteristic of schizophrenia.

IMPLICATIONS OF PHENOMENA FOR NORMAL

In the context of the schizophrenic functioning I have described, what can we say about the nature of normal psychological function?

Before trying to deal with this central question, I should perhaps first clarify what I mean by "normal." When I use the term, it is not meant in the sense of "ideal" performance—what might be considered, in the terminology I have long used, as performance at "capacity" level. I refer rather to the upper limits of functional ability under ordinary day-by-day conditions: the "capability" level. The normal person may on occasion slip into less adequate behavior, sometimes even performing at the level of a schizophrenic, but he characteristically performs at what I have called his capability level. The schizophrenic, on the other hand, may on rare occasions perform at his underlying capability level, but ordinarily he performs at a level far below. It is essential to keep this concept of *characteristic* performance in mind since individual and group variability are so great, particularly in the schizophrenic, that there are bound to be occasional overlaps between schizophrenic and normal performance. A normal person does not always perform "normally." The final criterion in evaluating both normal and pathological subjects has to be their characteristic day-by-day performance. The problem raised by the rare optimal performance sometimes found in schizophrenia is, of course, another question. It is related to that of underlying capacity level, which has important theoretical implications for the basic nature of the psychosis.

We must also keep in mind that we are dealing with a wide range of performance levels represented by the different individuals in our sample. This is, of course, true of our normal subjects as well as of our schizophrenic patients. So when we say "normal" or "schizophrenic" we are talking about a kind of abstract average person working at his characteristic level, who is roughly representative both of himself and of a range of his own class members.

In the context of the general transactional model I have presented, our findings on normal subjects, who were studied concurrently with the patient groups and compared with the schizophrenics at various stages of the process, yield a quite different picture from that of the chronic patients. Allowing for the obvious range of functioning it seems fair to sketch the normal's portrait for the present purposes in the following simplified way.

The normal person manifests curiosity and seeks out novelty in his environment. He demonstrates a depth of spontaneity which is qualitatively different from the superficial reactivity and fitful pseudopodic contacts of the schizophrenic, and his alertness to new activities is appropriate. He is infrequently disturbed by the irrelevant; that is, he is able to respond to the focal stimulus and disregard the peripheral. His perception and discrimination are realistic and close to the veridical.

The normal person habituates easily and is relatively free from perseveration. He demonstrates an appropriate balance between stability and flexibility, being neither too rigid nor too loose. He generalizes readily, at a conceptual level that is quite different from the superficial syncretic fusion of the schizophrenic.

The responses made by normal persons achieve a nice balance between communality (a similarity to others) and an originality (a difference from others) which does not have a bizarre quality. They also manifest an ability to distinguish between the personal and impersonal—to evaluate situations correctly, both avoiding the impersonalization of the personal and the personalization of the impersonal. And finally, the normal person is able to judge situations in the context of their probabilities, to approach uncertainty on an "as if" basis.

THEORETICAL IMPLICATIONS OF INFERENCES MADE ABOUT SCHIZOPHRENIC AND NORMAL CHARACTERISTICS

What can be said, in the light of theory, about the contrasting behaviors of schizophrenic and normal persons? Although I shall concentrate on schizophrenic behavior, I will make several explicit as well as implicit references to the normal. Without providing a specific description of the actual physiological or psychological structures of the schizophrenic, I will summarize certain general principles based on my own thinking while incorporating some of the insights provided by the work of other theorists.

In schizophrenia one sees a distinct weakening of the control center that serves the integrating, organizing function and provides the base for the establishment of what I have called "generalized" or "major" sets in the normal person. Actually this inability to establish and maintain major sets may, in the schizophrenic, be the secondary result of a direct, positive need to establish minor sets, to segmentalize both external and internal environments. This trend toward segmentalization appears to develop through the following stages: first, there is a tendency in the patient for individuated patterns to split off, followed by a reactive exaggerated strengthening effort on the part of the central control mechanism to regulate and to regain control of these split-off systems. (Among paranoid patients we quite frequently see such attempts to regain control leading to over-control.) This is usually unsuccessful and is followed by a diminution of the directing of energy to the outside environment. Finally, a kind of equilibrium is established through the dominance of the segmental, essentially regressive, patterns.

A variety of both experimental and clinical manifestations are associated with these stages. Thus, in the experimental realm we find the marked variability of response reflected in the low correlation coefficients in schizophrenics across a wide range of psychological functions; the inability to maintain set, which is particularly evident in reaction time studies; the slowing of response time as well as of adaptation and learning time; the difficulties with sustained and conceptual thinking; the weak goal behavior; the unrealistic nature of schizophrenic perception; the idiosyncrasy of response. These varieties of performance appear to be evidences of the tendency toward segmentalization, or, on occasion, of the attempt to overcome it.

We see another aspect of this tendency in the physiological realm. Thus, in our Worcester studies, we obtained significantly higher correlation coefficients for schizophrenic as compared with normal subjects on such measures as individual systolic with diastolic blood pressure, .62 as opposed to .43 (23), and of oral with rectal readings of body temperature, .73 as opposed to .56 (33). We may interpret this as a kind of "robotization." Such findings appear to be reflections of a process of segmentalization that removes such functions from normal adaptive and modulating control. These processes become "independent" and less amenable to the central control needed for most effective adaptation, whereas in the normal person this dependence is continually maintained.

It may be profitable at this point to leave our experimental data and turn briefly to the clinical symptomatology of the schizophrenic. These symptoms appear to have a similar segmental quality and can, in part, be explained within the framework of our underlying need-tension model. The schizophrenic patient seems to establish minor sets in an indirect effort to attain the satisfaction of primitive, fundamental needs which, in contrast with the normal person, have never been adequately satisfied. These early needs have to express themselves through a body and nervous system which have inexorably continued their natural physical growth. This is even more complicated by the fact that with the chronological growth of the developing organism, the schizophrenic finds himself in an environment which, because of his increasing age, is organized to provide fewer and fewer outlets for the infantile or childish needs which he still has to satisfy. And on the other side, the environment has demands of its own which the schizophrenic is expected to at least attempt to fulfill.

The schizophrenic's anachronistic cravings cannot be satisfied while total integrated control, the structure which insists on the maintenance of major sets, holds sway. Integrated control is therefore abandoned and the automatically matured devices are pervertedly used to satisfy these needs. There is a preoccupation with ordinarily unconscious bodily processes, with the mechanics of processes rather than with their ends; there are peculiar and magical uses of the thinking process, and numerous other distinctive schizophrenic symptoms. (Consider, for example, the schizophrenic patient who acquires knowledge by writing "Harvard" on a scrap of paper and swallowing it, or who acquires the courage he knows he lacks by swallowing a slip on which he has written "Lawrence.") Most, if not all, of the immense variety of such symptoms may be viewed as different expressions of only partial integration or individuation or breakdown of major sets—in other words, of segmentalization. In the defensive goal-seeking of the schizophrenic, integration may range from almost total disintegration to highly organized, integrated, but I must emphasize, distinctly *partial and localized* patterns of integrated behavior. It is, however, *rarely* total integration in the Coghillian (7) sense or of the expression of the establishment of major sets, the qualities which are so characteristic of the normal person.

In the schizophrenic there is an increased awareness of, and preoccupation with, the ordinarily disregarded details of existence, the details that normal people spontaneously forget, or train themselves, or are rigorously trained, to disregard. These, rather than the biologically adaptive functional aspects of the situation, appear to take on a primary role. As I once characterized it, the schizophrenic's activity might appropriately be described as "centipedal." He is, as in the paradoxical case of the centipede of the fable, so deeply concerned about the way his feet move that he loses sight of where they should be going. Even more profoundly disturbed than the centipede, the schizophrenic frequently appears to believe that to reach his goal he has merely to study his feet's movements. The normal person, on the contrary, is goal- rather than process-oriented.

In addition to the discrepancy between the need and the means available for its gratification, there is the segmentalization of the process of attaining the satisfaction of the need. If there is any creature who can be accused of not seeing the forest for the trees, it would appear to be the schizophrenic. If he is of the paranoid persuasion, he sticks to the path through the forest even more closely than the normal person, examining not only each tree along the way with meticulous care, but each tree's leaves as well. (As I have already indicated, this may possibly be a reaction to the underlying fundamental trend toward disorganization.) If, at the other extreme of the schizophrenic continuum, he falls into the hebephrenic pattern, he acts as though there were no paths and strays off the established trail entirely. He is attracted not only visually, but olfactorily and gustatorily as well, not only to the trees but even to the undergrowth and floor of the forest, all in a superficial, flitting way, apparently having forgotten his destination.

If we were to try to epitomize the schizophrenic individual's system in the most simple language, we might say that he has two major difficulties. First, he reacts to old situations as if they were new ones—he fails to habituate or automatize—and to new situations as if they were recently past ones—he perseverates. Second, he overresponds when the stimulus is relatively small, and he does not respond enough when the stimulus is great. With regard to reactivity, the chronic schizophrenic is certainly not a "seething caldron," as he has at times been described. He resembles rather the "simmering pot" on the back of the stove which perpetually simmers at such a low level that it never reaches the stage of producing even a savorless *pot-au-feu*.

In this attempt to account for at least part of the range of the phenomena in schizophrenia, I have deliberately limited myself to the chronic patient. Our data on acute patients are meager and insufficient for any secure theorizing. It may be useful, however, to place the acute patient in theoretical context, even if on more speculative grounds. To continue with the earlier metaphor, my impression is that the acute patient in the same forest undergoes a multitude of thrilling new experiences, reacting highly affectively, for instance, to novel and unusual patterns of light on the leaves or to unusual and subtle patterns of form in the branches. These are presumably expressions of the perceptive-associative processes which among normal persons, even when they are activated, are held under central control. In acute psychotic conditions, however, they are permitted to take over. Once experienced, these exciting impressions are so satisfying that they are often persisted in, despite any concurrent awareness that as far as one's obligations to the real world are concerned, one is dawdling, one is not getting on through the forest. The experiences appear so novel, so exciting, so seductive, that to ignore them appears impossible.

Here we *do* seem to have a "seething caldron." Even when kept well-covered, the contents of the pot frequently spill over onto the stove—the outside world—in an eruptive way. As seen, for instance, in catatonic excitement, this contact is not adaptive but rather explosive, overwhelming and catastrophic. I would guess that in those schizophrenics who turn instead toward the chronic, such integrated, yet segmental acts lose their strong affective permeation. The exciting content is increasingly replaced by more formal properties with gradually reduced affect, by segmental acts of the kind mentioned earlier in my description of the extremes of the paranoid and the hebephrenic. In the passage from the acute to the chronic state, one sees, as it were, the shift from paleophobia to neophobia and from hyperpathy to apathy, the extremes of the two closely intertwined parameters of cognition and affect. It is somewhere toward the center of each of these parameters that the normal person naturally falls.

There is little doubt that the schizophrenic's system is inefficient and unmodulated, full of affective "noise," and indeterminate figure-ground relationships. What a confusing world must be his when such fundamental modes of relating to reality are so seriously disturbed!

Although I have already outlined our basic findings on normal subjects, I would now like to add a few explicit comments. Our concurrent studies of both schizophrenics and normals have given us a good perspective from which to evaluate the qualities characteristic of normal functioning. The composite picture of the normal person compiled from our findings is that of a steady individual who deals with situations in a task-oriented fashion and maintains a proper balance and integration between himself and his environment. His involvement is measured and appropriate to the situation. He performs reasonably close to his capacity level and is much less burdened by irrelevant factors—those I have termed "remorating."

Man has appropriately been called a "time-binder" which, in the widest sense of the term, is what distinguishes him from the rest of the animal kingdom. But even in a narrow sense, the characterization is also apt, for "time-binding" typically calls for acts in the present that are based on the past and directed to satisfying present but, particularly, future needs. The schizophrenic, it would appear, acts in the present in the attempt to gratify some immediate urgent needs, but predominantly to satisfy past needs. Indeed, he gives the impression of not really having any future basic needs. The normal person acts essentially in a "time-binding" way. He does this most effectively when he is free from narcissism. For this discussion, I am expanding the usual definition of narcissism to include other, less immediately personal, derivative irrelevancies to which narcissists become cathected. When one knows the schizophrenic, one realizes how fortunate the normal person is in having achieved to at least a moderate degree this blessed state of freedom!

SOME COMMENTS ON THE RELATION BETWEEN ABSTRACT ATTITUDE AND GENERALIZED SET

In the general context of my theoretical discussion of normality in the light of schizophrenia, I want now to compare briefly Goldstein's concepts of the abstract and concrete attitudes with the theory I have proposed of generalized and segmental set. Although there is much that is similar in the two approaches, I believe that some basic differences exist.

Goldstein characterized the optimal response of the "total personality" as the ability to adopt the "abstract attitude." He indicated that this categorical attitude had the following potentialities:

"1. To assume a mental set voluntarily.
2. To shift voluntarily from one aspect of the situation to another.
3. To keep in mind, simultaneously, various aspects.
4. To grasp the essential of a given whole; to break up a given whole into parts, and to isolate them voluntarily.
5. To abstract common properties; to plan ahead ideationally; to assume an attitude toward the 'mere possible,' and to think or perform symbolically.
6. To detach our ego from the outerworld."

> "The abstract behavior is the more active one, whereas the concrete is the more passive one. For the concrete behavior, the above mentioned potentialities are not prerequisite" (17, p. 263).

My own views regarding normal as well as schizophrenic functioning are based on a theory of "major" or "generalized" set, by which I mean a state of readiness to respond to a coming stimulus, a condition of integrated organization and attention which facilitates the optimal response called for by a given situation. Sometimes this requires a readiness to respond to a specific stimulus, sometimes a readiness to respond to a generalization from a group of stimuli. At still other times preparation to respond to the last in a series of stimuli requires a person to organize himself in time, whether in a matter of milli-seconds or for extended periods. This state of preparation may be voluntary or involuntary, verbalized or unverbalized, temporary or relatively permanent; it may involve awareness, or be without awareness. In whatever situation, the major set stands in conflict with many possible intruding minor or segmental sets and predominates over them.

Specifically the major set involves:

1. Total integrated control in which the higher centers assume authority as needed. This demands the use of high central nervous and autonomic systems activity levels in goal-directed situations, and lower central nervous and autonomic systems activity levels to deal with peripheral or irrelevant stimulation;
2. Curiosity, receptivity to novelty, and generalized readiness to respond;
3. An appropriate balance between task- and ego-orientation. It calls for both a selective involvement with the task/environment and with the ego. With respect to the latter it reflects a characteristic which we call "ego strength";
4. Low perseveration and ready habituation; rapid automatization;
5. An ability to see the specific in the context of the general; realistic and modulated response—perceptually, motorically, and affectively;
6. An ability to deal with probabilities.

I am sure that you will have already noticed the considerable similarities between Goldstein's abstract attitude and my generalized set. I do not, however, accept Goldstein's emphasis on the *voluntary* because my definition of "set" includes the importance of the involuntary and nonvoluntary. Methodologically, I also disagree with his rejection of the contributions made by the investigation of single psychological functions for the understanding of total function. It is just such single-function studies that have led us to formulate theories like that of generalized set. I believe it was Goldstein's strong identification with the organismic point of view that led him to have a "certain blindness," to borrow a Jamesian phrase, for what he characterized as "single" approaches. (I hasten to add that these blindnesses were rare!) The findings of modern neurophysiology certainly raise a question of how "single," single approaches are. While I am in this mildly questioning mood I might also suggest that abstract and concrete behavior may be viewed as instances of generalized and segmental set.

Although I am quite sympathetic with many aspects of the organismic point of view, my own "conservative" predilections make me wonder whether Goldstein did not overemphasize "total" response at the cost of what on the surface appeared "partial" response. I recognize, however, that no theoretical formulation can be proposed which does not include many implicit assumptions that are rarely made explicit. So perhaps all that one may appropriately say is that the two theoretical views are not very far apart.

Having mentioned modern neurophysiology, let me add a few words about the correlation of the psychological with the physiological and anatomical, areas with which Goldstein was so involved. Although I have occasionally slipped into the use of physiological terms, I have tended on the whole to use them in a psychological manner. The problem of the correlation of the two still remains difficult at our present stage of knowledge. However, modern neurophysiology is opening new vistas for correlation of the phenomena we have been discussing (52), with its extensive uncovering of neural areas apparently having crucial relationships to emotion and attention, its acceptance of a dynamic, constantly active complex of units and interconnecting systems, its emphasis on the high degree of interrelationship between the phylogenetically old and the neocortex, and the evidence it has brought to our attention for the existence of important internal (largely inhibitory) control mechanisms which are to be found throughout the system. The braver among us have, however, already taken steps toward examining these scenes from a closer vantage point.[5]

CONCLUSION

In concluding, I must confess to underlying feelings of guilt. In my concern for clarity of exposition, I have unavoidably over-emphasized class membership and neglected the very substantial differences that exist across individuals in both the normal and schizophrenic groups. An intimate acquaintance over my whole life with at least reasonably normal persons and an equally close association over four decades with a great variety of schizophrenic persons make me uneasy about having disregarded the vivid individualities represented in both groups. And my underlying sympathies for Goldstein's general point of view, but particularly as a confirmed Jamesian, only multiply these feelings. So let me at least partially salve my conscience by ending with a quote from the latter's *Varieties* (30, p. 9): "Probably a crab would be filled with a sense of personal outrage if it could hear us class it without ado or apology as a crustacean, and thus dispose of it. 'I am no such thing,' it would say; 'I am MYSELF, MYSELF alone.' " I close therefore with *both* the ado *and* the apology!

[5] The work of Hernández-Péon and his associates (22), of Lindsley and his (34) are some examples. That of Callaway and his (5) are more closely linked to the theory of segmental set.

REFERENCES

1. Altman, Charlotte H., and Shakow, D. A comparison of the performance of matched groups of schizophrenic patients, normal subjects and delinquent subjects on some aspects of the Stanford-Binet. *J. educ. Psychol.*, 1937, *28*, 519–529.
2. Angyal, A. F. Speed and pattern of perception in schizophrenic and normal persons. *Charac. & Pers.*, 1942, *11*, 108–127.
3. Bennett, G. Structural factors related to the substitute value of activities in normal and schizophrenic persons: II. An experimental investigation of central areas of the personality. *Charac. & Pers.*, 1942, *10*, 227–245.
4. Broadbent, D. E. *Perception and Communication.* New York: Pergamon Press, Inc., 1958.
5. Callaway, E., Jones, R. T., and Layne, R. S. Evoked responses and segmental set of schizophrenia. *Arch. gen. Psychiat.*, 1965, *12*, 83–89.
6. Cannon, W. B. *The Wisdom of the Body.* New York: W. W. Norton & Co., Inc., 1963, pp. 302–304.
7. Coghill, G. E. The neuro-embryologic study of behavior: Principles, perspective and aim. *Science*, 1933, *78*, 131–138.
8. Cohen. L. H., and Patterson, M. Effect of pain on the heart rate of normal and schizophrenic individuals. *J. gen. Psychol.*, 1937, *17*, 273–289.
9. Cromwell, R., Rosenthal, D., Shakow, D., and Zahn, T. P. Reaction time, locus of control, choice behavior, and descriptions of parental behavior in schizophrenic and normal subjects. *J. Pers.*, 1961, *29*, 363–379.
10. Dempsey, E. W. Homeostasis. In S. S. Stevens (Ed.), *Handbook of Experimental Psychology.* New York: John Wiley & Sons, Inc., 1951, pp. 209–235.
11. Freud, S. (1920), Beyond the pleasure principle. *Standard Edition.* Vol. 18. London: Hogarth Press, 1955, pp. 1–64.
12. Freud, S. (1927), Fetishism. *Standard Edition.* Vol. 21. London: Hogarth Press, 1955, pp. 152–157.
13. Freud, S. (1937), Analysis terminable and interminable. *Standard Edition.* Vol. 23. London: Hogarth Press, 1955, p. 235.
14. Freud, S. (1940), An outline of psycho-analysis. *Standard Edition.* Vol. 23. London: Hogarth Press, 1955, pp. 195–204.
15. Freud, S. (1940), Splitting of the ego in the process of defense. *Standard Edition.* Vol. 23. London: Hogarth Press, 1955, pp. 275–278.
16. Goldstein, K. *The Organism: A Holistic Approach to Biology Derived from Pathological Data in Man.* New York: American Book Co., 1939.
17. Goldstein, K. The significance of psychological research in schizophrenia. *J. nerv. ment. Dis.*, 1943, *97*, 261–279.
18. Goldstein, K. *Human Nature in the Light of Psychopathology.* Cambridge, Mass.: Harvard University Press, 1940. Also, New York: Schocken Books, 1963.
19. Grinker, R. R. (Ed.) *Toward a Unified Theory of Human Behavior.* New York: Basic Books, 1956.
20. Hart, B. *The Psychology of Insanity.* London: Cambridge University Press, 1920.
21. Head, H. *Studies in Neurology.* Vol. 1. London: Oxford University Press, 1920, pp. 3–287.
22. Hernández-Péon, R. Psychiatric implications of neurophysiological research. *Bull. Menninger Clin.*, 1964, *28*, 165–185.

23. Hoskins, R. G., and Jellinek, E. M. The schizophrenic personality with special regard to psychologic and organic concomitants. *Proc. Assoc. Res. nerv. ment. Dis.*, 1933, *14*, 211–233.
24. Huston, P. E. Sensory threshold to direct current stimulation in schizophrenic and in normal subjects. *Arch. Neurol. Psychiat.*, 1934, *31*, 590–596.
25. Huston, P. E. The reflex time of the patellar tendon reflex in normal and schizophrenic subjects. *J. gen. Psychol.*, 1935, *13*, 3–41.
26. Huston, P. E., and Shakow, D. Studies of motor function in schizophrenia: III. Steadiness. *J. gen. Psychol.*, 1946, *34*, 119–126.
27. Huston, P. E., and Shakow, D. Learning in schizophrenia: I. Pursuit learning. *J. Pers.*, 1948, *17*, 52–74.
28. Huston, P. E., and Shakow, D. Learning capacity in schizophrenia: With special reference to the concept of deterioration. *Amer. J. Psychiat.*, 1949, *105*, 881-888.
29. Huston, P. E., Shakow, D., and Riggs, L. A. Studies of motor function in schizophrenia: II. Reaction time. *J. gen. Psychol.*, 1937, *16*, 39–82.
30. James, W. *Varieties of Religious Experience.* London: Longmans, Green & Co., 1902.
31. James, W. *Memories and Studies.* New York: Longmans, Green & Co., 1917, pp. 227–264.
32. James, W. *Collected Essays and Reviews.* New York: Longmans, Green & Co., 1920, pp. 384–385.
33. Linder, F. E., and Carmichael, H. T. A biometric study of the relation between oral and rectal temperature in normal and schizophrenic subjects. *Hum. Biol.*, 1935, *7*, 24–46.
34. Lindsley, D. B. Attention, consciousness, sleep and wakefulness. In J. Field (Ed.), *Handbook of Physiology,* Section 1: *Neurophysiology,* Vol. III. Washington: American Physiological Society, 1960, pp. 1553–1593.
35. Perry, R. B. *The Thought and Character of William James.* Vol. II. *Philosophy and Psychology.* Boston: Little, Brown & Co., 1935.
36. Rickers-Ovsiankina, Maria. Studies on the personality structure of schizophrenic individuals: I. The accessibility of schizophrenics to environmental influences. *J. gen. Psychol.*, 1937, *16*, 153–178.
37. Rickers-Ovsiankina, Maria. Studies on the personality structure of schizophrenic individuals: II. Reaction to interrupted tasks. *J. gen. Psychol.*, 1937, *16*, 179–196.
38. Rickers-Ovsiankina, Maria. The Rorschach test as applied to normal and schizophrenic subjects. *Brit. J. med. Psychol.*, 1938, *17*, 227–257.
39. Rickers-Ovsiankina, Maria. Studies on the personality structure of schizophrenic individuals: III. Substitute activities after interruption. Unpublished data.
40. Rodnick, E. H. The effect of metrazol shock upon habit systems. *J. abnorm. soc. Psychol.*, 1942, *37*, 560–565.
41. Roe, Anne, and Shakow, D. Intelligence in mental disorder. *Ann. N.Y. Acad. Sci.*, 1942, *42*, 361–490.
42. Rose, J. E., and Mountcastle, V. B. Touch and kinesthesis. In J. Field (Ed.), *Handbook of Physiology,* Section 1: *Neurophysiology,* Vol. I. Washington: American Physiological Society, 1959, p. 391.
43. Rosenthal, D., Lawlor, W. G., Zahn, T. P., and Shakow, D. The relationship of some aspects of mental set to degree of schizophrenic disorganization. *J. Pers.*, 1960, *28*, 26–38.

44. Rosenzweig, S. Further comparative data on repetition-choice after success and failure as related to frustration tolerance. *J. genet. Psychol.*, 1945, *66*, 75–81.
45. Rosenzweig, S., and Shakow, D. Mirror behavior in schizophrenic and normal individuals. *J. nerv. ment. Dis.*, 1937, *86*, 166–174.
46. Rosenzweig, S., and Shakow, D. Play technique in schizophrenia and other psychoses. II. An experimental study of schizophrenic constructions with play materials. *Amer. J. Orthopsychiat.*, 1937, *7*, 36–47.
47. Sands, S. L., and Rodnick, E. H. Concept and experimental design in the study of stress and personality. *Amer. J. Psychiat*, 1950, *106*, 673–679.
48. Schnack, G. F., Shakow, D., and Liveley, Mary L. Studies in insulin and metrazol therapy: II. Differential effects on some psychological functions. *J. Pers.*, 1945, *14*, 125–149.
49. Shakow, D. The nature of deterioration in schizophrenic conditions. *Nerv. ment. Dis. Monogr.*, 1946, No. 70, 1–88.
50. Shakow, D. Some psychological features of schizophrenia. In M. L. Reymert (Ed.), *Feelings and Emotions.* New York: McGraw-Hill, 1950, pp. 383–390.
51. Shakow, D. The psychological system. In R. R. Grinker (Ed.), *Toward a Unified Theory of Human Behavior.* New York: Basic Books, 1956, pp. 27–35.
52. Shakow, D. How phylogenetically older parts of the brain relate to behavior: 5. Some implications for psychology. Presented as part of a Symposium, How phylogenetically older parts of the brain relate to behavior. Held at the annual meeting of the AAAS, December 29, 1958, Washington, D. C.
53. Shakow, D. Segmental set: A theory of the formal psychological deficit in schizophrenia. *Arch. gen. Psychiat.*, 1962, *6*, 1–17.
54. Shakow, D. Psychological deficit in schizophrenia. *Behav. Sci.*, 1963, *8*, 275–305.
55. Shakow, D. The role of classification in the development of the science of psychopathology with particular reference to research. *Bull. Menninger Clin.*, 1966, *30*, 150–160.
56. Shakow, D., and Huebner, Dorothy M. Effects of repetition on the association test in schizophrenic and normal subjects. Unpublished data.
57. Shakow, D., and Huston, P. E. Studies in motor function in schizophrenia: I. Speed of tapping. *J. gen. Psychol.*, 1936, *15*, 63-106.
58. Shakow, D., and Jellinek, E. M. The composite index of the Kent-Rosanoff Association Test. *J. abnorm. Psychol.*, 1965, *70*, 403–404.
59. Shakow, D., and Radlo, G. Aspiration level in schizophrenia. Unpublished data.
60. Shakow, D., and Radlo, G. The effect of group competition on performance in schizophrenic subjects. Unpublished data.
61. Shakow, D., and Rapaport, D. The influence of Freud on American psychology. *Psychological Issues*, No. 13. New York: International Universities Press, 1964, pp. 67–68.
62. Shakow, D., Rosenzweig, S., and Hollander, L. Auditory apperceptive reactions to tautophone stimuli of schizophrenic and normal subjects. *J. nerv. ment. Dis.*, 1966, *143*, 1–15.
63. Walshe, F. M. R. The anatomy and physiology of cutaneous sensibility: A critical review. *Brain*, 1942, *65*, 48–112.
64. Wegrocki, H. J. Generalizing ability in schizophrenia: An inquiry into the disorders of problem thinking in schizophrenia. *Arch. Psychol.*, No. 254, 1940.

65. Weiss, P. Deformities as cues to understanding development of form. *Perspectives in Biology and Medicine*, 1961, *4*, 133–151.
66. Zahn, T. P. Autonomic reactivity and behavior in schizophrenia. *Psychiat. Res. Rpts.*, 1964, *19*, 156–173.
67. Zahn, T. P., Rosenthal, D., and Lawlor, W. GSR orienting reactions to visual and auditory stimuli in chronic schizophrenic and normal subjects. *Psychophysiology Newsletter*, 1963, *9*, 43–51.
68. Zahn, T. P., Rosenthal, D., and Shakow, D. Effects of irregular preparatory intervals on reaction time in schizophrenia. *J. abnorm. soc. Psychol.*, 1963, *67*, 44–52.
69. Zahn, T. P., Rosenthal, D., and Shakow, D. Reaction time in schizophrenic and normal subjects in relation to the sequence of series of regular preparatory intervals. *J. abnorm. soc. Psychol.*, 1961, *63*, 161–168.

Presented in part at the Kurt Goldstein Memorial Meeting, held at the 37th Annual Meeting of the Eastern Psychological Association on April 16, 1966, in New York City. An overlapping version of this paper was also presented in part at the "Conference on New Directions in Research on Normal Subjects" held at the Psychosomatic and Psychiatric Institute of the Michael Reese Hospital in Chicago on September 30 and October 1, 1966, and is being published separately.

V

THE PERSON

14

The Still Life as a Personal Object—A Note on Heidegger and van Gogh

by Meyer Schapiro
New York, New York

In his essay on *The Origin of the Work of Art* (3, 4), Martin Heidegger interprets a painting by van Gogh to illustrate the nature of art as a disclosure of truth.[1]

He comes to this picture in the course of distinguishing three modes of being: of useful artifacts, of natural things, and of works of fine art. He proposes to describe first, "without any philosophical theory . . . a familiar

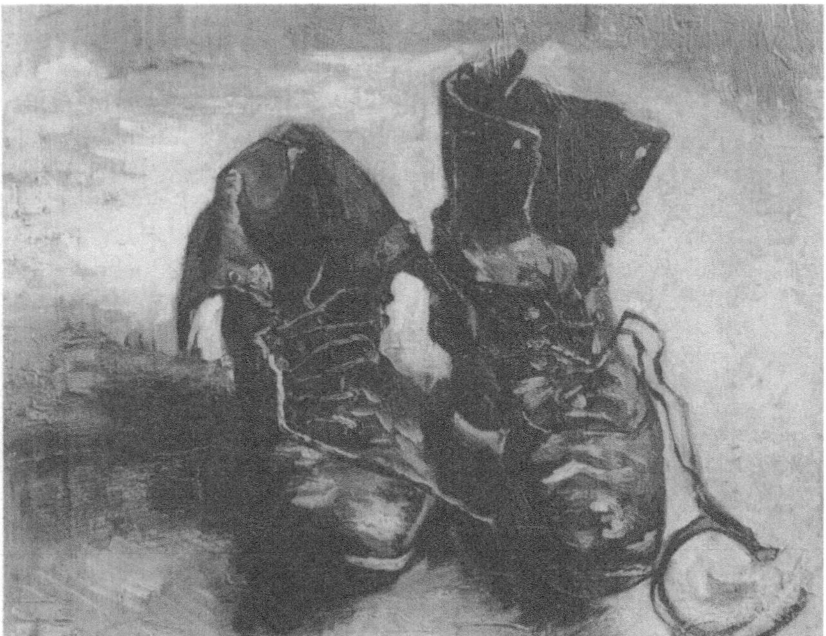

Figure 1. Vincent van Gogh, *Old Shoes*. Reproduced by kind permission of the Stedelijk Museum, Amsterdam.

[1] It was Kurt Goldstein who first called my attention to this essay, presented originally as a lecture in 1935 and 1936. All quotations are from the excellent translation by A. Hofstadter (4) and are reprinted by permission of Harper & Row, Publishers, Inc., New York, N. Y.

sort of equipment—a pair of peasant shoes"; and "to facilitate the visual realization of them" he chooses "a well-known painting by van Gogh, who painted such shoes several times." But to grasp "the equipmental being of equipment," we must know "how shoes actually serve." For the peasant woman they serve without her thinking about them or even looking at them. Standing and walking in the shoes, the peasant woman knows the serviceability in which "the equipmental being of equipment consists." But we,

> "as long as we only imagine a pair of shoes in general, or simply look at the empty, unused shoes as they merely stand there in the picture, we shall never discover what the equipmental being of equipment in truth is. In van Gogh's painting we cannot even tell where these shoes stand. There is nothing surrounding this pair of peasant shoes in or to which they might belong, only an undefined space. There are not even clods from the soil of the field or the path through it sticking to them, which might at least hint at their employment. A pair of peasant shoes and nothing more. And yet.
>
> "From the dark opening of the worn insides of the shoes the toilsome tread of the worker stands forth. In the stiffly solid heaviness of the shoes there is the accumulated tenacity of her slow trudge through the far-spreading and ever-uniform furrows of the field, swept by a raw wind. On the leather there lies the dampness and saturation of the soil. Under the soles there slides the loneliness of the field-path as the evening declines. In the shoes there vibrates the silent call of the earth, its quiet gift of the ripening corn and its enigmatic self-refusal in the fallow desolation of the wintry field. This equipment is pervaded by uncomplaining anxiety about the certainty of bread, the wordless joy of having once more withstood want, the trembling before the advent of birth and shivering at the surrounding menace of death. This equipment belongs to the *earth* and it is protected in the *world* of the peasant woman. From out of this protected belonging the equipment itself rises to its resting-in-self." (4, pp. 662–663).[2]

[2] Heidegger refers again to van Gogh's picture in a revised lecture of 1935, translated and reprinted in (5). Speaking of Dasein (being-there, or "essent") he points to a painting by van Gogh. "A pair of rough peasant shoes, nothing else. Actually the painting represents nothing. But as to what is in that picture, you are immediately alone with it as though you yourself were making your way wearily homeward with your hoe on an evening in late fall after the last potato fires have died down. What is here? The canvas? The brush strokes? The spots of color?" (5, p. 29).

Professor Heidegger is aware that van Gogh painted such shoes several times, but he does not identify the picture he has in mind, as if the different versions are interchangeable, all presenting the same truth. A reader who wishes to compare this account with the original picture or its photograph will have some difficulty in deciding which one to select. Eight paintings of shoes by van Gogh are recorded by de la Faille in his catalogue of all the canvasses by the artist that had been exhibited at the time Heidegger wrote his essay (cf. 6, no. 54, Fig. 60; no. 63, Fig. 64; no. 255, Fig. 248; no. 331, Fig. 249; no. 332, Fig. 250; no. 333, Fig. 251; no. 461, Fig. 488; no. 607, Fig. 597). Of these only three show the "dark openings of the worn insides" which speak so distinctly to the philosopher (6, nos. 255, 332, 333). They are clearly pictures of the artist's own shoes, not the shoes of a peasant. They might be shoes he had worn in Holland, but the pictures were painted during van Gogh's stay in Paris in 1886–87; one of them bears the date: "87" (6, no. 333; it is signed "Vincent 87"). From the time before 1886 when he painted Dutch peasants are two pictures of shoes—a pair of clean wooden clogs set on a table beside other objects (6, nos. 54 and 63). Later in Arles he represented, as he wrote in a letter of August 1888 to his brother, "une paire de vieux souliers" which are evidently his own (6, no. 461; 8, Vol. III, p. 291, Letter no. 529). A second still life of "vieux souliers de paysan" is mentioned in a letter of September 1888 to the painter Emile Bernard, but it lacks the characteristic worn surface and dark insides of Heidegger's description (6, no. 607; 8, Vol. IV, p. 227).

In reply to my question, Professor Heidegger has kindly written me that the picture to which he referred is one that he saw in a show at Amsterdam in March 1930.[3] This is clearly de la Faille's no. 255 (see Figure 1); there was also exhibited at the same time a painting with three pairs of shoes (6, no. 250), and it is possible that the exposed sole of a shoe in this picture inspired the reference to the sole in the philosopher's account. But from neither of these pictures, nor from any of the others, could one properly say that a painting of shoes by van Gogh expresses the being or essence of a peasant woman's shoes and her relation to nature and work. They are the shoes of the artist, by that time a man of the town and city.

Heidegger has written: "The art-work told us what shoes are in truth. It would be the worst self-deception if we were to think that our description, as a subjective action, first imagined everything thus and then projected it into the painting. If anything is questionable here, it is rather that we experienced too little in contact with the work and that we expressed the

[3] Personal communication, letter of May 6, 1965.

experience too crudely and too literally. But above all, the work does not, as might first appear, serve merely for a better visualization of what a piece of equipment is. Rather, the equipmental being of equipment first arrives at its explicit appearance through and only in the work.

"What happens here? What is at work in the work? Van Gogh's painting is the disclosure of what the equipment, the pair of peasants' shoes, *is* in truth" (4, p. 664).

Alas for him, the philosopher has indeed deceived himself. He has retained from his encounter with van Gogh's canvas a moving set of associations with peasants and the soil, which are not sustained by the picture itself but are grounded rather in his own social outlook with its heavy pathos of the primordial and earthy. He has indeed "imagined everything and projected it into the painting." He has experienced both too little and too much in his contact with the work.

The error lies not only in his projection which replaces a close and true attention to the work of art. For even if he had seen a picture of a peasant woman's shoes, as he describes them, it would be a mistake to suppose that the truth he uncovered in the painting—the being of the shoes—is something given here once and for all and is unavailable to our perception of shoes outside the painting. I find nothing in Heidegger's fanciful description of the shoes represented by van Gogh that could not have been imagined in looking at a real pair of peasants' shoes. Though he credits to art the power of giving to a represented pair of shoes that explicit appearance in which their being is disclosed—indeed "the universal essence of things" (4, p. 665), "world and earth in their counterplay"[4]—this concept of the metaphysical power of art remains here a theoretical idea. The example on which he elaborates with strong conviction does not support that idea.

Is Heidegger's mistake simply that he chose a wrong example? Let us imagine a painting of a peasant-woman's shoes by van Gogh. Would it not have made manifest just those qualities and that sphere of being described by Heidegger with such pathos?

Heidegger would still have missed an important aspect of the painting: the artist's presence in the work. In his account of the picture he has overlooked the personal and physiognomic in the shoes which made them so

[4] "Truth happens in van Gogh's painting. This does not mean that something is rightly portrayed, but rather that in the revelation of the equipmental being of the shoes that which *is* as a whole—world and earth in their counterplay—attains to unconcealment. . . . The more simply and essentially the shoes appear in their essence . . . the more directly and fascinatingly does all that *is* attain to a greater degree of being along with them" (4, p. 680).

absorbing a subject for the artist (not to speak of the intimate connection with the peculiar tones, forms, and brush-made surface of the picture as a painted work). When van Gogh depicted the peasant's wooden sabots, he gave them a clear, unworn shape and surface like the smooth still life objects he had set beside them on the same table: the bowl, the bottles, etc. In the later picture of a peasant's leather slippers he has turned them with their backs to the viewer (6, no. 607, Fig. 597). His own shoes he has isolated on the floor and he has rendered them as if facing us, and so individual and wrinkled in appearance that we can speak of them as veridical portraits of aging shoes.

We come closer, I think, to van Gogh's feeling for these shoes in a paragraph written by Knut Hamsun in the 1880's in his novel *Hunger*, describing his own shoes:

"As I had never seen my shoes before, I set myself to study their looks, their characteristics, and when I stir my foot, their shapes and their worn uppers. I discover that their creases and white seams give them expression—impart a physiognomy to them. Something of my own nature had gone over into these shoes; they affected me, like a ghost of my other I—a breathing portion of my very self" (2, p. 27—quoted by permission of Alfred Knopf, Inc., New York, N. Y.).

In comparing van Gogh's painting with Hamsun's text, we are interpreting the painting in a different way from Heidegger's. The philosopher finds in the picture of the shoes a truth about the world as it is lived by the peasant without reflection; Hamsun sees the real shoes as experienced by the self-conscious contemplating wearer who is also the writer. Hamsun's personage, a brooding, self-observant drifter, is closer to van Gogh's situation than to the peasant's. Yet van Gogh is in some ways like the peasant; as an artist he works, he is stubbornly occupied in a persistent task that is for him his inescapable calling, his life. Of course, van Gogh, like Hamsun, has also an exceptional gift of representation; he is able to transpose to the canvas with a singular power the forms and qualities of things; but they are things that have touched him deeply, in this case his own shoes—things inseparable from his body and memorable to his reacting self-awareness. They are not less objectively rendered for being seen as if endowed with his feelings and revery about himself. In isolating his own worn shoes on a canvas, he turns them to the spectator; he makes of them a piece from a self-portrait, that part of the costume with which we tread the earth and in which we locate the strains of movement, fatigue, pressure, heaviness—the burden of the erect body in its contact with the ground. They mark our inescapable position on the earth. To "be in someone's shoes" is to be in his predicament or his station in life. For a painter to represent his worn shoes as the main subject of a picture is for him to express a concern with the fatalities of his social being. Not the shoes as an instrument of use, though the landscape painter as a worker in the fields shares something of the peasant's life outdoors, but the shoes as "a portion of the self" (in Hamsun's words) are van Gogh's revealing theme.

Gauguin, who shared van Gogh's quarters in Arles in 1888, sensed a personal history behind his friend's painting of a pair of shoes. He has told in his reminiscences of van Gogh a deeply affecting story linked with van Gogh's shoes.

"In the studio was a pair of big hob-nailed shoes, all worn and spotted with mud; he made of it a remarkable still life painting. I do not know why I suspected that there was a story behind this old relic, and I ventured one day to ask him if he had some reason for preserving with respect what one ordinarily throws out for the rag-picker's basket.

" 'My father,' he said, 'was a pastor, and at his urging I pursued theological studies in order to prepare for my future vocation. As a young pastor I left for Belgium one fine morning, without telling my family, to preach the gospel in the factories, not as I had been taught but as I understood it myself. These shoes, as you see, have bravely endured the fatigue of that trip.'

"Preaching to the miners in the Borinage, Vincent undertook to nurse a victim of a fire in the mine. The man was so badly burned and mutilated that the doctor had no hope for his recovery. Only a miracle, he thought, could save him. Van Gogh tended him forty days with loving care and saved the miner's life.

"Before leaving Belgium I had, in the presence of this man who bore on his brow a series of scars, a vision of the crown of thorns, a vision of the resurrected Christ."

Gauguin continues: "And Vincent took up his palette again; silently he worked. Beside him was a white canvas. I began his portrait. I too had the vision of a Jesus preaching kindness and humility" (7, p. 53).[5]

It is not clear which of the paintings with a single pair of shoes Gauguin had seen at Arles. He described it as violet in tone in contrast to the yellow walls of the studio. It does not matter. Though written some years later, and with some literary affectations, Gauguin's story confirms the essential fact that for van Gogh the shoes were a piece of his own life.

[5] There is an earlier version of the story in (1). These two texts were kindly brought to my attention by Professor Mark Roskill.

REFERENCES

1. Gauguin, P. Natures Mortes. *Essais d'art libre*, 1894, *4*, 273–275.
2. Hamsun, K. *Hunger*. Translated by G. Egerton. New York: Knopf, 1941.
3. Heidegger, M. Der Ursprung des Kunstwerkes. In *Holzwege*, Frankfurt a.M.: Klostermann, 1950, pp. 7–68. Reprinted as a book, with an introduction by H.-G. Gadamer, Stuttgart: Reclam, 1962.
4. Heidegger, M. The origin of the work of art. Translation of (3) above by A. Hofstadter. In A. Hofstadter and R. Kuhns, *Philosophies of Art and Beauty*, New York: Random House, 1964, pp. 649–701.
5. Heidegger, M. *An Introduction to Metaphysics*. Translated by R. Manheim. New York: Anchor Books, 1961.
6. La Faille, J. B. de, *Vincent van Gogh*. Paris, 1939.
7. Rotonchamp, J. de, *Paul Gauguin 1848—1903*. Paris: G. Crès, 1925, 2nd edition.
8. Van Gogh, Vincent. *Verzamelde brieven van Vincent Van Gogh*. Amsterdam, 1952–1954. Four volumes.

15

The Delphic Oracle as Therapist

by Rollo May
New York, New York

On a plateau in the mountains at Delphi stands a shrine which for many centuries had a signal importance for the Greeks. Here they found help in meeting their anxiety. In this temple Apollo gave counsel through his priestesses during the chaotic archaic age and down through classical times. Even Socrates was to receive there his famous dictum, "Know Thyself," which has become the central touchstone for psychotherapy ever since. The sensitive Greek, anxious about himself, his family and his future in the upset, archaic times, could find guidance here, for Apollo knew the meaning of "the complicated games the gods play with humanity. . . . The Greeks believed in their Oracle, not because they were superstitious fools, but because they could not do without believing in it." (1, p. 75). Professor Dodds, in his excellent study of the irrational in ancient Greek culture, emphasizes the crucial assurance an "omniscient counselor could give . . . to a people burdened with the crushing sense of human ignorance and human insecurity, the dread of divine *phthonos*, the dread of *miasma*." (*Ibid.*).

The anxiety which the archaic Apollo helped people meet was that which accompanies a formative, fermenting, powerfully expanding period. It was not the neurotic anxiety characterized by withdrawal, inhibition, and the blocking off of vitality. The archaic Greek period was the period of emergence and vital growth, fraught with distress that resulted from the chaos of expanding outer and inner limits. Greeks were experiencing the anxiety of new possibilities that were forced upon them whether they wished it or not.

The shrine at Delphi rose to prominence at a time when the old stability and order of the family was crumbling, and the individual soon would have to be responsible for himself. In Homeric days, Odysseus' family in Ithaca could carry on with his wife Penelope and son Telemachus, whether Odysseus was there or at the wars in Troy or tossed for ten years on the "wine-dark sea." But now, in the archaic period, families must be welded into cities, and each young Telemachus felt himself standing on the brink of the time when he would have to choose his own future, and find his own place as part of a new city. The late contemporary writer Thomas Wolfe refers often to Telemachus as the myth of the search for the father, which was Wolfe's search as truly as the ancient Greek's. But it is indeed the hard and cold fact that Telemachus, like Thomas Wolfe himself, could not "go home again."

The city-states were struggling in anarchy, tyrant followed by tyrant (a term which in Greek does not have the usual destructive connotation it carries in English[1]), as the upsurging leaders tried to weld the new power into some order. In such a period of change and growth, *emergence* is often experienced by the individual as *emergency*, with all its attendant stress. This *anxiety of new possibilities* which preceded the classical age in ancient Greece was not unlike the anxiety in our own Renaissance which preceded our modern classical age; it was a similar period of radical upheaval of inner worlds, with new ethical and religious freedom for the individual. Not only in political and family relationships, but also in art, and religion and morality, the Greeks were struggling to find some order and structure.

Now it is important to remember that Apollo is the god of *form*, the god of reason and logic. Thus it is no accident that his shrine became the important one in this chaotic time and that through this god of proportion and balance the citizens sought "assurance that behind the seeming chaos there was knowledge and purpose" (1). Form and proportion and the golden mean of reason were essential if these men were to control their deep passions, not to tame their drives but to turn to constructive use the daimonic powers that the Greeks knew so well in nature and in themselves. Apollo is the god also of art, inasmuch as form—elegance—is an essential characteristic of beauty. Indeed, the name "Parnassus," the mountain at Delphi on which Apollo's shrine stood, has become a symbol in all western languages for devotion to the positive virtues of the mind.

We see more of the rich meaning carried in such a myth when we note that Apollo was also the god of "light"—not only the light of the sun, but the light of the mind, the light of reasonableness, the light of insight. He is often called Helios, the literal word in Greek for "sun," and "Phoebus Apollo," the god of brightness and radiance. In his youth, he is said to have slain the Python, the demon of darkness and illness. Finally, we note the most cogent point of all: Apollo is the god of healing, the sun which

[1] The word "tyrannos" refers simply to absolute ruler, of the type normally spawned in eras of political ferment and change. Some of these "tyrants," like Peisistratus, the "tyrant of Athens" in the late sixth century, are regarded as benefactors by historians and also by modern Greeks. I well recall my surprise when I first heard the boys of the college in Greece in which I taught speak of "Peisistratus, the tyrant of Athens," with the same quality of admiration, if not the same quantity, as boys in this country speak of George Washington.

brings light and life and health to people, and his son Aesculapius was to become the patron saint of medicine.

All of these attributes of the god Apollo, which were created by collective unconscious processes in the mythology of the dark pre-Homeric centuries before the archaic period, are interwoven with fantastic literal as well as figurative significance. How consistent and meaningful it becomes that this god is the god of good counsel, of psychological and spiritual insight, who will give guidance to a highly vital, formative age! A Greek man, setting out from Athens to go to Delphi to consult Apollo, would be turning over in his imagination, at almost every step during the two-day walk, this figure of the god of light and healing. Thus he would be proleptically participating in his own cure. Spinoza adjured us to "hold in imagination and fix our attention upon the desired virtue," and we would thus tend to acquire it. Our Greek would be doing this on his trip, and the psychological processes of anticipation, hope and faith would already be at work. His conscious intentions and his deeper intentionality were already committed to the event about to take place. This illustrates how symbols and myths carry, for the one who participates in them, their own healing power.

We can see in the superb statues of Apollo carved at this time—the archaic figure with his strong straight form, his calm beauty of head, the ordered features which are eloquent with controlled passion, even down to the slight "knowing" smile on his almost straight mouth—we can well see how this Apollo could be the symbol in which the Greek artists as well as other citizens of that period perceived their longed-for order. There is a curious feature in the statues of the archaic Apollo I have seen: the eyes are dilated, made more open than is normal in the head of a living man or in the classical Greek statues. (What a contrast to the relaxed, almost sleepy eyes of the familiar head of Hermes of Praxiteles of the fourth century!)

The dilated eyes of the archaic Apollo are characteristic of apprehension. They express the anxiety—the excessive awareness, the "looking about" on all sides to see what might happen—that goes with living in a fomenting age. There is a remarkable parallel between these eyes of the archaic Apollo and the eyes in the figures of Michelangelo, painted in our own formative period, the Renaissance: almost all of Michelangelo's human beings, powerful and triumphant as they appear at first glance, present, on closer inspection, the dilated eyes which are a tell-tale sign of anxiety. And as if to demonstrate that he is expressing the inner tensions not only of his age but of himself as a member of his age, Michelangelo in his self-portraits paints eyes which are again markedly distended in the way that is typical of apprehension.

The poet Rilke also was struck by Apollo's prominent eyes with their quality of seeing deeply. In his *Torso of an Archaic Apollo*, he speaks of "the eyes' apples slowly ripened," and continues,

> ". . . . . Yet
> his torso glows: a candelabrum set
> before his gaze which is pushed back and hid,
> restrained and shining. Else the curving breast
> could not thus blind you, nor through the soft turn
> of the loins could this smile easily have passed
> into the bright groins where the genitals burned . . .
> nor would this star have shaken the shackles off,
> bursting with light, until there is no place
> that does not see you. You must change your life" (4).

In this vivid picture we note how well Rilke catches the essence of *controlled passion*, not inhibited or repressed passion, as was to be the goal, during the later Hellenistic age, of some Greek teachers who had become afraid of vital drives.[2] Rilke shows the sense of the archaic period even in that curious last sentence which seems at first, but only at first, to be a *non sequitur:* "You must change your life."

How the shrine of Apollo functioned, and where the advice it gave came from, are of course fascinating questions. But unfortunately little seems to be known. The shrine was veiled in secrecy; those who directed it could not only give counsel to others, but could also keep their own. Plato tells us that a "prophetic madness" overcame the Pythia, the priestess who served as mouthpiece for Apollo. From this experience there emerged some "creative insight," so Plato believed, which represented deeper-than-normal levels of consciousness. Apollo spoke in the first person through the Pythia. Her voice changed and became husky, throaty and quavering like

[2] What a far cry is Rilke's interpretation from the inhibition and repression of drives of our own Victorian age. These early Greeks gloried in passion and eros and the daimonic. They wept and made love and killed with zest. Patients nowadays in therapy often remark at the strange spectacle in ancient Greece that it is the *strong* man, like Odysseus or Prometheus, who weeps. But the Greeks knew also that these powers—like Plato's horses in the myth of the chariot—must be directed and controlled. It is the essence of a man of virtue (arete) that he choose his passions rather than be chosen by them. Somewhere in this dialectic lies the explanation of why they did not need to go through the self-castrating practice of denying eros and the daimonic, as is the protective strategy of modern western man.

that of a modern medium; the god was said to come into her at the very moment of *enthusiasm*, as the root of the term, en-theo, literally suggests.

The counsel was generally given in poetry. Before the "séance," the priestess went through several ritualistic acts, such as special bathing, and perhaps drinking from a sacred spring, presumedly with the customary autosuggestive effects. But the oft-repeated statement that she breathed vapors issuing from a fissure in the rocks of the shrine which induced a hypnotic effect, is disposed of summarily by Professor Dodds:

> "As for the famous 'vapours' to which Pythia's inspiration was once confidently ascribed, they are a Hellenistic invention . . . Plutarch, who knew the facts, saw the difficulties of the vapour theory, and seems finally to have rejected it altogether; but like the Stoic philosophers, nineteenth century scholars seized with relief on a nice solid materialist explanation."[3] (1, p. 73).

Dodds goes on to remark pithily that "less has been heard of this theory since the French excavations showed that there are today no vapors, and no 'chasm' from which vapors could once have come." Such explanations are needless, Dodds avers with good sense, in view of the present-day evidence of anthropology and abnormal psychology. (*Ibid.* pp. 73–74).

The Pythian priestesses themselves seemed to be simple, uneducated women; Plutarch tells of one who was the daughter of a peasant. But modern scholars have a high respect for the intelligence system of the shrine. The "history of Delphi shows sufficient traces of a consistent policy to convince one that human intelligence at some point could play a deciding role in the process." (3). Though Apollo committed some notorious blunders in his predictions and advice, especially during the Persian wars, the people, with an attitude like many a patient in psychotherapy toward today's therapist, evidently forgave him because of the useful advice and help he had given at other times.

The point that interests us most here is the function of the shrine as a communal symbol which had the power to draw out the subconscious and unconscious collective insights of the Greeks. A genuine symbol, with its accompanying ceremonial rite, always becomes the mirror that reflects insights into new possibilities, new wisdom, and other psychic phenomena that the individual cannot experience on his own. He cannot for two reasons: The first is his own anxiety: the new insights often, and we could even say, typically, would frighten him too much were he to take full and

[3] I am grateful to Mr. Thomas Laws of Columbia University for first bringing this to my attention.

lonely responsibility for them. In an age of foment, such insights require more psychological and spiritual responsibility than most individuals are prepared to bear. In dreams people can let themselves do things, such as killing a parent; or they can think, for instance, "my mother wanted to abort me before I was born"; these they would be horrified to think or say in ordinary "rational" speech. Patients in therapy hesitate even to think these and similar things in daydreams, since such phantasies are felt to carry more individual responsibility. But if you can have a dream say it, or have Apollo in his shrine say it, you can be much more frank about your new truth.[4] Also, you escape hybris: Socrates could assert that Apollo at Delphi had pronounced him the wisest man then living, a claim he could never have made on his own.

The sayings of the priestess were not only couched in poetry, but, like mediumistic statements and dreams of all periods, they were sufficiently cryptic to require interpretation, and were susceptible to several possible meanings. This fact demanded that the recipient of the counsel not receive it merely passively, but put himself into the message. In the *Apologia* we are told how Socrates tried to puzzle out what the god meant by the famous maxims addressed to him. Ever since, thoughtful men like Nietzsche and Kierkegaard have been trying to fathom the god's advice to Socrates, and everybody still finds new meaning in "Know thyself."

But there is another reason why a shrine can be significant as the embodiment of the unconscious collective insights of the group. A symbol or myth acts like a projective screen in drawing out the insight. Like Rorschach cards, or Murray's Thematic Apperception Test, the shrine and its ceremonies are a screen that invites you and stimulates you to conceive of new possibilities.

Now I must hasten to insert a caution. The process going on at such a shrine may be called "projection," but we must insist that it is not "projection" in any pejorative meaning, neither in the psychoanalytical sense that you "project" what is "sick" in you or what you cannot face; nor in the empirical psychological sense that implies the process is simply subjective, and that the cards or TAT pictures have nothing to do with the result. In my judgment, both of these pejorative senses of projection result from the common failure of western men to understand the nature of symbol and myth.

The "screen" is not merely a blank mirror. It is, rather, *the objective pole necessary for calling forth the subjective processes of consciousness.* The

[4] A symbolic rite thus functions like a collective dream.

Rorschach cards *are* definite and real forms of black and color, even though no one ever before has "seen" in them the things you or I may see in them. Such "projection" is in no sense a "regression" by definition, or something less respectable than being able to say what you want to say in rational sentences without the cards. This process goes on all the time in art. The paint, the canvas, are objective things which have powerful and exciting influences on the artist in bringing out his ideas and visions. The artist is in a dialectical relation, indeed, not only with paint and canvas, but with the shapes he sees in nature, as the poet is with the words of his inherited language. The artist, the poet, and the musician dare to bring forth new forms, new kinds of vitality and meaning. They are, at least partially, protected from going "crazy" in this process of radical emergence, by the form lent by the media, namely the paints, the marble, the words, the musical notes.

I propose that the shrine of Apollo can be seen best as a communal symbol. We can postulate, then, that its insights come by a communal symbolic process involving both subjective and objective factors in a dialectical relation with each other. The symbol and myth, by their nature, are distinguished by their capacity to unite subjective and objective processes. For anyone who participates in the shrine, new forms, new ideal possibilities, new ethical and religious structures, may be born from levels of experience which underlie and transcend the individual's customary waking consciousness. Plato, we have noted, calls this process the ecstasy of prophetic madness. "Ecstasy" means "standing outside one's self," (ex-stasis), which is a time-honored method of transcending our ordinary consciousness, and for arriving at insights we could not attain otherwise. An element of ecstasy, however slight, is part and parcel of every genuine symbol and myth; for if we genuinely participate in it, for that moment we are taken "out of" and "beyond" ourselves.

The psychological approach to the myth is only one of several possible avenues. In taking this approach I do not with to "psychologize away" the myth's religious meaning. From the religious aspect, the insight which comes in the dialectical interplay of the subjective elements in the individual with the objective fact of the shrine is seen as revelation. To the genuine believer, the myth is never purely psychological; it always has an element of revelation, whether from Apollo, or Yahweh in the Hebrew religion, or Being in oriental religious terms. If we completely psychologize away this religious element, we shall be unable either to appreciate the power with which Aeschylus and Sophocles write their dramas, and even unable to understand what they are talking about. Aeschylus, Sophocles and the other dramatists could write great tragedy because of the religious dimensions of the myths, which gave strength to their belief in the dignity of man and the ultimate meaning of his destiny.

Quotations from Dodds (1) and Rilke (4) reprinted by permission of the University of California Press.

REFERENCES

1. Dodds, E. R. *The Greeks and the Irrational.* Berkeley, California: The University of California Press, 1964.
2. Guerber, H. A. *The Myths of Greece and Rome.* London: G. G. Harrap & Co., 1907.
3. Parke, H. W. *History of the Delphic Oracle.* Cited by Dodds (1).
4. Rilke, R. M. *Selected Poems.* Translated by C. F. MacIntyre. Berkeley, California: University of California Press, 1964.

16

Some Varieties of Psychological Organization

by Silvan S. Tomkins

New York, New York

Let me state at the outset that I consider man's primary motives to consist of eight innate affects, or feelings. These are the positive affects of excitement, enjoyment and surprise, and the negative affects of distress, anger, fear, shame and contempt. These are innate. One does not learn to smile in enjoyment nor to cry in distress. However, the objects of each affect are *both* innate and learned. A baby does not learn the birth cry. It is an innate response to the excessive stimulation attendant upon being born. He will later cry when he is hungry or tired or exposed to too loud sounds. None of these are learned responses. But eventually he *will* learn to cry about many things about which he was initially unconcerned. He may learn to cry in sympathy when others are in distress, and cry. But if the crying of others may be learned to evoke one's own distress cry, so may it also be learned to evoke contempt or shame rather than sympathy. There is thus nothing under the sun which some human beings have not learned to enjoy, to fear, or to hate, to be ashamed of, or to which to respond with excitement or contempt or anger. It is the innate plasticity of the affect mechanism, which permits the investment of any type of affect in any type of activity or object, that makes possible the great varieties of human personalities and societies. Cultural diversity rests upon the biological plasticity of the affect system in man. Puritanism, or negative affect about pleasure, and masochism, or positive affect about pain, are extreme examples of the plasticity of affect investment. The theoretical possibilities of the variety of profiles of activation, maintenance, and decay of each affect are without limit. I may be happy as a child and very sad as an adult, or conversely. I may be angry for a moment, for an hour, for a day, or always, or never. I may be frightened only occasionally, or I may be anxious all my life. I may feel mildly ashamed for myself or deeply humiliated. I may feel ashamed because I have shown my feelings too publicly, or because I was unable to show my feelings toward someone who needed my sympathy. In short, the object, the duration, the frequency, and the intensity of affect arousal and investment are without limit. It is this capacity of the individual to feel strongly or weakly, for a moment or for all his life, about anything under the sun, and to govern himself by such motives, that constitutes his essential freedom.

Personality is an aggregate of many types of organizations. Consider the heterogeneous nature of biological man. With respect to his height, he grows to a maximum in early adulthood and then stops growing. With respect to his weight, there is a parallel development, but he may continue to grow heavier while he remains the same height. He has only one set of eyes all his life. But he has baby teeth which fall out, and then a second set which he may keep the rest of his life or which he may also lose. With respect to pigmentation he may be blonde as a child, brunette as an adult and gray or bald in his later years, or blonde throughout his life. His eyes may be blue throughout his life, or blue as a child and brown as an adult. Some of his tissues can regenerate. Some will not, and so on. Heterogenity in structure and in profile of development is the rule and not the exception. At the psychological level where learning plays so dominant a role, it would be surprising if there were less heterogeneity of basic structures. Psychological structures vary critically, we think, in *ideo-affective density*, in *stability*, and in their *rate and direction of change*. Consider first the varieties of ideo-affective densities. We may define affect density as the product of its intensity times its duration. We now introduce a derivative concept: ideo-perceptual-memorial-action-affect density. By this we mean the product of the intensity multiplied by the duration of all the capacities for involvement which the individual possesses. At one time his involvement may be primarily ideational, at another time primarily affective, or primarily overtly behavioral, or primarily perceptual, or memorial, or any combination of these. For purposes of brevity we will henceforth refer to this as *ideo-affective density*, and use the term *ideation* to refer to the variety of non-affective cognitions as well as to action. We do not mean by this to imply in any way that we regard action as a type of thinking, or in any way to blur the differences between perception, memory and thinking. We will use the term simply as a convenient abbreviation for the density of involvement of all of the critical sub-systems which together constitute a human being. Bearing in mind this special usage of the words *ideo-* and *ideation*, we will now define ideo-affective density as the product of the intensity and duration of affect and the concurrent ideation about the object of the affect. Low ideo-affective density refers to those experiences which generate little or no affect, and little or no ideation, or, if the affect and ideation are intense, they do not last long. High density occurs whenever the individual has both intense feelings and ideation which continue at a high level over long periods of time. In such a case there is a monopolistic capture of the individual's awareness and concern. Low and high densities represent two ends of a continuum of organizations of motive, thought and behavior which are critical for the understanding of commitment.

We wish to distinguish two gross segments of an ideo-affect density continuum—the low and high density segments.

Let us first consider the low end of the continuum. We distinguish two different kinds of organization, both of which are characteristically low density organizations. Further, each type of organization may be primarily positive or negative in affect. One organization is *transient, casual* and the other is *recurrent, habitual.*

Consider first a transitory positive, low density ideo-affective organization. Such is the laughter in response to a joke. The experience might be extremely enjoyable but nonetheless of very low density, because it recruited no continuing ideation or affect beyond the momentary experience. An example of a transitory negative low density ideo-affective organization is a cut incurred while shaving which occasioned a brief stab of pain and distress, but no further thought or feeling beyond this isolated experience. Each individual's life-time contains thousands of such relatively casual, transient encounters. Collectively they may sum to a not inconsiderable segment of the life span. Nonetheless, they constitute an aggregate of isolated components without substantial impact on the personality of the individual.

The recurrent, habitual types of low density ideo-affective organizations characteristically begin with considerable intensity of affect and ideation but end with minimal involvement. Consider first the negative recurrent habitual case. Everyone learns to cross streets with minimal ideation and affect. We learn to act as if we were afraid, but we do not in fact experience any fear once we have learned how to cope successfully with such contingencies. Despite the fact that we know that there is real danger involved in our daily walking across intersections, and that many pedestrians are in fact killed, we exercise normal caution with minimal attention and no fear. It remains a low density ideo-affective organization, despite daily repetition over a lifetime. Successful avoidance strategies remain low density organizations because they do not generalize or spread. They do not spread just because they are successful. It should be noted that these organizations, though we have called them recurrent habitual, are far from being simple motor habits. They are small programs for processing information with relatively simple strategies, but one may nonetheless never repeat precisely the same avoidance behaviors twice in crossing the street. These simple programs generate appropriate avoidant strategies for dealing with a variety of such situations, and caution is nicely matched to the varying demands of this class of situations, with a minimum of attention and affect. Every individual, including the psychotic, possesses hundreds of such avoidance and escape low density organizations. (It is a surprise on first exposure to psychotic patients to discover—as my friend Edward Engel confided to me one day—that a schizophrenic, when eating soup for lunch, does not put the soup into his eye!) This is not to say that crossing the street was always a low density ideo-affective organization. The earliest such experiences may well have been high adventures for the daring child, or they may have been the occasion of severe punishment at the hands of an anxious parent, terrified at the sight of his toddler walking in front of a speeding automobile. Both the excitement and the pain, or distress, or fear which might have been suffered at the hands of a parent do not long continue. Quickly all children learn some caution in this matter, and it ceases to claim either much ideation or feeling. Such attenuation of feeling and thought necessarily depends upon the success of problem solutions. Paradoxically, human beings are least involved in what they can do best: once problems are solved, they remain solved. Man as a successful problem-solver ceases to think and to feel about successful performance and turns ideation and affect to the continuing, or new, unsolved challenges.

This is so whether the original affect which powered problem solving was positive or negative. Just as we experience no terror in confronting traffic at the curb, so too with positive, low density ideo-affective organizations we experience no positive enjoyment or excitement in the daily recurrent performance which once delighted. As I finish my daily shaving I rarely puff with pride and think, "There, I've done it again!" I act in this case, as in crossing the street, *as if* I experienced an affect, and had a wish to achieve this goal. I do indeed achieve my intention—to shave—but the positive affect behind this ritual has long ceased to be emitted concurrently with the action. Like the low density avoidance strategy of crossing the street, it may be done daily—repeated several thousand times during a lifetime—with little or no effect on other action, or affect, or memory, or perception.

What then of the high density ideo-affective organizations? By definition they can be neither transitory nor recurrent but must be enduring. Whether predominantly positive or negative in tone, they must seize the individual's feelings and thoughts and actions to the exclusion of almost all else. Consider first negative monopolism of thought and feeling. If successful and continuing problem solution is the necessary condition of the low density organization, *temporary* problem solution is the necessary condition of the negative high density organization. Consider our man on the curb. He is normally cautious but not overly concerned because his solution to the problem has always worked. But suppose that one day a passing motorist loses control of his car and seriously injures our hero. After his return from the hospital he is a bit more apprehensive than before, and now stands back a little farther from the edge of the curb than he used to. He may continue his somewhat excessive caution for some time, and, as he notes a car approaching with what appears a little too much speed, may even begin to wonder, with occasional fear, whether such an accident might ever happen again. But if all goes well this increase in density of ideation and affect will pass, and, before long, he will be indistinguishable from any other casual pedestrian. But in our tragedy all does not go well. Uncannily a drunken driver pursues our hero, and he is hit again. This time it is more serious, and so we see the beginnings of a phobia. Our hero stations himself inside a building, peering up and down the street, before he will venture out to dare negotiate the crossing. By now his preoccupation with, and fear of, the deadly vehicle has grown to invade his consciousness even when he is far from the scene of potential danger. In the last act of this drama it is a bulldozer which penetrates his apparent fortress.

What next? Will he be safe in the hospital? His ideation and affect have now reached a point of no return. He will henceforth generate possibilities which no reasonable man would entertain, and these phantasies will evoke affects proportional to their extremity. He will now begin negative ideo-affective creativity. Such a high density ideo-affective organization is capable of providing a lifetime of suffering and can resist reduction through new evidence. This happens if, and only if, there has occurred a sequence of events of this type: threat, successful defense, breakdown of defense and re-emergence of threat, second successful new defense, second breakdown of defense and re-emergence of threat, third successful new defense, third breakdown of defense and re-emergence of threat, and so on; until an expectation is generated that no matter how successful a defense against a dread contingency may seem, it will prove unavailing and require yet another new defense, *ad infinitum*. Not only is there generated the conviction that successful defense can be successful only temporarily, but also, as new and more effective defenses are generated, the magnitude of the danger is inflated in the imagination of the harried one. We have defined this dynamic as a *circular incremental magnification*. It is circular and incremental since each new threat requires a more desperate defense, and the successive breakdown of each newly improved defense generates a magnification of the nature of the threat and the concurrent affect which it evokes. We have defined such a circular incremental magnification series as a set of $- + -$ triads in which negative affect is defended against, and replaced, by positive affect, but then breaks down and again produces negative affect. In comparison with the analogous low-density organization, it is the continuing uncertainty of permanent problem solution which is critical in monopolizing the individual's ideation and affect. Paradoxically, it is just the fact that the individual is *not* entirely helpless in dealing with a given situation which continually magnifies both the apparent nature of the threat and his skill in coping with it. In this respect the individual may be likened to a tennis player who is first defeated by a poor opponent, and who then practises sufficiently to defeat that opponent. But his triumph proves short-lived since his opponent now also improves and in turn defeats him. This then leads our hero to improve his skill so that once again he defeats his adversary, but this leads to yet another defeat when the latter improves his skill, and so on and on.

Let us now examine the structure of the positive, high density ideo-affective organization. Instead of a series of $- + -$ triads, here it is a series of $+ - +$ triads which is responsible for the circular incremental magnification. Instead of increasing concern with warding off a threat, it is rather the magnification of a positive affect and the ideation about its object which is involved. Although there is negative affect sandwiched in between two positive affects in this type of triad, the individual is primarily concerned with attaining the object of positive affect. Let us consider two types of such positive ideo-affective organizations.

First, consider what we will define as psychological addiction. The addicted cigarette smoker will serve as an example. Individual A enjoys smoking a cigar or a cigarette after dinner. This is an unadulterated reward. At other times of the day he is unaware both of the enjoyments of smoking and of any suffering because he is not smoking. Individual B does not enjoy smoking *per se*, but rather uses cigarettes as a pacifier or sedative whenever he becomes distressed or anxious. Smoking at such times reduces his suffering and makes him feel better. It is not only that the function of smoking is here limited to the reduction of negative affect, but also that such negative affect arises from some source other than smoking. He is *not* disturbed simply because he is not smoking, but rather is disturbed because something else went wrong in his life. So, when everything goes well for B, he does not miss smoking, because the only function which smoking serves is to reduce other kinds of suffering. B does not think of smoking when he is not smoking—except for those occasions when he is disturbed. If he is not disturbed he has concerns other than smoking. Individual C is an addicted smoker. Like A he too enjoys smoking and like B he uses smoking to reduce all types of suffering. But here the resemblances end.

C first of all is *always* aware of not smoking whenever this occurs. Second, he always responds to this awareness with negative affect which continues to increase in intensity until he can smoke. Third, he will always drop all competitors for his attention and try to get a cigarette; and fourth, upon getting a cigarette and beginning to smoke he will respond with intense enjoyment at the reduction of his suffering of negative affect. Like A he enjoys smoking, and like B he also reduces his suffering by smoking, but the suffering which he *must* reduce is the suffering he experiences (and has created) just because he is not smoking. No matter how well his life goes, he is unable to be unaware of not smoking, whenever this occurs. Contrary to B he may be able to tolerate many other types of suffering without resort to sedation by smoking. So long as he has a cigarette in hand he may be quite courageous in confronting innumerable problems other than that of not-smoking. B in similar circumstances might have had resort to smoking to leave the field, to sedate himself into comfort rather than to confront his problem. In addiction, too, there is circular incremental magnification produced by an ever-accelerating suffering in the absence of a cigarette and an ever-increasing rewarding experience of positive affect upon the reduction of the suffering of negative affect.

The hold of cigarette smoking or any other high density addiction arises from the intolerability of the ever-mounting negative affect which is experienced whenever the addict attempts to break his addiction. As his suffering mounts he becomes more and more unable to tolerate the absence of smoking and extrapolates into the future a vision of an increasingly intolerable suffering, till in panic at this prospect he succumbs to his longing. It is a series of painful longings reduced by smoking which increases both the suffering of negative affect and the intensity of positive affect while smoking, in an accelerating circular incremental magnification.

Psychologically this process is similar to the mourning experience of the bereaved. The lost love object is magnified in value because of the conjoint suffering and longing which makes vivid to the bereaved his hitherto not entirely appreciated dependence on the lost love object. It is the barrier to ever again enjoying the presence of the beloved which reveals and *creates* a new appreciation. Although addiction is thereby heightened in mourning, and though longing and suffering may be intensified to the point of intolerability, the mourner ultimately is freed from his heightened dependence because he is forced to endure the abstinence suffering until it no longer increases in intensity, and then begins slowly to decline in intensity, until finally there is minimal suffering and no *awareness* that the lost love object has been lost. In this respect the mourner is returned to the state of someone who has been able to overcome his addiction to smoking. The addicted cigarette smoker will not willingly suffer through such abstinence suffering, because it seems to him, as to the bereaved, that he will never be able to tolerate the loss of the love object. In addiction, it should be noted, we are dealing with the lure of the familiar and the positive affect which is involved in enjoyment. It is the return to the familiar, heightened in value by the suffering of separation which creates the magic of reunion, be that reunion with an old friend, an old place or an old activity such as smoking. In contrast to commitment, as we will presently see, there is here much less involvement of exploration, of novelty and of created challenge.

In commitment the positive high density ideo-affective organization also involves the reward of the positive affect of enjoyment, but in addition the positive affect of excitement becomes more prominent. Let us consider two examples of commitment, one characteristically abortive commitment which ends either by transformation into an addiction at somewhat less than maximal density, or ends in disenchantment; the other a high density commitment which for some extends over the entire life span. We refer in the first instance to romantic love and in the second to the committed scientist.

Consider first the *romantic lover* who intends to commit himself for life to his beloved. As we distinguished cigarette smokers, A, B, and C, we may distinguish A in this domain as one who very much enjoys his contacts with his lady friend, but who does not miss her when he is otherwise occupied. B has a lady friend he does not miss when all goes well. But he always turns to her for comfort when he becomes disturbed. She does in fact always bring him tranquility, and having been mothered back into peace of mind, he is prepared again to pick up his life, and to forget his benefactress with gratitude but no regret, for the time being. Not so with C, the romantic lover. He is forever aware of the absence of his beloved, and of their enforced separation, to which he responds with intense suffering and longing. Every time he is separated he dies a little and thereby, like the true mourner, comes to appreciate more and more his dependence upon the beloved who grows increasingly desirable in her absence. Upon reunion with the beloved, the intensity of his enjoyment and excitement is proportional to his prior suffering, and there is begun a circular incremental magnification. If the beloved becomes more valuable when she brings to an end the intolerable suffering and longing that preceded reunion, so much the greater will the next suffering of separation become, since the beloved has by now become even more wonderful than before. Just as the nature of the threat is magnified in the negative high density series of $- + -$ triads, so here is the nature of the positive object magnified in the series of + − + triads. In contrast to the ever-increasing negative threat, the beloved does not necessarily continue to support indefinite magnification of her magical qualities. Romantic love imposes separation and uncertainty which increases the period of time over which longing for the love object can occur; but with the transition to the honeymoon and marriage, the prolonged intimacy and mutual exploration eventually produce a sufficient reduction in novelty and uncertainty so that excitement can no longer be indefinitely maintained. When, under these conditions of continuing contact, the beloved will no longer support the indefinite magnification of wonder and excitement, there may appear disenchantment or boredom, or an ideo-affective organization of reduced intensity and duration, with excitement replaced by the enjoyment of the familiar and deepening relationship. But the husband will no longer miss his wife throughout the working day even though he deeply enjoys his reunion with her at each day's end. We have traced this potential high density ideo-affective organization, which may be short-circuited by marriage, to better illuminate the nature of enduring high density commitment.

Consider next the varieties of *committed scientists*, and those who are interested but not committed. Scientist A enjoys tremendously both the discovery of truth and the search for truth. He likes to putter around the laboratory. He likes to run experiments. He enjoys it when they succeed. But he is a nine-to-five scientist. When he goes home it is to another world. He does not take his scientific troubles home with him. Indeed, he experiences a minimum of suffering in his role as scientist. He is in this respect like the person who loves to smoke after dinner, and like the person who enjoys the company of his lady friend, but who do not miss their enjoyment or suffer in the interim. Individual B, on the other hand, uses science as a sedative. Whenever he becomes depressed he turns to reading science or watching TV programs concerning the latest advances in science. However, as soon as his life becomes more rewarding, his interest in science flags, like the person who smoked to comfort himself, and like the individual who sought out his lady friend to ease his suffering, but, once mothered back into peace of mind, forgot his benefactress. Consider now scientist C who is committed for a lifetime to the pursuit of truth. Like the addicted smoker he is always aware of the absence of his longed-for ideal object—ultimate, permanent truth. Like individual A, he enjoys the scientific way of life. He enjoys puttering with laboratory equipment and running experiments. But underlying all his enjoyment is a continuing unrest and suffering over the possibilities of error, and over the possibility of missing the main chance. When everything works as planned he is deeply excited and enjoys briefly the fruits of his labor. But his contact with truth is ordinarily as brief as it is sweet. Truth is a mistress who never gives herself completely or permanently. She must be wooed and won arduously and painfully in each encounter. With each encounter she deepens both the scientist's suffering and then his reward. It is a love affair which is never entirely and deeply consummated. Immediately following each conquest, the victory is always discovered to have been less than it appeared, and the investigation must now be pursued with more skill and more energy than before.

The set of triads + − + is in some respects similar to the negative set of triads − + −. In both cases skill must constantly be improved, and in both cases the effectiveness of achieved skill is only temporary. The difference is that in the negative high density ideo-affective organization the individual is pursued by a threat, whereas in positive commitment he pursues an object of ever-increasing attractiveness. In both cases circular incremental magnification is responsible for the *creation* of an idealized object. The magic of truth exists in such a magnified form only in the mind of one who will pursue truth despite increasing suffering, so that each encounter becomes both more bitter and more sweet. There is minimal uncertainty in the familiar object of addiction, and there is a finite uncertainty in the romantic love affair which is almost entirely explored during the honeymoon. In the scientific commitment, however, there is sufficient continuing uncertainty so that endless circular incremental magnification of the + − + triad can be sustained indefinitely if the individual has become committed. Thus, a scientist who has made a major discovery and thereafter elects to rest on his laurels has ceased to be a committed scientist, with high density of ideation and affect about science. It is a critical feature of high density commitment that there can be no *enduring* positive affect in having attained the pursued finite object. Rather, the object is continually redefined, so that a newer version of the quest can be mounted. The same dynamic appears in the pursuit of money or power. These are also capable of committing the individual to an endless insatiable quest for an object which is put out of reach almost immediately after it is attained.

Let us turn now to yet another group of the committed—the reformer and those he reforms. Why and how do individuals and societies become committed to ideologies and to social movements? We will examine four abolitionists, Garrison, Phillips, Weld, and Birney, as committed reformers.

The commitment of Garrison, Phillips, Weld, and Birney to abolitionism proceeded in a series of steps consistent with our general theory of commitment. The critical role of adult experience in the spiral stepwise triads of + − + affects which gradually deepen commitment is underlined by the early resonance of each of these leaders to ways of life quite diverse from each other, and from their future way of life. No one could have predicted with any confidence that these four young men would eventually provide the leadership for the abolitionist movement. Garrison was first attracted to writing and to politics as a way of life. Phillips led the life typical of the Boston Brahmin of his time: attendance at Harvard College, Harvard Law School and then the opening of a law practice. Weld first gave a series of lectures on mnemonics, the art of improving the memory. Birney was twice suspended from Princeton for drinking, though he was each time readmitted, and graduated with honors. He, like Phillips, became a gentleman lawyer, priming himself for a political career. After an early failure in politics he became a planter and lived the life of the young Southern aristocrat, drinking and gambling to excess. Paradoxically, of the four, he was the earliest to interest himself in the slaves, but the last to commit himself to their emancipation as his way of life.

The stages in the development of their commitment to abolitionism may be summarized briefly as follows: first, a resonance to the general idea of the salvation of others; second, risk is ventured on behalf of those who need to be saved; third, as a consequence of the risk which has been taken, there is punishment and suffering; fourth, as a consequence of such suffering, resonance to the original idea of the necessity of salvation is deepened, and identification with the oppressed is increased, as is hostility toward the oppressor; fifth, as a result of increased density of affect and ideation, there will be an increased willingness to take even greater risks and more possible punishment and more suffering; sixth, increased risk taking does indeed evoke more punishment and more suffering; seventh, there is an increasing willingness to tolerate suffering which follows risk taking, concomitant with a proportionately increasing intensity and duration of positive affect, and ideation, in identification with the oppressed and with fellow abolitionists, and an increasing negative affect toward the enemy whose apparent power and undesirability is magnified as the density of affect and ideation increases. The + − + triad alternates between resonance and risk taking (+), punishment and suffering (−), increased density of positive affect and ideation (+), resulting in increased risk taking (+), so that the entire triad is endlessly repeated. This cumulatively deepens commitment until it reaches a point of no return—when no other way of life seems possible to the committed reformer. The spiral, composed of + − + triads, is therefore a + − +, + − + set rather than a + − + − + sequence. The increased density of positive affect and ideation at the end of the + − + results in an increased positive affect invested in more *risk*, the + in the next + − + triad.

It should be noted that the pathway from early resonance to final commitment is not necessarily without internal conflict. Some of the suffering comes from within as well as from the enemy. Each of these men was to suffer doubt at some point whether he should give himself completely to abolitionism as a way of life.

CONCLUSION

We have said that psychological structures vary critically in ideo-affective density, in stability, and in their rate and direction of change.

We have seen that habitual rituals are stable organizations—they remain stable because they work. Commitment and negative monopolism are examples of growing organizations which continue to grow. They grow because there is a preponderance of positive affect interrupted by negative affect in commitment, and because there is a preponderance of negative affect interrupted by positive affect in negative monopolism. In each case preponderant affect is heightened by its antithesis. If a joke is a rapidly growing and rapidly dying organization, a brief love affair is an example of an organization which grows over a longer period and dies at a slower rate. Mourning or disenchantment are examples of dying psychological organizations which previously had attained high ideo-affective density, and which eventually are radically reduced in ideo-affective density.

There is no necessary relationship between the ideo-affective density of an organization and its stability, rate or direction of change. Weak organizations may be stable or unstable. Weak organizations may grow and strong ones may die. An affair may grow into a stable marriage. A heretofore stable marriage may lead to divorce after many years. Just as the personality possesses structures which vary in ideo-affective density, so too do they vary (independently) in their stability and in their rate and direction of change.

This paper was presented at the Kurt Goldstein Memorial Meeting, held at the 37th Annual Meeting of the Eastern Psychological Association on April 16, 1966, in New York City. The writer's work is supported *in toto* by a U.S. Public Health Service Career Research Award from the National Institute of Mental Health, 1-K6-MH-23, 797-d.

17

The Present Crisis in Psychoanalysis

by Erich Fromm

New York, New York

There is little doubt that psychoanalysis finds itself in a mounting state of crisis which has become increasingly visible in the last ten years. This crisis pertains both to the theoretical and the clinical aspects of psychoanalysis.

On theoretical grounds alone the concepts of the libido theory and the pleasure principle are widely held to be outmoded, not only by psychoanalysts outside the Freudian organization, but also by many authors within the Freudian establishment. This is true especially of the now-leading group of Freudian theoreticians, the ego psychologists, some of whom admit that these tenets contradict the more recent findings of neurophysiology. At the same time the concepts governing the second phase of Freud's work since the early twenties, i.e., those dealing with the life and death instinct, were never properly coordinated with the earlier theories, neither by himself, nor by his pupils; thus they remained a theoretical torso, despite the fact that they represented important progress over the initial instinct theory.

Aside from these theoretical failures, competition with psychoanalysis increased in various other fields. On the one hand, neurophysiology made discoveries which, together with the treatment of mental illness by means of psycho-active drugs, constituted an enormous theoretical and therapeutic advance in psychiatry. On the other hand, academic experimental and animal psychology (with their application to human behavior) have also advanced considerably. Kurt Goldstein, Jean Piaget, L. S. Vygotsky and Konrad Lorenz, are among the most outstanding contributors to modern psychological theory.

Simultaneously with the theoretical standstill of classical psychoanalysis, a marked disappointment with its therapeutic results can be observed. Given an unaltered and outmoded theory, an almost unchanged therapeutic procedure, and a background of over-optimistic claims for therapeutic possibilities, psychoanalysts began to have doubts, often only unconsciously, and to lose faith in their method. At the same time the number of disappointed patients also grows. For several reasons this phenomenon is not as visible as it might be; many of the therapeutic gains are not based on the effects of the uncovering of the unconscious, but on faith in the correct "interpretation" of the analyst, and the wish not to have wasted a considerable investment in money and time. These results can be compared to the cures effected by a placebo, i.e., "transference cures," provided the condition is amenable to suggestion. Furthermore, many patients do not really want to change. They want to talk to somebody, somebody who does not criticize or scold them, and whose theory, to the extent that it explains the secret of mental life, becomes a substitute for religion, philosophy or politics. Among the people who are thus particularly attracted are the lonely or very narcissistic on the the one hand, and, on the other hand, the urban middle and upper middle class who have lost faith in God, in a moral law derived from God, and in political progress; for these psychoanalysis constitutes a frame of orientation and even devotion, thus fulfilling a universal human need.

The critique of Freud's theory began with Adler, who criticized the overemphasis on sex and stressed aggression, the wish for power and the effects of organic inferiority. He represented the superficial optimism of the new lower middle classes who were victorious and hopeful for a time just before and after 1918. He was extremely clever in discovering the "tricks" of the mind, but he lacked the profundity of Freud, and certainly his genius.

Jung, more gifted and brilliant than Adler, came from the opposite direction. He was the true heir of romantic anti-rational and anti-rationalistic thought, in some respects the heir of Friedrich Nietzsche, Nicolai Hartmann and Ludwig Klages. It is an ironical fact that Freud and Jung thought for a while that they had the same goals. In reality they were like two men going in opposite directions, meeting at some point along their separate roads, and talking together. For a while they may forget that they are not headed in the same direction, and that their common interest is but a momentary one. For Freud the unconscious was essentially irrational; yet he wanted to understand it in order to dissolve it or to control it. Jung, for whom the unconscious was a source of deep wisdom, wanted to get in touch with it in order to increase the deepest sources of man's vitality.

What was common to both Adler and Jung was the wish to found a school of their own, and this wish necessitated that they emphasize and blow up the points of their revision, and minimize the fundamental discoveries of Freud. Adler could not stand in Freud's shadow; Jung could not stand Freud, and his kind of thinking. For the anti-rationalist, reactionary romantic, the rationalism and intellectual sincerity of Freud became unbearable.

I shall not discuss Rank here; one of the most gifted of Freud's pupils, he, in many ways like Jung, had a profound understanding of mythology and symbolism. The history of his "defection" is complicated, and it would require more detailed research to arrive at a conclusion as to the real causes for his final split with Freud.[1]

The second group of revisions were made by authors who remained within the Freudian camp. The one to be mentioned first is Freud himself. A great deal of brilliant and intelligent effort has been applied lately by men like David Rapaport, Robert Holt, George Klein and others, to trace in minute detail the history of Freud's thought, and the development and change of his ideas. They did this not only out of sheer historical interest, but also in order to show that ego psychology had its roots already in Freud's earliest work. However, their detailed history is more brilliant than useful. Freud suffered from what one might call the tendency to over-theorize. He was deeply impressed by his teacher, E. Brücke, and the methods of the physiological laboratory. He hoped to formulate a psychological theory which would have the same accuracy and complexity as those of the physiologists of the time. In addition, it was a personal trait of his to spend a great deal of energy in making and re-making constructions, often only in loose connection with the empirical material. Freud's systematic change from the conscious/unconscious dichotomy to the tripartite ego/id/super-ego organization has been described as a fundamental revision of great significance. I believe that it was a rather small change in terminology and theoretical outlook, and that the essential assumptions remained the same. If one compares the early writings of Freud with the *Outline of Psychoanalysis* (5) which he wrote in the last year of his life, and with his 1937 paper, "Analysis Terminable and Interminable" (4), one sees how little Freud changed his basic concept and how much the fundamental points developed at the beginning of his scientific career remained unaltered to the end. There is only one substantially important change, and that is the one proposed in the twenties. It culminated in the assumption that the basic conflict in man is that between the life instinct (Eros)—including what was once called the ego instinct —and the destructive instinct, (death instinct). Perhaps under the impact of the unexpected outburst of destructiveness during the First World War, perhaps also as a result of certain disappointments with the libido theory, Freud revised his theory on this central point. He assumed

---

[1] Ernest Jones, in his biography, makes the point that Rank suffered from a psychosis and implies that this was the reason for his defection. I have tried to refute this version by quoting evidence that contradicts Jones' absurd statement (cf., 6).

that the drive for destruction, death, disintegration, etc., was as strong as Eros, the drive for integration and unification. Unfortunately he never succeeded in unifying the old and the new theories. The libido of the first epoch was the energy of the sexual drive arising from chemical processes within the organism; when too much tension was built up it created distress and the need for the reduction of tension (pleasure principle). The libido was supposed to have its base in certain erogenous zones (oral, anal, and finally, genital), while the life instinct, Eros, did not have such physiological roots. Rather, it was a general biological principle. Its aim was to unify and integrate, not to build up tension which, under normal conditions, was to be reduced in the sexual act. Nor was there any further clarification of the death instinct; it had no roots in any particular bodily zone. Moreover, it was applied to very distinct phenomena, such as aggression, hostility, sadism and destructiveness that cannot all be subsumed within the same category. Unfortunately most psychoanalysts did not bother to refine the new concept. Some refused to accept it altogether. Others simply used it as a new terminology for what had previously been called libido, sadism, aggressiveness, etc.[2] Thus, while Freud had undertaken a basic revision of his theory, this revision by-passed the problem of the real contradictions between his first and his second theoretical phases.

A number of other authors undertook thorough revisions of the Freudian theories and remained within the establishment of the Freudian organization. Among the most important of these were Frieda Fromm-Reichmann, S. Rado, A. Kardiner, F. Alexander and, more recently, R. Spitz and E. Erickson. Their theoretical revisions were often of a fundamental and far-reaching nature. They usually expressed them in such a way that the psychoanalytic bureaucracy did not take any steps against them.

The third group of authors who tried to revise Freud's theory are different from those described heretofore. They neither wanted to form new schools to compete with "psychoanalysis," nor did they want to restrict their formulations and teaching according to the dictates of the psychoanalytic bureaucracy. When organization pressure became too great and their positions untenable, they left the psychoanalytic societies to which they belonged. This group, often called "neo-Freudians," or "culturalists," were represented primarily by H. S. Sullivan, Karen Horney and E. Fromm.

[2] I have tried to connect the theory of the death instinct with Freud's earlier instinctual theory, and to show that the so-called "death instinct" is not a biological principle parallel to the life instinct, but a pathological phenomenon representing affinity to death, destruction, decay, and all that is not alive—in fact, it is the extreme form of what Freud had described as the anal libido (*cf.*, 7).

These three authors of the so-called "neo-Freudian school" had in common mainly two views: First, they could not accept Freud's libido theory any longer; and, secondly, they placed greater emphasis on cultural factors than the Freudian orthodoxy did. Actually, Freud himself had been much more concerned with social influences than were the "Freudians." Moreover, the rejection of the libido theory and the greater emphasis on social and cultural factors constituted a revision of Freud's theory which is no more drastic than that of many critics within the Freudian camp, for instance that of Kardiner, and, especially, that of the ego psychologists. The only difference is, perhaps, that the three afore-mentioned writers expressed their critiques earlier than their colleagues inside the Freudian organization, and with a great deal less interest in smoothing over the differences by appropriate verbiage. At the same time, however, there were many differences among them, and they should not be classified together in one "school." Sullivan's theory of interpersonal relations grew out of a most minute study of child development and the pathological processes of later life, particularly with regard to the more severe forms of mental illness. For him the central concepts are those of interpersonal relations and of the need of the individual to defend himself against anxiety. Horney's deviation began with her critique of Freud's theory of feminine development. She went on to emphasize many factors of great importance, such as the role of anxiety, the differentiation between neurotic and basic anxiety, the role of the self-image, of hostility and competition. Fromm differs from Sullivan and Horney in his concept of culture. He sees society in the dynamic sense of Marxist theory, and tries to understand how a particular practice of life resulting from the basic elements of social structure molds human passions in such a way that they become useful for the function of that particular social structure ("social character"). Fromm is not primarily concerned with what the ego psychologists call the ego function. Instead, his concern is with drives. He tries to establish a theory of drives based not on Freud's earlier mechanistic-physiological model, but on man's multiple possibilities to mould his energies as he relates himself to the world, through processes of assimilation and socialization. Aside from this more detailed and dynamic view of social influence, he also has tried to demonstrate man's need for a frame of orientation and devotion.

The fourth group to be discussed in this brief survey is a real "school" again, but one which has been formed within the orthodox movement, and, in fact, has become the leading exponent of present-day official psychoanalytic theory. I am referring to the school of "ego psychology," represented mainly by H. Hartmann, R. M. Loewenstein, G. Klein, E. Kris, B. Gill, D. Rapaport, R. H. Holt and R. W. White. While the views of the members of this group differ to some extent from each other, they represent, in essence, the same basic orientation, one which constitutes a revision of Freud's psychoanalysis. This revision is perhaps more drastic than the revision of any of the previously mentioned writers, with the exception of those of Jung and Adler. Their basic alteration revolves around the idea that, in order to become a general system of psychology, psychoanalysis must stress the function of the ego much more than was ever done by Freud. This sounds innocent enough if taken literally. Closer study, however, shows that the ego psychologists tend to substitute the interest in ego development for the earlier interest in the instinctual drives, although they never say that the Freudian instinctual drive is obsolete. They see the ego and the id no longer as polarities, but as a continuum. With the exception of the most archaic elements in the psychic apparatus, every psychic act may be regarded from two points of view, and may thus be seen as arising from the ego and the id, respectively. The same holds true for the fundamental differentiation Freud made between "primary" and "secondary" processes. They too are seen as part of a continuum, and no longer as two opposite modes of functioning. As far as energy is concerned, much is made of neutralized, de-sexualized energy, which is at the disposal of the ego. Freud's theory of the death instinct is utilized to account for the increased amount of neutralized energy on the assumption that the de-sexualized energy is complemented by energy stemming from the aggressive instincts, but in a de-aggressivized form. The ego psychologists assume a conflict free, autonomous ego sphere, and emphasize the ego apparatuses which include motility, learning, etc. Much of what they say is undoubtedly true, but the fact that there are many psychic functions which are not the result of libido or destructiveness is a discovery only for orthodox Freudians; they alone had believed that almost everything in mental life is the result of instinctual drives and conflicts. In their attempt to establish the importance of a "conflict-free," autonomous ego sphere, the ego psychologists even give up important positions in psychoanalysis. They do not investigate the impact of drives on learning and other ego functions, although they do not deny it. They question libido theory as inconsistent with recent findings in neurophysiology, but they do not attempt to revise the concepts of instinctual drives; they neglect the whole sphere of irrationality, always with proper assertions of their continuity with Freudian thought. They defend the legitimacy of their revision by an attempt to show that ego psychology appears already in the work of Freud prior to

1897, and by great emphasis on Anna Freud's book *The Ego and the Mechanisms of Defense* (3).[3] These comparisons are deceptive. It is perfectly true that, in the course of his work Freud became increasingly interested in the unconscious sectors of the ego, and that he and Anna Freud began to study the defensive functions of the ego more and more, as did others—for instance, Wilhelm Reich. But theirs was an altogether different undertaking from that of the ego psychologists, who try to show to what extent an autonomous and conflict-free ego is responsible for behavior, not only in the sense of defense, but in the sense of motivation.

David Rapaport gives an excellent summary of those parts of Freudian theory which are likely to last, and those whose survival is in doubt, according to the ego psychologists. Among the latter he mentions: 1) the specific drives, e.g., sex, aggression, love and death instinct, etc.; 2) the concepts of cathexis, bound and free energy, and neutralization; 3) the concepts of id, ego and super-ego; and 4) the concept of libido development. If these concepts are in doubt, then indeed concepts which the Freudians have supposed to be fundamental for Freudian analysis are in doubt, and the present revisions are no less drastic than those proposed by the so-called "revisionists." Not that I disagree with some of these revisions, nor do I believe that Horney or Sullivan would have disagreed. The crucial difference, however, is that Horney, Sullivan and I tried to find a more adequate frame of reference for the theory of irrational drives, while the ego psychologists de-emphasize what was most significant in Freud's contribution, and over-emphasize those aspects which had never been doubted by non-Freudian academic and experimental psychology. It seems that the ego psychologists are trying to stick formally to Freudian thought, especially to his *method* of thinking. At the same time, they deprive analysis of its radical character, namely, the unmasking of false consciousness, ideologies and rationalizations through the discovery of their irrational motivations. There is certainly a great deal of subtle and brilliant thinking in the theorizing of the ego psychologists; yet they hardly do more than attempt to make psychoanalytic theory respectable, especially in the eyes of academic psychology and from the standpoint of neurophysiological findings. If one considers the work of J. Piaget, L. S. Vygotsky, K. Bühler and many others, and their excellent and profound statements on child development, on the development of perception, cognition, etc., then the ego psychologists seem to be rather sterile, restricted to the demonstration that they too know the importance of these

[3] *cf.*, David Rapaport's introduction to Erickson (2).

phenomena, which academic and experimental psychology have handled quite successfully for many years.

The threat to psychoanalysis by ego psychology is in a way much greater than that which arose from Jung and Adler. Ego psychology emasculates psychoanalysis, that is, the basic discoveries of Freud. These were the discovery of the unconscious, irrational forces which determine the behavior of man; the discovery of resistance which is aroused in the attempt to uncover the repressions; the discovery of rationalization and symptoms which maintain the repression; and the discovery of the liberating and energizing effect on the whole personality if the unconscious is made to become conscious. Freud's theory was a radical critique of consciousness, not a theory which gave much importance to the role of an autonomous ego. It was the theory of a radical liberal whose specific object was a critique of Victorian sexual morality, and who based his theory on the assumption that the most important and most repressed motivations of man were the sexual drives in conflict with instincts seeking the preservation of the individual, i.e., ego instincts. From a sociological standpoint it is not difficult to see that Freud's radical concept was a narrow one. It stemmed from the culture of Victorian middle class society and, furthermore, it was dominated by the methods of mechanistic materialism which nowhere in the world had found as radical an expression as in the work of Brücke and Helmholtz. With the social changes that occurred after the First World War, especially in the face of the successful sexual revolution and the beginning of a highly alienated consumer culture, Freud's earlier assumptions lost much of their force. Given the altered social circumstances and the new findings of neurophysiology, the model of the libido theory and the pleasure principle had become outdated, and had lost much of their usefulness. But in the ensuing years, the liberal radicalism of Freud was transformed into a conservative liberalism and conformism which was to be characteristic of the psychoanalysts who formed the bureaucracy of the psychoanalytic movement.

The era after the First World War showed the strength of other irrational forces, and the importance of other human problems. First of all, it demonstrated the strength of aggressive, hostile and destructive forces in man, a fact which, as mentioned before, impressed Freud very much during the last part of his life. While the repression of sexual impulses is due essentially to specific norms and ideologies in a given society (and is not to be found in many other societies, be they primitive or highly developed), the repression of destructiveness is much more fundamental, because destructiveness and the love of death contradict life in all its forms and threaten any individual and social structure. Still other problems came to the fore. In a bureaucratic, industrialized society, man becomes progressively more alienated, has no contact with others, no genuine interests and feelings and transforms himself more and more into a thing. He becomes frightened and anxious, and he must try to repress his anxiety and the feeling of meaninglessness of his life. Indeed, his ego functions have developed marvelously, but these are not the problems that confront modern man. The shift of emphasis to the study of ego functions may gain for psychoanalysis the respectability, although not the achievement, of academic psychology. At the same time, such a shift deprives psychoanalysis of its radical, critical, and indeed, revolutionary character. In other words, it loses its identity as one of the most fruitful and profound discoveries in the field of the human mind.

This danger presented by the ego psychologists has been recognized by orthodox analysts such as Robert Waelder. In a critique of a paper by A. Kardiner, A. Karush and L. Ovsey (8), Waelder (10) expresses the view that "adaptionist" psychodynamics is a doctrine of radical rationalism and environmentalism that eliminates the inner frontier. More specifically directed against the ego psychologists is the critique by S. Nacht in a symposium on *The Mutual Influences in the Development of Ego and Id* (9). Nacht writes: "The attempt to raise psychoanalysis toward the heights of general psychology . . . as Hartmann, Odier and de Saussure among others . . . would like to do, seems to me sterilizing and a regressive step, to say the least, if it is aimed at a change of our methodology" (9, p. 55.) While I differ from psychoanalysts like Waelder and Nacht in that I believe that the classic concepts of Freud are in need of thorough revision, I share with them the conviction that the ego psychological school constitutes a retreat from the essence of psychoanalysis.

It would go far beyond the scope of this essay to outline the direction in which I see the future development of psychoanalysis. A few remarks must suffice here. The future of psychoanalysis, in my opinion, lies in the constructive revision of the theory of irrational drives, especially the examination of the destructive passions in man, a continuation of Freud's work on the death instinct, beyond the point where he left it. Closely related to the study of destructiveness is the study of the indifference to life which becomes ever more marked in contemporary industrial-bureaucratic society. Man ceases to love life, is attracted by organization, by all that is mechanical, and he is ready to sacrifice life to the demands of organization and gadgets. This indifference to life, and this attraction to what is not alive, is perhaps the most dangerous psychic factor threatening all our humanist values and, in the last analysis, our survival (*cf.*, 7).

Almost all of Freud's discoveries must be looked at afresh, freed of their framework of his "physiologizing" psychology. The concepts of ties to mother, the nature of the Oedipus complex, narcissism, love, anxiety, stand in need of revision. In addition, man's need for a frame of orientation and devotion (including a value system), and problems such as alienation and identity must be studied thoroughly. Eventually, the study of the economic, social and political structure of the society in its role of determining character, and also as a function of character, must be continued beyond its present status, especially through empirical socio-psychological research. Some authors have begun such revisions based on existentialist philosophy;[4] others, including myself, on the basis of Marx' humanism.

The study of the irrational motivations of man is only one of the tasks which confront psychoanalysis. Another is the study of the phenomenon of repression, especially, its individual and social causes. We still need to know a great deal more about the causes of repression, beyond the factors of castration fear, fear of abandonment, etc.; for example, the phenomenon of social isolation must be studied, the deepest fear, perhaps, which man has *qua* man. We know even less about the process of making the unconscious conscious, of conscientiation[5] or de-repression. What are the individual and social conditions for conscientiation, and why does conscientiation have the energizing, creative effect we so often observe? Since the theory of ab-reaction has been discarded no truly satisfactory explanation has been developed.

In connection with all these problems, a thorough revision of analytic technique seems to be indicated. The reality of the relationship between analyst and patient has been underestimated by the exaggerated use of the concept of transference. Too much emphasis has been placed on the genetic view of the repetition of early experiences. While this significance of early experience cannot be doubted, it is always necessary to look at psychic phenomena from a *functional* viewpoint. We must come to understand at each moment what goes on in the unconscious of a patient, even if we know nothing about his childhood. His dreams are like an X-ray picture of the person, and their analysis will remain, indeed, the "royal road" to the unconscious. It will prove even more fruitful once it is freed from too

---

[4] *cf.*, the work of L. Binswanger, R. May, and others.

[5] I use this word for "the making conscious" from the Spanish usage. It corresponds to the noun "repression" and is a badly needed term in all discussion on the effect of making the unconscious conscious.

much reliance on associations, and when the significance of universal symbols ceases to be underestimated. Freud's philosophical and physiological orientation imposed certain restrictions on his theory. I believe that if the theory is freed of these restrictions, his findings will be the basis for a new and fruitful development of psychoanalysis.

There is one condition for such a development which must be mentioned, even though briefly. Great harm has been done to psychoanalysis by transforming it into a "movement" administered by bureaucracies who control the members and determine what are the right and the wrong ideas. Thus, analysis as a science has been transformed into an ideology. It is clear that if people want to discuss problems they must have certain points of view in common, but what is common to psychoanalysis should have a much broader range than that which seems permissible to the present-day bureaucracy of the psychoanalytic organization. Indeed, this bureaucratic machinery has become absurd; even such issues as whether the patient lies on the couch or sits on a chair, whether he is seen five times or only twice a week, have been made to serve as the criterion of what is to be called psychoanalysis and what is not. An organization of psychoanalysts who share the interest in the study of unconscious strivings and processes, and who practice a therapy based on conscientiation is useful as long as it remains a loose, scientific organization that does not aim to determine who is a psychoanalyst, nor to control theory and therapy. Psychoanalysis would undoubtedly have had a much healthier and more productive development if it had dissolved itself as a 'movement' after Jung's secession in 1913. Eitingon, one of the seven members of the unofficial leading body of the movement, had the insight to express this very clearly in 1913 to Lou Andréas-Salomé, a most gifted and admired student of Freud's. Eitingon said to her in a conversation about the Munich Congress: "The best thing now would be for the whole association to blow up; in that way like minds could find one another honestly, and Freud would not be forced to go to war against attacks from his own camp, or to protect those who stand with him without being able to give full guarantee for their correctness (i.e., inferior supporters)" (1).

If pyschoanalytic theory and therapy are to overcome their present crisis, psychoanalysis must return to being once more a radical theory, not in terms of the year 1900 but in those of present day society. It must become critical of the ideologies which in personal and social life mask the increasing de-humanization and alienation of man. It must not try to be respectable except to the keenest minds in its own ranks, and the ranks of other scientists, and then not in terms of vested scientific interests and institutions. Freud dared to be impervious to the conventional thought of his time, but the kind of thought that was daring in 1900 is innocent and conventional today. In fact, paradoxical as it may sound, a scientific theory which remains essentially unchanged during sixty years ceases to be the same theory, even if it continues to use the same words.

To conclude: Though I am critical of the present situation of psychoanalysis, I am by no means skeptical about its future. If psychoanalysis becomes once again a radical, humanistic theory, its contribution to the understanding of human behavior, to the therapy of individual mental disturbances and to the "pathology of normalcy" will constitute significant progress in both theory and therapy. But a critique is a condition for constructive work.

This paper is a short summary of a chapter in a larger work in preparation under the tentative title *Humanist Psychoanalysis*, supported in part by Research Grant 5ROI MH 13144-02 from the National Institute of Mental Health, U.S. Public Health Service. I also want to express my sincere appreciation for the cooperation of Dr. Jerome Brams.

REFERENCES

1. Andréas-Salomé, Lou. *Freud Journal of Lou Andréas-Salomé*. Stanley A. Leary, ed. New York: Basic Books, 1964.
2. Erickson, E. H. Identity and the life cycle. *Psychol. Issues*, 1959, *1*, Monogr. 1. New York: International Universities Press.
3. Freud, Anna. *The Ego and the Mechanisms of Defense*. New York: International Universities Press, 1964.
4. Freud, S. Analysis terminable and interminable. *Internat. J. Psychoanal.*, 1937, *18*, 373. Reprinted in *Collected Papers*, Vol. 5, (J. Strachey, ed.) London: Hogarth Press, 1950, pp. 316–357.
5. Freud, S. *An Outline of Psychoanalysis*. New York: W. W. Norton, 1949.
6. Fromm, E. *Sigmund Freud's Mission*. New York: Harper & Row, 1959.
7. Fromm, E. *The Heart of Man*. New York: Harper & Row, 1964.
8. Kardiner, A., Karush, A. and Ovsey, L. A methodological study of Freudian Theory. I. Basic concepts. *J. nerv. ment. Dis.*, 1959, *129*, 11–19.
9. Nacht, S. Discussion of 'The mutual influences in the development of Ego and Id.' Symposium held at the 17th Congress of the International Psycho-analytical Association in Amsterdam, Holland, on August 8, 1951. Reprinted in *The Psychoanalytic Study of the Child. Vol. VII*. New York: International Universities Press, 1952.
10. Waelder, R. Adaptational view ignores 'Drive.' *Internat. J. Psychiat.*, 1966, *2*, 569–575.

VI

CONTRIBUTIONS TO METHODOLOGY

18

The Structure of Experimental Thought

by Walther Riese
Glen Allen, Virginia

In a general and somewhat vague fashion we tend to assert that the ancients did not understand the art of experimenting. To my knowledge J. Barthélémy Saint-Hilaire (1) was the first among modern thinkers who insisted that in antiquity experiments as well as observations were made. To be sure, the same author states in his preface that experimentation was but in its embryonic stage in the writings of Aristotle and the ancient naturalists. In a similar vein, we learn from L. Bourgey (8) that the authors of the *corpus hippocraticum*—who were not themselves members of the authentic Hippocratic school—used experimentation as the criterion of truth, even though their experiments served to illustrate and imitate a phenomenon rather than to reproduce it. Bacon is considered the father of experimental philosophy, and the history of medicine regards William Harvey as the first experimental physiologist. It is true that all these men conducted experiments. However, making experiments is not the same as the *experimental method*. The credit for having created this belongs to Claude Bernard.[1]

This eminent scholar defined his method on repeated occasions. In his *Introduction to the Study of Experimental Medicine* we read: "The experimenter tries to apply *determinism;* with the help of reasoning and of experiment he tries to connect natural phenomena with their necessary conditions or, in other words, with their immediate causes. By this means, he reaches the law which enables him to control phenomena. All natural philosophy is summarized in *knowing the law of phenomena*. The whole experimental problem is reduced to *foreseeing and directing phenomena*" (3, p. 57).

In this definition, reasoning serves the ultimate goal, namely the knowledge of controlling phenomena.

However, in the definition given in the *Cahier rouge* (5) the function of reasoning is no longer that of a tool ("with the help of which" one tries to connect the natural phenomena with their immediate causes); instead, reasoning has become the supreme goal, even the only goal, the true essence

[1] We read in Goldstein's autobiography (9) that his confidence was enhanced when he learned that his basic (i.e., holistic) concept was "so much in accordance with the theoretical interpretation of the French physiologist Claude Bernard . . ."

of the method. "What characterizes the experimental method is not so much the manner of obtaining the facts as the manner of reasoning with and about them" (5, p. 41).

Thus, a shift of emphasis has taken place in Bernard's thought. The stress is no longer on the artificial procedures of experimentation; instead, it is on the experimenter's reasoning. This shift of emphasis is even more pronounced in the definition given in Claude Bernard's posthumously published work: ". . . The experimental method does not consist in the indispensable use of certain experimental procedures, but rather in the employment of a certain intellectual process or rather of a mode of reasoning applied to the facts in order to elicit from them the truth" (6, p. 229).

Claude Bernard thus remained convinced that "for the experimental method, as everywhere else, *the only true criterion is reason*" (2, p. 122).

And so, in the last analysis, thought becomes the criterion of the experimental method. Bernard's method is a method of reasoning rather than of manipulation, a method of operating with the mind rather than with the hand. We must therefore recognize, in Bernard's method, a basic though unadmitted[2] "Copernican" element. He tried to see if one could not account better for the possibility of truth if one were to admit that the object gravitates around the subject, and not vice versa. My thesis derives strong reinforcement from significant passages in the posthumous work and the *Philosophie, manuscrit inédit* of Claude Bernard (4). We read in the *Principes de Médecine Expérimentale:* ". . . the mind of humanity taken as a whole advances like the mind of a single man; the same is true when man's mind is being applied to the development of the sciences; it progresses like the mind of a scientist dedicated to the solution of a special and isolated question" (6, p. 80).

This passage appears at the beginning of a chapter entitled *The development of the sciences in general represents the natural progress of the human*

[2] I agree with the conclusion of Reino Virtanen that Claude Bernard did "not recognize the novel character of the Copernican Revolution which Kant instituted . . ." and, in general, that Kant did not play a decisive role in the development of Bernard's thinking. (14, pp. 40–42).

However, the passages cited here and in my earlier paper on the same subject (13) leave no doubt concerning the existence of a Kantian element *implicit* in the experimental method. In fact, experimental reasoning rests on "absolute determinism" of the phenomena, and such determinism implies causal thought, i.e., one of Kant's pure conceptions of the understanding, or categories. Kant referred to his Copernican Revolution as to a new *method of thought* which is based on the principle that we only cognize in things *a priori* that which we ourselves place there. But he also referred to the new method of thought as to an *experiment,* thus shedding light at an early hour on the experimental reasoning uncovered in my paper and considered to be at the root of Claude Bernard's experimental method.

mind. There follows this paragraph: "Despite the seeming disorder and the infinite variety of circumstances that appear in the history of sciences we can, by analysis, bring order into this chaos, and we can always trace it back to the physiological laws of thinking; which proves that the history of science cannot be separated from the history of the human mind" (*ibid*).

This is no mere passing comment or extravagant idea (of which, in any case, there is hardly a trace in the writings of Claude Bernard); the same idea recurs in *Philosophie, manuscrit inédit.* "All these (i.e., religion, philosophy, science itself) constitute the reasoning of humanity which is analogous to the reasoning of each individual . . ." (4, p. 2).

Let us not commit the error and injustice of attributing this idea to romantic sources. The idea that the whole man embodies humanity was indeed dear to certain philosophers of the (German) romantic school who had always in view the unity, even the identity, of nature and spirit. Claude Bernard was violently opposed to such gratuitous speculations. In truth, the above cited passages disclose an undeniably rational character. Actually, it is the reasoning of the individual (scientist) that is shared by humanity and which the history of science reveals to us. The apparent chaos of the history of science is linked up with the laws of reasoning and thus made intelligible. Now we understand the importance of that other view of Bernard's according to which "the order of events and their rational linkage, that is to say, their cause-effect relations" are implied in the history of philosophy. And the eminent physiologist concludes: "Without this last point of view, history represents only simple annals or mémoires. That is to say, these are the mere raw material of history" (4, p. 3).

Thus it is that the great doctrines conceived as so many theories of experience, appear as *methods* for the scientist rather than as successive and independent phases of the irreversible course of the *historical* evolution of thinking humanity.

Now we understand Bernard's conclusion that experimental science finally arrives through "successive oscillations." "After an all too precipitous anticipation of rationalism (that is to say, of an hypothesis or a theory) one abandons rationalism, returns to the facts and then, having gathered a number thereof, one comes back to rationalism all the more willingly . . ." (6, p. 80).

What was important for him was "that rationalism and empiricism be well balanced in the progress of science."

The idea of oscillations recalls the groping of an experimenter towards an hypothesis. Claude Bernard described this state most eloquently: "One must project one's hypothesis forward as a snail projects his feelers to explore and palpate the space ahead. As soon as he perceives some obstacle he withdraws them, only to extend them anew towards the side . . ." (6, p. 78).

The passages cited show that the investigator's progress is cyclical, and that *experimental research passes through stages* (such as rationalism and empiricism) *which, when taken separately, are mutually exclusive; but when they are understood as methods of one and the same experimental reasoning, they complement each other*. To return to the "successive oscillations," we need to establish which one is the final stage. Is it rationalism, i.e., the hypothesis, or is it empiricism, i.e., the facts?

Claude Bernard did not leave this very important question unanswered. According to him, we are on experimental terrain as long as our theories are simply the expression of what we know, without being at all absolute. We lean on these theories to advance the cultivation of science, always careful to verify experimentally such new facts as we deduce from these theories (6, p. 79). Thus, we enlarge the theory through experiment which, to all appearances, has the last word.

The constancy of experimental results is the vulnerable element of the experimental method. Claude Bernard recognized the *individuality* of the living being, and he breaks this up into the individuality of external circumstances, of the inner environment, of the species, idiosyncratic, i.e., personal individuality, the individuality stemming from hereditary variation, from age, body build, sex, nutritional state and psychical influence. To these he added variation of effects according to time and repeated action of the agents (6, pp.156–157) among which we now recognize the modifying influences upon the result of electrical excitation of the cerebral cortex, thanks to the work of Sherrington, Dusser de Barenne, *et al.*

How can we then maintain the constancy of effects which is, after all, linked intimately to the idea of determinism so dear to Claude Bernard? I have turned to the repetition of individual phenomena in the thought of the experimenter who uses reasoning by analogy. The constancy of the effects can then be maintained intellectually, even if not factually (12, p. 91). In my analysis of the logical structure of experimental counterproof I arrived, in analogous fashion, at the conclusion, that the experimental work which comes to a halt in *reality* continues in the *thought* of the experimenter. The latter, believing that he has fulfilled the demands of determinism once he has furnished a proof followed by counterproof, or a series of proofs and counterproofs, anticipates the results of an infinite number of *virtual* proofs and counterproofs, a result which cannot be distinguished from that based on *real* experiments provided they are made, or imagined to be made, under the same conditions. The experimenter, who passes from individual results to their *generalization*, interprets the results of experiments he had *not* done by analogy with the results of experiments *actually completed*. At the very heart of experimental reasoning we find, therefore, *reasoning by analogy*.

Hence, if it is true that the experimenter who seeks a constant experimental effect despite infinite individual conditions and variations must fall back on reasoning by analogy as the ultimate criterion, then the experimental method itself emerges, once more, as a method of *reasoning*, leading from the initial reasoning of the preconceived idea to the final reasoning by analogy.

SUMMARY

There are to be found in Claude Bernard's writings several definitions of the experimental method. The author tries to derive from the classical texts and the posthumous writings of Claude Bernard the authentic meaning of his experimental method. It does not consist in the indispensable use of certain experimental procedures, but in the use of a certain intellectual procedure or, rather, in a mode of reasoning intended to derive truth from facts. However, due to never-lacking individual conditions and variations, the experimenter in search of a constant experimental result must refer to reasoning by analogy as the ultimate criterion of the experimental method, which thus emerges as a method of *reasoning* leading from the initial reasoning implied in the preconceived idea to the final reasoning implied in analogy.

REFERENCES

1. Barthélémy Saint-Hilaire, J. B. *Psychologie d'Aristote*. Opuscules (Parva Naturalia). Paris: Damont, à l'Institut, 1847.
2. Bernard, C. *Introduction à l'étude de la médecine expérimentale*. Preface by Jean-Louis Faure. Paris: 1926. Collection "L'intelligence."
3. Bernard, C. *An Introduction to the Study of Experimental Medicine*. Trans. Henry Copley Greene. With an introduction by Lawrence J. Henderson. New York: Macmillan, 1927.
4. Bernard, C. *Philosophie, manuscrit inédit*. Paris: Boivin & Cie, 1937.
5. Bernard, C. *Le cahier rouge*, 4th edition. Paris: Gallimard, 1942.
6. Bernard C. *Principes de médecine expérimentale*. Paris: Presses Universitaires de France, 1947.
7. Binet, L. *Esquisses et notes de travail inédits de Claude Bernard*. Recueillies et commentées par Léon Binet. Paris: Masson & Cie, 1952.
8. Bourgey, L. *Observation et expérience chez les médecins de la collection hippocratique*. Paris: Vrin, 1953.

9. Goldstein, K. Autobiography. W. Riese, (ed.). In *A History of Psychology in Autobiography,* Vol. V. New York: Appleton-Century-Crofts, 1967.
10. Riese, W. Le déterminisme de Claude Bernard et ses rapports avec la neurologie contemporaine. *L'encéphale,* 1934, *29,* 661–675.
11. Riese, W. Claude Bernard in the light of modern science. *Bull. Hist. Med.,* 1943, *14,* 282–294.
12. Riese, W. *La pensée causale en médecine.* Paris: Presses Universitaires de France, 1950.
13. Riese, W. La structure logique de la contre-épreuve expérimentale. (Interprétation d'une page de Claude Bernard). *Acta Biotheoretica,* 1958, *12,* 188–194.
14. Virtanen, R. *Claude Bernard and his place in the history of ideas.* Lincoln, Neb.: University of Nebraska Press, 1960.

Translated from the French by Marianne L. Simmel and revised by the author. This paper was supported by U.S. Public Health Service Research Grant MH-04011 from the U.S. Department of Health, Education, and Welfare, U.S. Public Health Service.

19

Dimensions of Knowledge

by Paul Oppenheim
Princeton, New Jersey

1

It is a common observation in methodological writings that a scientist can expend a given amount of intellectual effort in several ways. A scientist's knowledge is said to be abstract or concrete,[1] broad or deep, theoretical or observational, typifying or individualizing, specialistic or universalistic, nomothetic or idiographic, more or less balanced, strong or weak in terms of the total intellectual effort.

If we assume that the application of these terms to types of mentality is a derivative one, and that their primary application is to scientific "publications" (in a very broad sense, including, for example, verbal communications), we are led to the problem of constructing precise definitions of these concepts for a set of sentences while reserving the psychological terms for illustrative purposes. In doing so we follow a well-established tradition: concepts such as rational belief have already found definitions in formalized languages as properties of, or relations between, sets of sentences.

In this sense, it is the purpose of this essay to give a rational reconstruction for concepts used widely, and for a long time, in the literature of philosophy of science. We propose to construct a number of fundamental measures that are applicable to any publication, and which seem capable of being interpreted as "dimensions of knowledge." All of these measures are defined with the aid of two basic ones, namely *extensity* and *strength,* with the result that a high degree of systematization is achieved.

The concept of strength of a sentence, and hence of a set of sentences, has been explicated independently by Kemeny (10), and, under the name "Amount of Information" by Bar-Hillel and Carnap (1). Under another name, the concept of extensity has also been explicated by Goodman (5, chapter III; 6) and by Kemeny (11). We intend to show how certain other measures can be defined in terms of these two basic magnitudes, and how a scientific publication can be described with their aid. An account of strength and extensity will be given subsequently.

Our principal results may be anticipated here: it will develop that while

[1] As is well known, the distinction between "abstract" and "concrete" played an important role in Goldstein's work. For his application to scientific knowledge, *cf.* (4), especially pp. 63, 234–235.

a large number of formal measures of scientific publications can be defined in terms of our two basic concepts of extensity and strength, three other measures (described below) play, by their very nature, a fundamental role. The values of these three measures for a given publication can be considered as constituting its coordinates in a three-dimensional "logical space." Furthermore, they are independent; when the value of two of these "dimensions" is given, the value of the third is still completely open. Contrariwise, the other measures which are described later on, are not independent in the above sense.

The possibility of computing absolute or relative values of the various measures should not be rejected on *a priori* grounds, provided these values are mathematically well-defined. Individual judgments might differ, of course, as to the adequacy of our procedure. We realize that the constructions in this paper rest on severe simplifications. This is unavoidable when the first steps are taken in unexplored territory.

2

The concepts of strength and extensity belong to deductive logic. If our magnitudes are to have precise (syntactical) definitions, we must imagine that our language (i.e., the language of science, since we wish to speak about scientific publications) has somehow been formalized; that its syntax and semantics have been precisely specified. If all the meaning postulates (3, 12) are given when the language is formalized, then syntactical definitions can be given for our fundamental notions of strength and extensity, and, as a result, for all of the derivative notions that we shall introduce.

We shall not assume that the extra-logical constants of this language (which we shall call L) are logically independent, as has very often been assumed in the philosophy of science. (Many of Carnap's explications of logical truth and degree of confirmation presuppose this.) On the contrary, we assume that all terms in standard scientific use are admitted in L (after suitable clarification, where necessary). "Definitions" will be construed simply as meaning postulates of L.

In short, we assume, as have many serious writers on the logic of science, that the whole language of science has been formalized in *some* consistent way (20). But we will try to make our results independent of any specific assumptions about the *manner* of formalization. Then publications must be characterized in terms of conjunctions of assertions in our formal language. Since we are concerned only with empirical science, we may even say, "of *synthetic* assertions in our formal language." However, essential characteristics of publications would be lost if a publication were regarded *merely* as a conjunction of statements. If it could be, then, since a conjunction of sentences is itself a sentence, we could identify "publication" and "sentence," and say that we shall be concerned with *sentences* in a formalized language.

In general, however, a publication reports certain observations. These observations cannot be identified as such on the basis of the vocabulary they contain. On the one hand, an observation may be reported in theoretical terms, e.g., "I saw NaCl dissolve in H_2O"; and, on the other hand, an observational term may be used in a statement which is not a report of something that was actually observed. For example, "black" and "crow" are terms of the kind called "observation terms" in the recent literature of the philosophy of science: then "all crows are black" contains only observation terms, but it would certainly not be an observation report. Even the sentence, "In the tree there is a black crow" could function either as a report of an observation, or as an hypothesis.

Thus two publications might contain the same sentences, but might differ with respect to which of those sentences are taken as reports of observations, and which as theory. For this reason we shall think of a publication as an ordered pair of sets of sentences. The first set, O, consists of the observational part of the publication; the second set, T, consists of the theoretical part.

However, certain of our measures would become unreasonable if a further division were not made. A publication will, in general, consist not only of observational and theoretical statements, but will also make reference to "auxiliary theories," that is, to accepted theories from the literature of science. A publication which actually asserts very little in the way of theoretical statements might contain an extended reference to Newton's theory of gravitation. Counting this as part of the theory of publication would yield a result indicative of a highly theoretical publication, which is extremely counter-intuitive. For this reason, we divide a publication into three parts: the observational part; the auxiliary part; and the theoretical part. For the purposes of the measures to be defined in this paper, the auxiliary part will, in a sense, be neglected: it will be as if we considered a publication to consist of just O and T.

3

We wish to indicate briefly the nature of our two fundamental concepts, strength and extensity. At least one explication of each of these concepts exists in the literature. The discussion to follow will not presuppose that any particular explication for these two concepts is accepted, but only that some explication which is acceptable has been found, or can be found.

We may begin with the concept of *strength* which is intended to mean "amount of information." The term has been precisely defined by Kemeny (10). Since any statement can be expressed as a truth-function (which may be infinite) of atomic sentences, we may define strength of a basic sentence as unity, i.e., we say that any basic sentence has a strength of 1. Then a conjunction of independent basic sentences will have a strength which is simply the sum of the strengths of the particular sentences; e.g., a conjunction of three independent basic sentences would have the strength 3. Using the principle that the strength of a conjunction of independent sentences is the sum (and using certain other principles of a more technical nature), it has proved possible to define strength not only for restricted languages, but even for languages formalized within higher order predicate calculi. While we shall not presuppose any particular explication for the concept of strength, the features just mentioned might be taken as criteria of adequacy to be met by any explication of the concept. Clearly, a conjunction of independent assertions conveys an amount of information which is the sum of the amounts of information conveyed by the conjuncts.

The concept of *extensity* may be clarified by the following two remarks:

1. Extensity is an explicatum for "breadth of subject matter." The extensity of a publication depends on the number of predicates it uses, and also on the number of argument-places. It is, therefore, the formal opposite of Nelson Goodman's concept of "simplicity" (6); in fact, it may also be referred to as "complexity of vocabulary." Like strength, it has been defined for predicates of any degree and kind; and Kemeny has shown (11) that the definition may be extended to higher predicate calculi.

2. We may illustrate the concept with the numerical result for a special case. If a publication contains only independent one-place predicates, then its extensity is simply the number of these predicates. For example, a publication referring to "cat—non-cat," "black—non-black," and "carnivorous—non-carnivorous," uses as its primitive vocabulary three one-place predicates; it has ,therefore, the extensity 3. We will not even attempt to outline a general definition for extensity. That is necessarily very complicated because a publication in general contains dependent predicates, and we have to avoid counting a predicate too many times. For example, if a publication contains "male" and "parent," and also "father," then the predicate "father" does not add to the complexity of vocabulary of the

publication, since it can be defined in other terms occurring in the publication.

We must justify now our identification of the concept of "complexity of vocabulary" with the concept of extensity, or "breadth of subject matter." In the first place, the term "subject matter" has been used traditionally to indicate that the writers were thinking only of what we shall call the "taxonomic vocabulary." Thus, if one publication speaks of crows and another speaks of lions and dogs, normally one would answer the question "What are the subject matters of the respective publications?" by saying that the subject matter of the first publication is crows, and the subject matter of the second publication is lions and dogs. However, it seems to us that this notion of subject matter is overly simplified. Let us imagine a publication which speaks of a thousand species, but which, in each case, asks only one question: "Is there any correlation between the amount of salivation at the sight of meat, and the number of colds the animal gets during the year?" Normally someone would say, "Oh, that is really a very narrow publication. It is true that it speaks of many species, but it investigates such a limited question." Yet, we can also imagine that a publication about a single species, let us say ants, investigates so many aspects that we might be tempted to regard it as a comparatively broad publication. For this reason, it has seemed to us that in determining the breadth of subject matter of a publication, we must count the total vocabulary, that is, the total vocabulary of the observational and theoretical parts; the auxiliary part is neglected, as indicated above.

There remains the question as to *how* we should count. We believe that in the case of independent one-place predicates, simply counting each predicate as "one" is the most plausible suggestion. Thus, if a publication uses thirteen such predicates, it has a total breadth of subject matter, or extensity, of 13. It is further reasonable to say that in the case of dependent predicates in the publication, we should avoid "counting a predicate too many times" in the sense described above. In brief, there are not two distinct concepts, breadth of subject matter and complexity of vocabulary, but only one (16, p. 160).

While our primary interest is in the quantitative concept "breadth of subject matter," one may ask about the meaning of the term "subject matter," all the more since this term has been the occasion of some philosophical discussions. We take the *classes denoted by the predicates* in a publication as the *subject matter* of the publication. (One may also take "subject matter" in an intensional, rather than an extensional, sense. In this case, one takes the *attributes designated by the predicates*, instead of the classes denoted, as the subject matter.)

Since a publication may contain dependencies, its extensity number is not necessarily the same as the number of its classes or its predicates. If we are told that the extensity of a publication is 17, we cannot infer that it speaks of seventeen classes. But we can say that the classificatory power of its vocabulary is equivalent to the classificatory power of seventeen independent one-place predicates. We can make as *fine* a classification *as if* it spoke of just seventeen classes.

4

We have now introduced our basic magnitudes, extensity and strength. For many purposes, however, it will be more convenient to consider not the absolute strength of a publication, but its strength *relative* to its breadth of subject matter, which we shall call its *intensity*. If i stands for intensity, s for strength, and $ext(V)$ for the extensity of the vocabulary of a publication,

$$\text{D1.}\ i = s/ext(V).$$

Intensity or "amount of information per unit subject matter" may be thought of as representing the *thoroughness* with which a publication studies its subject matter. In view of its complementarity relation with breadth, we could also call it the "depth" of the publication; however, it seems to us that the term "intensity" expresses our concept better. The reader may regard the formal concept of intensity as an explicatum for one sense of the term "depth."

As we remarked at the outset, it is our intention to construct a "space" in which publications can be located. The *x-axis* of this space will be simply the extensity of the publication. Formally,

$$\text{D2.}\ x = ext(V).$$

We now turn to the magnitude just introduced, intensity or i. Intensity will not be one of our dimensions, because we have found that in giving an adequate description of the methodologically-relevant aspects of a publication, it is necessary to consider separately the intensity of the theoretical part and of the observational part of the publication. But let us temporarily treat i as if it were a separate dimension. We then have, so far, a two-dimensional "logical space" with coordinates i and x. In this space, any publication may be located: its position on the x-axis will indicate the breadth of its subject matter, and its position on the i-axis will indicate its depth or thoroughness.

From D1 and D2 we have immediately:

$$\text{T1. } xi = s,$$

that is, extensity multiplied by intensity equals strength. (See Figure 1.) We may call the curves of constant strength (the equilateral hyperbolas $s = ix =$ constant) *equistrength* curves. And we might picture a scientist arriving at a given strength of publication, i.e., at a given equistrength curve, by having travelled along various paths, if we allow his course to be charted by the locations of possible publications corresponding to the various stages in the preparation of his actual publication. If a publication exhibits great intensity, i.e., great strength per predicate, but comparatively few predicates—it has comparatively small extensity—then its location on an equistrength curve indicates relative concentration of its strength; if it has comparatively small intensity in proportion to its extensity, then its location indicates relative deployment of its strength. As a further step, we should like to indicate the course by which a given

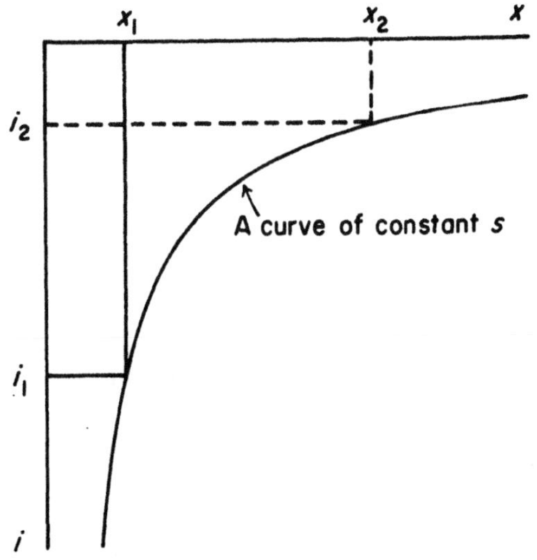

Figure 1. Dotted line represents accomplishment of broad and shallow publication. Solid line represents equal accomplishment of narrow and deep publication. $x_1i_1 = x_2i_2$

publication has arrived at its location on the equistrength curve by a specification of direction. For this purpose we might take the angle φ_1 (see Figure 2). However, as this has no direct logical interpretation, let us consider its tangent, the ratio of intensity to extensity,

$$\text{D3.}\ \gamma = i/x.$$

A curve of constant γ is a ray going through the origin. Hence this coordinate together with s, determines a polar-hyperbolic coordinate system (see Figure 2).

Figure 2 shows how we interpret Pascal's famous distinction between "fort et étroit" and "ample et faible." The more or less "ample" corresponds to high or low extensity. The more or less "fort" corresponds to high or low intensity. The direction angle, γ, indicates whether the scientist travels in the direction of being broad and weak, or in the direction of being narrow and strong. Thus we may refer to it as *the degree of concentration* of the strength of a publication.

This reflects only one of a number of possible interpretations of Pascal's statement. Our interpretation assumes that Pascal's distinction pre-

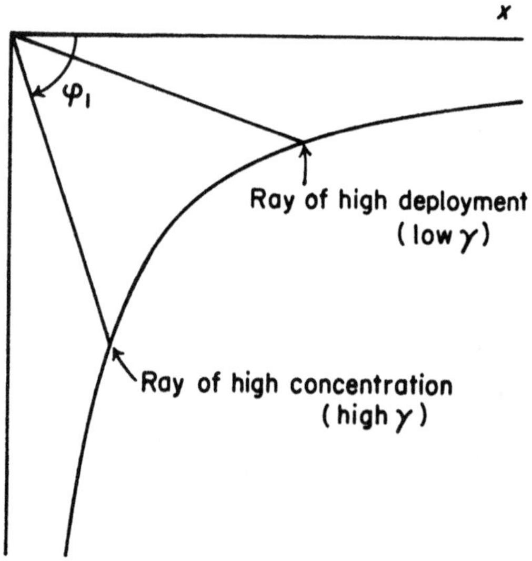

Figure 2

supposes a "constancy principle"; that is to say, that Pascal meant to compare only *publications of equal strength* (otherwise we would have had to consider also publications which are "broad and strong" and publications which are "narrow and weak"). Thus, we interpret Pascal as saying this: in a publication of *a given strength* the author can choose between two methods of allocating that strength: he may penetrate deeply into a small region, or he may thinly "blanket" a large region.

This is, of course, a dichotomous typology. Such typologies do not seem as useful as do magnitudes capable of degree (functors). Therefore, we have replaced this "Aristotelian dichotomy" by a *continuous* or graded conception (9) of degree of concentration.

Degree of concentration and extensity are independent. A publication may have a high degree of concentration and high extensity; but then it must have very great intensity (or it may have a low degree of concentration and very small extensity; but then it must have very low intensity).

We shall now extend the simple two-dimensional "logical space" to three dimensions. The new construction continues to rest on the assumption that there are two different but fundamentally equivalent ways of characterizing a given publication. These correspond to two different approaches to the geometry of a plane: The rectangular coordinate system and the polar-hyperbolic system. Thus, on the one hand, we may characterize a publication by its breadth of subject matter, or extensity, and its depth, or intensity; on the other hand, we may characterize a publication by its degree of concentration, that is to say, by the direction in which it moves, i.e., either in the direction of being more "fort et étroit," or in the direction of being more "ample et faible"; and by how far it moves in that direction, that is, by its strength, or the amount of information it conveys. One might intuitively feel that these are two somewhat different ways of characterizing a publication. It is indeed surprising to discover that the concepts stand, under our explication, in this neat geometrical relationship.

5

It would seem dangerously artificial, however, to proceed much beyond these remarks without taking account of the important distinction between theory and observation. Therefore, we now take up the distinction between the theoretical part of a publication and its observational part. Henceforth we shall locate a publication not in the plane of the diagrams previously given (Figures 1 and 2), but in three dimensions. A formulation in words follows the symbolic definitions:

D4. $y = O/x$ (the observational intensity),
D5. $z = T/x$ (the theoretical intensity), where
D6. $O = s_0$ (the observational strength),
$T = s - O$ (the theoretical strength).

That is, we take the x-coordinate to be the extensity itself, as before. The y-coordinate is the ratio of observational strength to extensity, while the z-coordinate is the ratio of theoretical strength to extensity. The observational strength of a publication is just the strength of its observational part. The theoretical strength is the difference between total strength and observational strength. It might seem more natural to let theoretical strength be the strength of the publication's theory, sT, but since O is normally relevant to T as factual support (13), it is not independent of it, and hence the strength of the theory plus the strength of the observations would be greater than the total strength of the publication. This is avoided by defining T as the difference between s and O, which cancels out the strength of the overlapping content.

With these definitions for a three-dimensional space, we have two principles as consequences of the single principle of our two-dimensional space, $ix = s$. These are $xy = O$ and $xz = T$. In other words, the extensity multiplied by observational intensity equals observational strength, and the extensity multiplied by theoretical intensity equals theoretical strength.

Let us proceed to the *units* for each of our cases. For simplicity's sake, we shall call an atomic sentence that is not an observation sentence an *atomic hypothesis*. Then we may say that the x-coordinate is measured in "imps" (independent monadic predicates), the y-coordinate is measured in atomic observation per predicate, and the z-coordinate is measured in atomic hypotheses per predicate.

Of course, this does *not* mean that a publication with the locus: extensity 17, theoretical intensity 3, observational intensity 3, is necessarily written with 17 independent one-place predicates, and contains 51 independent atomic hypotheses and 51 independent atomic observations. The sense is rather as follows: a) its vocabulary has the same *classificatory power* as a vocabulary of 17 independent monadic predicates (so that 17 is the *equivalent number* of "imps"); b) the strength of its theoretical part (having discarded any "overlapping content" with the observational part) is the same as the strength of 51 independent atomic sentences (so that 3 is the *equivalent number* of "atomic hypotheses per predicate"); c) the strength of the observational part is the same as the strength of 51 independent atomic sentences (so that 3 is the *equivalent number* of "atomic observations per predicate").

The z = zero plane is the locus of all purely observational or descriptive publications, such as publications by a historian who writes a mere chronicle, or a geographer who merely locates, or a mere recorder of "curiosa."

In our three-dimensional space, the loci of publications of equal strength are, of course, no longer curves but hyperbolic surfaces. To locate publications by strength and direction ,i.e., by the directions in which their writers have gone, and by their final accomplishments, we need another coordinate. Though we might choose angle φ_2 (see Figure 3), we prefer the tangent of the angle, and define degree of theoretization, θ, as the ratio of theoretical strength to observational strength.

$$\text{D7. } \theta = T/O$$

Although closely related to our z-coordinate, theoretical intensity, it is not the same. A weak and purely speculative publication could have an infinite degree of theoretization, θ, but would have a low z because of its low strength. Conversely, a publication with high or maximum z could

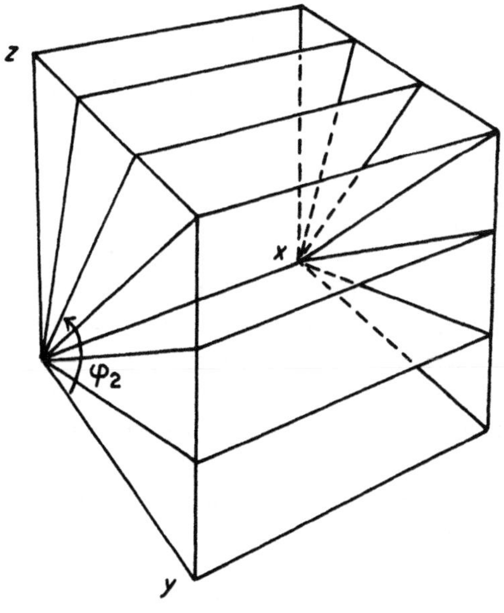

Figure 3

have considerably less than maximum degree of theoretization if it contained such observational material.

A publication's direction or tendency is now determined by two factors: its degree of concentration, and the extent to which it is theoretical, i.e., contains hypotheses which go beyond accepted observational facts. Thus γ and θ together determine a ray, giving the direction; s tells us how far to go in this direction. This is the natural generalization of the two-dimensional polar-hyperbolic system.

To see these and other features more clearly, we may examine the *transformation equations* connecting the x, y, z coordinates with the γ, θ, s coordinates (16, pp. 168–169).

With this we have completed the task of introducing our dimensions and of extending the result given for two dimensions to our whole "logical space."

Before leaving the subject of our fundamental dimensions, we wish to add a remark on the problem of "incidental material."

If a predicate conveys very little information, e.g., if the sentences containing it could be deleted without much decreasing the strength of the publication, it should be counted as contributing little or nothing to the extensity of the publication. This idea has been formalized (16, p. 172).

6

From this point forward, we shall be concerned mainly with the explication of the following three distinctions: 1) The distinction between the "universalist" and the "specialist," or rather, with the logical analogue of the psychological distinction between "universalistic" and "specialistic" publications; 2) the distinction between "typifying" and "individualizing" publications; and 3) the distinction between "nomothetic" and "idiographic" publications. In addition to defining three "indices" which will constitute syntactical counterparts of these three distinctions, we shall also define certain related or subsidiary concepts.

In the following sections, we make the usual divisions of the total vocabulary of our language L into individual-vocabulary (IV) and predicate-vocabulary. Furthermore, we have found it convenient to divide the predicate-vocabulary into taxonomic terms or taxonomic vocabulary, TV, and attribute-vocabulary, AV.

We begin with the concept "specialist." A scientist may be a specialist in different ways. Thus we might speak of an "attribute specialist," i.e., a scientist who studies very few attributes, in the limiting case only one; for example, a scientist who investigated only "blueness" would be an extreme attribute specialist. The opposite extreme is the scientist who is concerned with all attributes; such a scientist would be the extreme "attribute universalist."

Similarly, a scientist may investigate only one taxonomic group, or he may be concerned with an elaborate part of the taxonomic system. In general, the breadth, or its opposite, the narrowness, of the TV of a publication determines whether an author is a taxonomic universalist or specialist. This distinction between taxonomic and attribute-specialization—or universality—is useful in clarifying cases in which these concepts are confused in everyday language (16, p. 175).

Combining these two ideas, we find that the measure of total universality or specialization of a publication is simply its extensity, x. But since normalized measures are in this case more intuitive than non-normalized, we prefer to divide this by the extensity of the total vocabulary of L, x_L, (since this represents the maximum of any corrected or uncorrected extensity), to get U, our measure of "*degree of universality*":

$$\text{D8.} \quad U = x/x_L$$

U is thus a measure of total universality or specialization, without distinction between attribute-universality or -specialization, and taxonomic-universality or -specialization. But we may still distinguish other types of specialization and universality; if the publication has a relatively complex taxonomic vocabulary, compared to the complexity x_{TS} of the total taxonomic system, or if the quantity x_{TV}/x_{TS} is close to 1, the publication exhibits taxonomic-universality (and if the quotient is close to 0, taxonomic-specialization); similarly, if x_{AV}/x_{AVL} is close to 1, where x_{AVL} is the extensity of the total AV of L, the publication exhibits attribute-universality (and if the quotient is close to 0, attribute-specialization). In applying these latter indices, it is important that the publication be formalized in such a way that all species mentioned in it appear explicitly, e.g., "man" must be used, not "rational animal," etc.

The limits of U as defined by *D8.* are easily seen: The ideal "polyhistor" investigates every taxonomic group with respect to every predicate. Thus, he requires a vocabulary which is equivalent to (and therefore as broad as) the whole vocabulary of L. Hence in this case $U = 1$. Conversely, $U = 1$ only if the publication, when written in the simplest way one can find, requires the total vocabulary. At the other extreme is the publication which mentions one taxonomic group and one attribute. For such a publication, which may be regarded as the logical outcome of specialization carried to the limit, $U = 2/x_L$ (=0 approx.). In general, U will increase as the publication *either* studies more taxonomic groups, *or* investigates its taxonomic subject matter with respect to more attributes, or both.

In short, the measures of universality U is simply the extensity of the publication *normalized* by dividing by the extensity x_L of the total vocabulary.

The degree of universality of breadth of subject matter of a publication must be carefully distinguished from the *degree of concentration* of its strength, discussed above. A publication may be universalistic and still have a high degree of concentration; but then it must be very strong (or it may be specialistic and nevertheless have a low degree of concentration; but then it must be very weak). The difference is that universality and specialization depend on the absolute breadth of subject matter, i.e., ignoring strength, whereas the degree of concentration depends upon the strength, as well as upon the breadth of subject matter.

For publications of *the same strength*, degree of universality and degree of concentration are indeed correlated, as is stated by the following theorem.

T4. For publications of the same strength, U and γ are monotonically decreasing functions of each other.

Let us call $\delta = 1/\gamma$ the *degree of deployment*. Then, for publications of the same strength the following conditions are equivalent: extensity is large (or small), deployment is large (or small); and likewise, intensity is large (or small), concentration is large (or small):

T5. For publications of the same strength, x and δ, and i and γ, respectively, are monotonically increasing functions of each other and have simultaneously the same limits (zero and infinity).

In short, when one is comparing publications of the same strength, concentration and intensity are virtually the same magnitude, and likewise deployment and extensity (or universality). However, when the strengths are not the same, these magnitudes are quite independent.

The fact is that publications of the same strength, being "ample et faible" or "fort et étroit," can be characterized in a number of different ways, as a consequence of T5. This may explain why it is that Pascal's remark is open to a number of interpretations. Of course, there may be still other interpretations which cannot be expressed in terms of our dimensions.

7

As the extensity of the individual-vocabulary of a publication is always zero, one respect in which publications differ is the range of individuals they concern. While none of our basic measures, i.e., the dimensions, depends upon it, it seems interesting to seek a measure of the range of the individual-vocabulary of a publication. The most obvious suggestion is to take, as the measure in question, simply the number of members of IV, that is, the number of individual-names plus the individual-descriptions occurring in a publication.

With the aid of this measure, we can define an index which will perhaps formally correspond to a distinction which has been used almost as widely as the specialist-universalist distinction explicated above. We refer to the distinction between "individualizing" and "typifying" publications.

We introduce $x = ext(P)$ as the extensity of a publication. Hence x is a measure of the number of predicates employed in the publication. On the other hand, R is the range of the individual-vocabulary, just defined. Thus, the quotient, $\tau = R/x$ is the ratio of individual-names to predicates, or number of individual-names per predicate, and may be taken as the *degree of typification*. In other words, a publication which speaks of few individuals, but describes them by means of many predicates, is highly individualizing; whereas a publication which speaks of many individuals in terms of few predicates, is highly typifying. (This leads to the relation $R = \tau x$, between our measures for breadth of individual-vocabulary and for breadth of predicate-vocabulary.) Further, typification, in the present sense, is one kind of "abstractness," and individualization one kind of "concreteness."

For example, consider the following publications:

1) a_1 is a lion . a_2 is a lion . a_3 is not a lion . a_4 is a lion . a_5 is not a lion . . .
2) a_1 is a lion . a_1 is carnivorous . a_1 is intelligent . a_1 is large . a_1 is unfriendly . . .

The first classifies each individual ($a_1, \ldots an$) as a lion or not lion; hence it is highly typifying: the second uses many predicates for the individual; hence it is highly individualizing.

Under our formula $\tau = R/x$, we have for publication 1), $\tau = n$, while for 2) $\tau = 1/n =$ approx. 0 (for large n). Thus, the first publication receives a high, and the second a very low value of τ.

The measure of typification may be normalized, i.e., may be made to take on values from -1 to $+1$, by taking $\tau = (R - x)/(R + x)$. According to the normalizing formula, for publication 1) $\tau = (n - 1)/(n + 1) =$ approx. 1; while for publication 2) $\tau = (1 - n)/(1 + n) =$ approx. -1, which seems in accordance with our intuition. Note however, that this index in its present meaning has nothing to do with generalized sentences. Therefore, in its computation only the singular sentences of the publication may be considered.

8

Finally, let us turn to Windelband's (19, p. 145) distinction between "nomothetic" and "idiographic" scientific publications. A nomothetic work, in Windelband's sense, is one which contains mainly universal laws: the classic example is a work in theoretical physics; while an idiographic work is one in which individuals are studied in their uniqueness: the classic example would be a biography (*cf.* 16, pp. 182–184).

One might ask whether "nomothetic-idiographic" can be defined by a combination of theoretization and typification; i.e., that *necessary* and *sufficient* conditions for "nomothetic" are 1) high degree of theoretization, and 2) high degree of typification; while necessary and sufficient conditions for "idiographic" are 1) low degree of theoretization, and 2) low degree of typification. But we cannot agree with this.

A publication is idiographic if it consists of many statements about particular events or individuals. It is equally idiographic whether these statements belong to the O part or the T part of the publication; they could belong to either. Thus, a publication may be idiographic and have either a high or a low degree of theoretization.

Furthermore, a nomothetic publication is simply one that consists mainly of universal laws (including statistical laws). Thus, a nomothetic publication has a high degree of theoretization. If it refers to individuals, it can refer to many cases or to just one individual (for instance, if many hypotheses are being exemplified or tested by means of a single case). Thus, a publication may be nomothetic and have either a high or a low degree of typification.

In short, all we can say is this: *if* a publication is nomothetic, it must have a high degree of theoretization (but not conversely); and *if* a publication is idiographic, it must have a low degree of typification (but not conversely).

9

The measures discussed up to now are by no means the *only* ones which could be defined within the logical space developed here. Among other such measures, we mention three which have been dealt with in other publications: Degree of Confirmation (7 and 8, Article 10), Degree of Factual Support (13) and Systematic Power (14). Each of these concerns, in a sense, the relations between the observational and the theoretical parts of a publication.

In addition to these three measures the "logical space" developed here may have psychological implications as suggested at the beginning of this paper: One might define psychological traits corresponding to our syntactical measures of publications. That is, a publication by a scientist can itself be regarded as a "psychological test"; then the degree of theoretization, θ, (for example) would be the "score" on this "test." In this sense, the θ of his publications operationally defines a degree of theoretization for the *scientist.* As a matter of fact, Kling (15) and Ross (18) have used the method of factor analysis in order to investigate the value of these concepts for a psychological description of persons. Conversely, there may be many distinctions within psychology which could be explicated with the help of the concepts developed here.

It would be interesting to see if there are laws connecting psychological factors indicated by the location of a publication in our "logical space," e.g., a scientist's degree of theoretization, or his degree of concentration, with other psychological factors, perhaps factors of "personality" type—or with physiological factors. It seems strange to us that there are virtually no illustrations of this in the literature, even on a speculative level. The only illustration known to us is a remark by Carnap (2, p. 218), to the effect that introverts tend to be more abstract and theoretical, extroverts more concrete and observational in scientific work. Some debates between experimentalists and theoreticians, between typifiers and individualizers, between humanists and natural scientists, etc., might be revealed in this way as pseudo-conflicts, i.e., as clashes of intellectual personality types rather than as genuine doctrinal differences in scientific method.

The concepts developed here may be useful in still another respect: If one considers sciences as exemplified by scientific publications, our "logical space" can be extended to all of science. In particular, it seems possible that some of our basic measures can be used to provide a natural order of scientific disciplines (17).

An earlier, more extensive version of this paper was published in *Revue Internationale de Philosophie,* No. 40, 1957, Fascicule 2, pp. 151–191.

While the author alone takes the responsibility for the content of this article, he would not have been able to develop his ideas in the present form had it not been for Bohnert, H. G., Brody, N., Hempel, C. G., Kemeny, J. G., and Putnam, H., each of whom made very important suggestions and contributions to the final formulation. This is hereby acknowledged with sincere appreciation.

REFERENCES

1. Bar-Hillel, Y., and Carnap, R. Semantic information. *Brit. J. Philos. Sci.*, 1953, *4*, 147–157.
2. Carnap, R. *Logical Foundations of Probability.* Chicago: The University of Chicago Press, 1950.
3. Carnap, R. Meaning postulates. *Philos. Stud.*, 1952, *3*, 65–80.
4. Goldstein, K. *Human Nature.* Cambridge: Harvard University Press, 1940.
5. Goodman, N. *The Structure of Appearance.* Cambridge: Harvard University Press, 1950.
6. Goodman, N. Axiomatic measurement of simplicity. *J. Philos.*, 1955, *52*, 709–722.
7. Helmer, O., and Oppenheim, P. A syntactical definition of probability and of degree of confirmation. *J. Symb. Logic*, 1945, *10*, 25–60.
8. Hempel, C. G. *Aspects of Scientific Explanation.* New York: The Free Press, 1965.
9. Hempel, C. G., and Oppenheim, P. *Der Typusbegriff im Lichte der neuen Logik.* Leiden, 1936.
10. Kemeny, J. G. A logical measure function. *J. Symb. Logic*, 1953, *18*, 289–308.
11. Kemeny, J. G. Two measures of complexity. *J. Philos.*, 1955, *52*, 722–733.
12. Kemeny, J. G. A new approach to semantics. (Part I), *J. Symb. Logic*, 1956, *21*, 1–27.
13. Kemeny, J. G., and Oppenheim, P. Degree of factual support. *Philos. Sci.*, 1952, *19*, 307–324.
14. Kemeny, J. G., and Oppenheim, P. Systematic power. *Philos. Sci.*, 1955, *22*, 27–33.
15. Kling, F. R. An empirical study related to "Dimensions of Knowledge". *Rev. Internat. Philos.*, 1957, *40*, 194–205.
16. Oppenheim, P. Dimensions of knowledge. *Rev. Internat. Philos.*, 1957, *40*, 151–191.
17. Oppenheim, P. A natural order of scientific disciplines. *Rev. Internat. Philos.*, 1959, *49*, 354–360.
18. Ross, J. Three cognitive dimensions. *Psych. Rep.*, 1965, *17*, 291–300.
19. Windelband, W. *Präludien.* Vol. 2. Tübingen: J. C. Mohr (Paul Siebeck), 1915.
20. Woodger, J. H. *The Technique of Theory Construction.* Chicago: The University of Chicago Press, 1939.

VII

BIBLIOGRAPHY

20

Bibliography of the Published Writings of Kurt Goldstein

by JOSEPH MEIERS
New York, New York

INTRODUCTION

To our knowledge no complete bibliography of Kurt Goldstein's writings has been available heretofore. On four previous occasions the present writer has been engaged in compiling such a bibliography.

The first was intended as a modest offering to Goldstein, my teacher, for his seventieth birthday, in 1948, the year when his career as a physician and scientist comprised a span of forty-five years. That bibliography contained only about one hundred entries and was, of necessity, quite incomplete. At that time the writer was unable to consult the libraries in New York City; information was difficult to obtain from sources in West Germany, while communication with those in the Soviet zone was practically nil. In addition, this labor of love was to be a birthday surprise which precluded inquiries of the celebrant.

This surprise element continued to be a factor, though to a lesser degree, in the second bibliographical endeavor undertaken for Goldstein's eightieth birthday. In the interim, I had consulted his personal collection of reprints. This collection, however, was far from complete, since it contained of his earlier papers only those he had rapidly gathered on his departure from Germany in 1933. Among them were many of his shorter articles and some records of participation in symposia, discussions, etc. By that time communication with German sources had become more satisfactory, and some additional material was obtained from them.

This second bibliography (1903–1958) was arranged by topics, and within each topic, chronologically. Kurt Goldstein himself preferred such an arrangement as it was handier for readers and research workers.

The third compilation of Goldstein's publications was done by myself and Dr. Norbett Mintz during the winter of 1958–1959. This one was limited to the writings published after Goldstein's arrival in the United States, thus to the years 1936–1959. In many ways this task was easier than the earlier attempts had been, especially since almost all entries were in English, and the reference and bibliographical details readily available.

Goldstein heartily appreciated this bibliography, part of an offering for his eightieth birthday; it was published in the *Kurt Goldstein 80th Anniversary* issue of the *Journal of Individual Psychology*, May 1959; throughout his later years Goldstein used it frequently, especially in reply to inquiries that came to him from many places.

Additional items that had come to my attention were published after his death as a supplement accompanying a memorial article—a fourth step in this sequence of bibliographies. For the present contribution my aim has been a complete bibliography of the works of Kurt Goldstein. It includes more than fifty entries not contained in the previous compilations. Still, it is not impossible that some writings by Goldstein have remained undiscovered despite diligent and systematic search, both here and abroad. There are a few of his papers that are unpublished as yet.

Part II of this bibliography contains a selection of articles about Kurt Goldstein, and a listing of special issues of journals published in his honor. A more comprehensive bibliography of writing about Kurt Goldstein is on deposit at the American Documentation Institute.[1] It contains reviews, discussions, obituaries, etc.; by its very nature it remains as yet incomplete.

Mr. and Mrs. William Haudek have offered to assist scholars in quest of rare or hard-to-find writings by Kurt Goldstein. Almost all writings can be inspected upon request, and reprints of many articles are available. Inquiries and requests should be addressed to Mrs. William Haudek, 1080 Fifth Avenue, New York, N. Y., 10028.

It remains for me to express my gratitude to those many persons, both here and abroad, who greatly facilitated the compilation of this bibliography. Among them must be named: Dr. Agnes Stählin, librarian of the University of Erlangen, Germany; Dr. Marianne L. Simmel, the editor of this volume; Dr. Goldstein's daughter, Mrs. William Haudek; Ann D. Meiers; and others too numerous to be mentioned by name.

I should like to close this introduction with the words of Gotthold Ephraim Lessing—words with which Kurt Goldstein fully concurred:

"... We would rather be given less praise
And prefer to be read all the more!"

---

[1] This more comprehensive bibliography of writings about Kurt Goldstein has been deposited as Document number 9498 with the ADI Auxiliary Publications Project, Photoduplication Service, Library of Congress, Washington, D.C., 20540. A copy may be secured by citing the Document number and by remitting $2.50 for photoprints, or $1.75 for 35 mm. microfilm. Advance payment is required. Make checks or money orders payable to: Chief, Photoduplication Service, Library of Congress.

Part I: Writings by Kurt Goldstein

1903

1. Beiträge zur Entwicklungsgeschichte des menschlichen Gehirnes. I. Die erste Entwicklung der grossen Hirncommissuren und die "Verwachsung" von Thalamus und Striatum. (Vorläufige Mitteilung). *Anatomischer Anzeiger*, 1903, *22*, 415–417.
2. Beiträge zur Entwicklungsgeschichte des menschlichen Gehirnes. I. Die erste Entwicklung der grossen Hirncommissuren und die "Verwachsung" von Thalamus und Striatum. *Archiv für Anatomie und Physiologie, Anatomische Abteilung*, 1903, 29–60.
3. *Die Zusammensetzung der Hinterstränge. Anatomische Beiträge und kritische Übersicht.* Inaugural Dissertation, University of Breslau, 1903.
4. Die Zusammensetzung der Rückenmarkshinterstränge. *Monatsschrift für Psychiatrie und Neurologie*, 1903, *14*, 401–427.

1904

5. Die Abhängigkeit der Muskulatur vom Zentralnervensystem während der Embryonalzeit. *Archiv für Entwicklungsmechanik der Organismen*, 1904, *18*, 584–592.
6. Kritische und experimentelle Beiträge zur Frage nach dem Einfluss des Zentralnervensystems auf die embryonale Entwicklung und die Regeneration. *Archiv für Entwicklungsmechanik der Organismen*, 1904, *18*, 57–110.
7. Versuch einer Einteilung der Rückenmarkshinterstränge. *Deutsche Zeitschrift für Nervenheilkunde*, 1904, *25*, 456–464.
8. Zur Frage der Existenzberechtigung der sogenannten Bogenfurchen des embryonalen menschlichen Gehirns, nebst einigen weiteren Bemerkungen zur Entwicklung des Balkens und der Capsula Interna. *Anatomischer Anzeiger*, 1904, *24*, 579–595.
9. Zur vergleichenden Anatomie der Pyramidenbahn. *Anatomischer Anzeiger*, 1904, *24*, 451–454.

1905

10. Untersuchungen über das Vorderhirn und Zwischenhirn einiger Knochenfische. *Archiv für mikroskopische Anatomie und Entwicklungsgeschichte*, 1905, *66*, 135–219.

1906

11. Ein Beitrag zur Lehre von der Aphasie. *Journal für Psychologie und Neurologie*, 1906, *7*, 172–188.
12. Merkfähigkeit, Gedächtnis und Assoziation. Ein Beitrag zur Psychologie des Gedächtnisses auf Grund von Untersuchungen Schwachsinniger. *Zeitschrift für Psychologie und Physiologie der Sinnesorgane*, 1906, *41* (1. Abteilung), 38–47; 117–144.
13. Zur Frage der amnestischen Aphasie und ihrer Abgrenzung gegenüber der transcorticalen und glossopsychischen Aphasie. *Archiv für Psychiatrie und Nervenkrankheiten*, 1906, *41*, 911–950.

1907

14. Casuistische Beiträge zur Symptomatologie der Erkrankungen der motorischen Kernsäule. *Archiv für Psychiatrie und Nervenkrankheiten*, 1907, *42*, 1072–1085.
15. Ein Beitrag zur Lehre von den Alcoholpsychosen; nebst einigen Bemerkungen über die Entstehung von Halluzinationen. *Allgemeine Zeitschrift für Psychiatrie und psychisch-gerichtliche Medizin*, 1907, *64*, 240–285.
16. Einige Bemerkungen über Sprach-Halluzinationen. *Allgemeine Zeitschrift für Psychiatrie und psychisch-gerichtliche Medizin*, 1907, *64*, 713–714.

1908

17. Ein Fall von manisch-depressivem Mischzustand, (zugleich ein Beitrag zur Lehre von der Ideenflucht und den Hallucinationen). *Archiv für Psychiatrie und Nervenkrankheiten*, 1908, *43*, 461–504.
18. Intermittierendes Hinken eines Beines, eines Armes, der Sprach-, Augen- und Kehlkopfmuskulatur. Intermittierendes Hinken oder Myasthenie? *Neurologisches Centralblatt*, 1908, *27*, 754–762.
19. *Über das Realitätsurteil halluzinatorischer Wahrnehmungen.* Inaugural Lecture, University of Königsberg, 1908. Privately printed.
20. Zur Lehre von der motorischen Apraxie. *Journal für Psychologie und Neurologie*, 1908, *11*, 169–187; 270–283.
21. Zur Theorie der Hallucinationen. Studien über normale und pathologische Wahrnehmung. *Archiv für Psychiatrie und Nervenkrankheiten*, 1908, *44*, 584–655; 1036–1106.

1909

22. Ein Fall von Insuffisance pluriglandulaire. Zugleich ein Beitrag zur Lehre von der Meningitis serosa. *Deutsches Archiv für klinische Medizin*, 1909, *98*, 277–288.
23. Einige Bemerkungen über Aphasie im Anschluss an Moutier's "L'aphasie de Broca." *Archiv für Psychiatrie und Nervenkrankheiten*, 1909, *45*, 408–440.
24. Embolie der Arteria cerebelli posterior inferior. *Deutsche medizinische Wochenschrift*, 1909, *35*, 1125.
25. Der makroskopische Hirnbefund in meinem Falle von linksseitiger motorischer Apraxie. *Neurologisches Centralblatt*, 1909, *28*, 898–906.
26. Meningitis serosa. *Deutsche medizinische Wochenschrift*, 1909, *35*, 1946–1947.
27. Pathologische Anatomie der Dementia praecox. *Deutsche medizinische Wochenschrift*, 1909, *35*, 1169.
28. Über segmentäre Bauchmuskellähmung (bei Poliomyelitis acuta anterior und Kompression des Rückenmarks). *Deutsche Zeitschrift für Nervenheilkunde*, 1909, *38*, 93–108.
29. Zur Frage der cerebralen Sensibilitätsstörungen von spinalem Typus. *Neurologisches Centralblatt*, 1909, *28*, 114–120.
30. Zur pathologischen Anatomie der Dementia praecox, speziell der plötzlichen Todesfälle bei derselben. *Allgemeine Zeitschrift für Psychiatrie und psychisch-gerichtliche Medizin*, 1909, *66*, 702–703.
31. With G. Cohn. Weitere Beiträge zur Symptomatologie der Erkrankungen der motorischen Kernsäule. *Deutsche Zeitschrift für Nervenheilkunde*, 1909, *37*, 21–34.

1910

32. Einige prinzipielle Bemerkungen zur Frage der Lokalisation psychischer Vorgänge im Gehirn. *Medizinische Klinik*, 1910, *6*, 1363–1368.
33. Hydrocephalus. *Deutsche medizinische Wochenschrift*, 1910, *36*, 684.
34. Meningitis serosa unter dem Bilde hypophysärer Erkrankung. Zur Differentialdiagnose des Tumor cerebri und der Meningitis serosa. *Archiv für Psychiatrie und Nervenkrankheiten*, 1910, *47*, 126–153.
35. Polyzythaemie und Hirnerweichung. *Medizinische Klinik*, 1910, *6*, 1492–1495.
36. Über die aufsteigende Degeneration nach Querschnitts-Unterbrechung des Rückenmarks. (Tractus spino-cerebellaris posterior; tractus spino-olivaris; tractus spino-thalamicus). *Neurologisches Centralblatt*, 1910, *29*, 898–911.
37. Über die Lokalisation psychischer Vorgänge im Gehirn. *Schriften der physikal.-ökonomischen Gesellschaft* (*Sitzungsberichte, biologische Sektion*), 1910, *51*, 340–343.
38. Über eine amnestische Form der apraktischen Agraphie. *Neurologisches Centralblatt*, 1910, *29*, 1252–1255.
39. Ueber Aphasie. *Beihefte zur Medizinischen Klinik*, 1910, *6*, 1–32.
40. Zur pathologischen Anatomie der Dementia praecox. *Archiv für Psychiatrie und Nervenkrankheiten*, 1910, *46*, 1062–1090.

1911

41. Die amnestische und die zentrale Aphasie (Leitungsaphasie). *Archiv für Psychiatrie und Nervenkrankheiten*, 1911, *48*, 314–343.
42. Kretinismus. *Deutsche medizinische Wochenschrift*, 1911, *37*, 1004.
43. Über Apraxie. *Allgemeine Zeitschrift für Psychiatrie und psychisch-gerichtliche Medizin*, 1911, *68*, 741–745.
44. Über Apraxie. *Beihefte zur medizinischen Klinik*, 1911, *7*, 271–302.

1912

45. Ein Beitrag zur Lehre von der Cysticerkose des Gehirns und Rückenmarks, insbesondere der Meningitis cysticercosa. *Archiv für Psychiatrie und Nervenkrankheiten*, 1912, *49*, 742–793.
46. Die Halluzinationen, ihre Entstehung, ihre Ursachen und ihre Realität. In *Grenzfragen des Nerven- und Seelenlebens*, 1912, *13*, No. 86, pp. 72. Wiesbaden, J. F. Bergmann.
47. Hirntumoren. *Deutsche medizinische Wochenschrift*, 1912, *38*, 1762–1763.
48. Über die zentrale Aphasie. *Allgemeine Zeitschrift für Psychiatrie und psychisch-gerichtliche Medizin*, 1912, *69*, 766–767.
49. Ueber die zentrale Aphasie. Discussion abstract, Jahresversammlung des Deutschen Vereins für Psychiatrie. *Deutsche medizinische Wochenschrift*, 1912, *38*, 1440.
50. Die zentrale Aphasie. *Neurologisches Centralblatt*, 1912, *31*, 739–751.

1913

51. Demonstration zu den Erkrankungen der Drüsen mit innerer Sekretion. (Idiotie mit gleichzeitiger Hypoplasie der Drüsen). *Deutsche medizinische Wochenschrift*, 1913, *39*, 34–44.

52. Ein Fall von Akromegalie nach Kastration bei einer erwachsenen Frau. *Münchener medizinische Wochenschrift*, 1913, *60*, 757–759.

53. a) Rechtsseitige Hemiplegie, Aphasie, und linksseitige Apraxie.—b) Gehirn einer Patientin mit rechtsseitiger Hemiplegie, Aphasie, ideatorischer Apraxie und Agnosie.—c) Gehirn eines Mannes mit vollständiger Aufhebung der Sensibilität auf einer Seite (rechts) und Augenmuskellähmungen auf der anderen und der gleichen Seite. *Deutsche medizinische Wochenschrift*, 1913, *39*, 1074–1075.

54. *Über Rassenhygiene*. Berlin, 1913, Springer. Pp. 96.

55. Über Störungen der Schwereempfindungen bei gleichseitiger Kleinhirnaffektion. *Neurologisches Centralblatt*, 1913, *32*, 1082–1087.

56. Ueber die Störungen der Grammatik bei Hirnkrankheiten. *Monatsschrift für Psychiatrie und Neurologie*, 1913, *34*, 540–568.

57. Weitere Bemerkungen zur Theorie der Halluzinationen. *Zeitschrift für die gesamte Neurologie und Psychiatrie*, 1913, *14*, 502–544.

58. Zwei Geschwister mit Myxidiotie und vorhandener, sicher nicht grob veränderter, Schilddrüse. *Deutsche Zeitschrift für Nervenheilkunde*, 1913, *49*, 103–122.

59. With H. Baumm. Klinische und anatomische Beiträge zur Lehre von der Verstopfung der Arteria cerebelli posterior inferior. *Archiv für Psychiatrie und Nervenkrankheiten*, 1913, *52*, 335–377.

1914

60. Ein Beitrag zur Lehre von der Bedeutung der Insel für die Sprache und der linken Hemisphäre für das linksseitige Tasten. *Archiv für Psychiatrie und Nervenkrankheiten*, 1914, *55*, 158–173.

61. Einige Bemerkungen zu der Arbeit von Stertz: Die klinische Stellung der amnestischen und transkortikalen Aphasie usw. *Deutsche Zeitschrift für Nervenheilkunde*, 1914, *52*, 504–514.

62. Kleinhirnerkrankung. *Deutsche medizinische Wochenschrift*, 1914, *40*, 1594.

63. a) Transkortikale motorische Aphasie.—b) Subkortikale sensorische Aphasie.—c) Affektion des linksseitigen Kleinhirns. *Deutsche medizinische Wochenschrift*, 1914, *40*, 466–467.

64. Ueber Eunuchoide. Ueber familiär auftretende Entwicklungsstörungen der Drüsen mit innerer Sekretion and des Gehirns. *Archiv für Psychiatrie und Nervenkrankheiten*, 1914, *53*, 649–672.

65. With F. Reichmann. Über die körperlichen Störungen bei der Dementia praecox. (Vorläufige Mitteilung.) *Neurologisches Centralblatt*, 1914, *33*, 343–350.

1915

66. Die Ausfallserscheinungen bei Schussverletzungen des Gehirnes und ihre Behandlung. *Jahresbericht über die Leistungen und Fortschritte auf dem Gebiete der Neurologie und Psychiatrie*, 1915, *19*, XIV–XX.

67. Beobachtungen an Schussverletzungen des Gehirns und Rückenmarks. *Deutsche medizinische Wochenschrift*, 1915, *41*, 215–217; 250–254.

68. Ludwig Edinger. *Monatsschrift für Psychiatrie und Neurologie*, 1915, *62*, 1439–1442.

69. Ueber den zerebellaren Symptomenkomplex in seiner Bedeutung für die Beurteilung von Schädelverletzten. *Münchener medizinische Wochenschrift*, 1915, *62*, 1439–1442.

70. Zur operativen Therapie der Schussverletzungen der Wirbelsäule und des Rückenmarks. *Neurologisches Centralblatt*, 1915, *34*, 114–117.
71. With A. Wallenberg and C. U. A. Kappers. An Herrn Professor Edinger. *Deutsche Zeitschrift für Nervenheilkunde*, 1915, *53*, 423–424.

1916

72. Die Behandlung der Ausfallserscheinungen bei Kopfschussverletzungen. *Zeitschrift für ärztliche Fortbildung*, 1916, *13*, 597–602; 630–635.
73. *Schemata des Neurologischen Institutes zu Frankfurt a. M. zum Einzeichnen von Kopf- und Gehirnverletzungen*. Wiesbaden, 1916, J. F. Bergmann.
74. Über die Behandlung der "monosymptomatischen" Hysterie bei Soldaten. *Neurologisches Centralblatt*, 1916, *35*, 842–852.
75. Über corticale Sensibilitätsstörungen. *Zeitschrift für die gesamte Neurologie und Psychiatrie*, 1916, 33, 494–517.
76. Übungsschulen für Hirnverletzte. *Zeitschrift für Krüppelfürsorge*, 1916, *9*, 17–21.
77. Ueber die Behandlung der umschriebenen Ausfallssymptome bei den Schussverletzungen des Gehirns. *Fortschritte der Medizin*, 1916, *33*, 209–211.
78. Ueber die sekundären Erscheinungen nach Schussverletzungen peripherer Nerven. *Zeitschrift für orthopädische Chirurgie*, 1916, *36*, 358–369.
79. Uebungsschulen für Hirnverletzte. *Zentralblatt für chirurgische und mechanische Orthopädie*, 1916, *10*, 4–7.
80. With F. Reichmann. Beiträge zur Kasuistik und Symptomatologie der Kleinhirnerkrankungen (im besonderen zu den Störungen der Bewegungen, der Gewichts-, Raum-, und Zeitschätzung). *Archiv für Psychiatrie und Nervenkrankheiten*, 1916, *56*, 466–521.
80a. With F. Reichmann. Beiträge zur Kasuistik und Symptomatologie der Kleinhirnerkrankungen (im besonderen zu den Störungen der Bewegungen, der Gewichts-, Raum-, und Zeitschätzung). *Neurologisches Centralblatt*, 1916, *35*, 593–595.
81. . . . drei Typen kortikaler Sensibilitätsstörung. (Discussion of paper by O. Foerster.) *Deutsche Zeitschrift für Nervenheilkunde*, 1917, *56*, 188–190.

1917

82. Erfahrungen aus einem Lazarett für Hirnverletzte. *Neurologisches Centralblatt*, 1917, *36*, 683–684.
83. Die militärische Sachverständigentätigkeit auf dem Gebiete des Ersatzwesens und der militärischen Versorgung bei den Hirnverletzungen. In *Die militärische Sachverständigentätigkeit auf dem Gebiete des Ersatzwesens und der Versorgung*. Jena, 1917, G. Fischer. Pp. 194–232.
84. Neurosen nach Kriegsverletzungen. Discussion of papers by H. Oppenheim, M. Nonne and R. Gaupp. *Deutsche Zeitschrift für Nervenheilkunde*, 1917, *56*, 178; 188–190.
85. Die transkortikalen Aphasien. *Ergebnisse der Neurologie und Psychiatrie*, 1917, *2*, 349–629.
86. Über die ärztliche und fürsorgliche Behandlung der Hirnverletzten. *Die Kriegsbeschädigtenfürsorge*, 1917, *1*, 644–648.
87. Über die Behandlung der Kriegshysteriker. *Medizinische Klinik*, 1917, *13*, 751–758.

88. Über den heutigen Stand der Lehre von der Rindenblindheit. *Zeitschrift für die gesamte Neurologie und Psychiatrie*, 1917, Referatenband *14*, 97–115.
89. Ueber körperliche Störungen bei Hirnverletzten: 1. Mitteilung: Ueber den Einfluss der Hirnverletzung auf den Zuckerstoffwechsel. *Münchener medizinische Wochenschrift*, 1917, *64*, 1249.
90. Zur Lokalisation der Sensibilität und Motilität in der Hirnrinde. *Neurologisches Centralblatt*, 1917, *36*, 489–492.

1918

91. Die Aufgabe der Schwester bei der Behandlung der Hirnverletzten. *Die Schwester: illustrierte Monatsschrift*, 1918, *6*.
92. Gedenkrede auf Ludwig Edinger. (Reported by Hainbach). *Medizinische Klinik*, 1918, *14*, 427.
93. Konzentrische Gesichtsfeld-Einschränkung: (Discussion of paper by A. Saenger). *Deutsche Zeitschrift für Nervenheilkunde*, 1918, *59*, 199–216; 225.
94. Ludwig Edinger. *Zeitschrift für die gesamte Neurologie und Psychiatrie*, 1918, *44*, 114–149. (Reprinted in part, cf. #313.)
95. Rechtshändigkeit. *Die Umschau, Wochenschrift über die Fortschritte in Wissenschaft und Technik*, 1918, 147–148.
96. Über Behandlung und Fürsorge der Hirnverletzungen. *Deutsche medizinische Wochenschrift*, 1918, *44*, 783.
96a. Ueber Behandlung und Fürsorge der Hirnverletzungen. *Berliner klinische Wochenschrift*, 1918, *55*, 823.
97. Ueber körperliche Störungen bei Hirnverletzten. II. Ueber Störungen der Vasomotilität des Pulses, des Blutbildes, des Blutdrucks, der Temperatur bei Hirnverletzten. *Münchener medizinische Wochenschrift*, 1918, *65*, 104–106.
98. Die verschiedene Bedeutung der beiden Hirn-Hälften und ihre Beziehung zur Rechtshändigkeit. *Bericht der Senckenbergischen Naturforschenden Gesellschaft*, 1918, *41*, 77–78.
99. With A. Gelb. Psychologische Analysen hirnpathologischer Fälle auf Grund von Untersuchungen Hirnverletzter. I. Zur Psychologie des optischen Wahrnehmungs- und Erkennungsvorganges. *Zeitschrift für die gesamte Neurologie und Psychiatrie*, 1918, *41*, 1–142.
100. With A. Gelb. Das "röhrenförmige Gesichtsfeld" nebst einer Vorrichtung für perimetrische Gesichtsfelduntersuchungen in verschiedenen Entfernungen. (Vorläufige Mitteilung.) *Neurologisches Centralblatt*, 1918, *37*, 738–748.

1919

101. *Die Behandlung, Fuersorge und Begutachtung der Hirnverletzten. Zugleich ein Beitrag zur Verwendung psychologischer Methoden in der Klinik.* Leipzig, 1919, F. C. W. Vogel.
102. Ludwig Edinger: 13. April 1855—26. Januar 1918. *Bericht der Senckenbergischen Naturforschenden Gesellschaft*, 1919, *49*, 143–151.
103. Über die Rentenversorgung bei Folgen von Hirnverletzungen. In C. Adam (Ed.), *Dienstbeschädigung und Rentenversorgung.* Jena, 1919, G. Fischer. Pp. 93–120.
104. With F. Reichmann. Über corticale Sensibilitätsstörungen, besonders am Kopfe. *Zeitschrift für die gesamte Neurologie und Psychiatrie*, 1919, *53*, 49–79.

1920

105. With A. Gelb (Eds.), *Psychologische Analysen hirnpathologischer Fälle.* Leipzig, 1920, J. Barth. Vol. I. Pp. 561.

Contents (not numbered in the book)

106. (I) Gelb, A. and Goldstein, K. Zur Psychologie des optischen Wahrnehmungs- und Erkennungsvorganges. Pp. 1–142. *cf.* #99. Translated in part in W. D. Ellis, *Sourcebook of Gestalt Psychology,* London, 1938, Routledge, Kegan Paul. Selection 26, pp. 315–325.

107. (II) Gelb, A. and Goldstein, K. Das "röhrenförmige Gesichtsfeld" nebst einer Vorrichtung für perimetrische Gesichtsfelduntersuchungen in verschiedenen Entfernungen (Vorläufige Mitteilung). Pp. 143–156. *cf.* #100.

108. (III) Gelb, A. and Goldstein, K. Über den Einfluss des vollständigen Verlustes des optischen Vorstellungsvermögens auf das taktile Erkennen. Pp. 157–250. Later cited as II in this series. *cf.* #109.

(IV) Fuchs, W. Untersuchungen über das Sehen der Hemianopiker und Hemiamblyopiker. I. Teil: Verlagerungserscheinungen. Pp. 251–353. Later cited as III in this series. Published also in *Zeitschrift für Psychologie und Physiologie der Sinnesorgane. 1. Abteilung. Zeitschrift für Psychologie,* 1920, *84,* 67–169. Translated in part in W. D. Ellis, *op. cit.,* Selection 28, pp. 333–343.

(V) Gelb, A. Über den Wegfall der Wahrnehmung von "Oberflächenfarben." Pp. 354–418. Later cited as IV in this series. Published also in *Zeitschrift für Psychologie und Physiologie der Sinnesorgane. 1. Abteilung. Zeitschrift für Psychologie,* 1920, *84,* 193–257. Translated in part in W. D. Ellis, *op. cit.,* Selection 27, pp. 326–332.

(VI) Fuchs, W. Untersuchungen über das Sehen der Hemianopiker und Hemiamblyopiker. II. Teil: Die totalisierende Gestaltauffassung. Pp. 419–561. Later cited as V in this series. Published also in *Zeitschrift für Psychologie und Physiologie der Sinnesorgane. 1. Abteilung. Zeitschrift für Psychologie,* 1921, *86,* 1–143. Translated in part in W. D. Ellis, *op. cit.,* Selection 29, pp. 344–356.

A second volume in this series was evidently projected, but there is no evidence that it ever appeared. However, between 1922 and 1932 the following numbered articles were published under the general heading *Psychologische Analysen hirnpathologischer Fälle auf Grund von Untersuchungen Hirnverletzter*—occasionally abbreviated—and under the editorial byline of A. Gelb and K. Goldstein.

(VII) Gelb, A. and Goldstein, K. Über Gesichtsfeldbefunde bei abnormer "Ermüdbarkeit" des Auges (sog. "Ringskotome"). *Albrecht von Graefes Archiv für Ophthalmologie,* 1922, *109,* 387–403. *cf.* #120.

(VIII) Benary, W. Studien zur Untersuchung der Intelligenz bei einem Fall von Seelenblindheit. *Psychologische Forschung,* 1922, *2,* 209–297.

(IX) Gelb, A. Über eine eigenartige Sehstörung ("Dysmorphopsie") infolge von Gesichtsfeldeinengung. Ein Beitrag zur Lehre von den Beziehungen zwischen "Gesichtsfeld" and "Sehen." *Psychologische Forschung,* 1923, *4,* 42–63.

(X) Gelb, A. and Goldstein, K. Über Farbennamenamnesie, nebst Bemerkungen über das Wesen der amnestischen Aphasie überhaupt und die Beziehung zwischen Sprache und Verhalten zur Umwelt. *Psychologische Forschung,* 1925, *6*, 127–168. *cf.* #171.

(XI) Gelb, A. and Goldstein, K. Zur Frage nach der gegenseitigen funktionellen Beziehung der geschädigten und der ungeschädigten Sehsphäre bei Hemianopsie. (Mikropsie infolge der Vorherrschaft der Vorgänge in der geschädigten Sehsphäre.) *Psychologische Forschung,* 1925, *6*, 187–199. *cf.* #172.

(XII) Mäki, N. Natürliche Bewegungstendenzen der rechten und der linken Hand und ihr Einfluss auf das Zeichnen und den Erkennungsvorgang. *Psychologische Forschung,* 1928, *10*, 1–19.

(XIII) Hochheimer, W. Analyse eines "Seelenblinden" von der Sprache aus. Ein Beitrag zur Frage nach der Bedeutung der Sprache für das Verhalten zur Umwelt. *Psychologische Forschung,* 1932, *16*, 1–69.

(XIV) Siekmann, W. Psychologische Analyse des Falles Rat . . . (Ein Fall von sog. motorischer Aphasie.) *Psychologische Forschung,* 1932, *16*, 201–250.

109. With A. Gelb. Psychologische Analysen hirnpathologischer Fälle auf Grund von Untersuchungen Hirnverletzter. II. Abhandlung. Über den Einfluss des vollständigen Verlustes des optischen Vorstellungsvermögens auf das taktile Erkennen. *Zeitschrift für Psychologie und Physiologie der Sinnesorgane. 1. Abteilung. Zeitschrift für Psychologie,* 1920, *83*, 1–94. *cf.* #108.

110. With F. Reichmann. Über praktische und theoretische Ergebnisse aus den Erfahrungen an Hirnschussverletzten. *Ergebnisse der inneren Medizin und Kinderheilkunde,* 1920, *18*, 405–530.

1921

111. With A. Wallenberg (Eds). Ludwig Edinger's *Einführung in die Lehre vom Bau und den Verrichtungen des Nervensystems.* 3rd edition. Leipzig, 1921, F. C. Vogel.

1922

112. Der amyostatische Symptomenkomplex. (Discussion of paper by E. Pollak and A. Jacob.) *Deutsche Zeitschrift für Nervenheilkunde,* 1922, *74*, 98–99.

113. Klinische und anatomische Demonstration zur Frage der Parkinson-ähnlichen Erkrankungen bei Encephalitis epidemica. *Münchener medizinische Wochenschrift,* 1922, *69*, 29.

114. Psychologische Methoden zur Untersuchung der Hautsinne. In Abderhalden (Ed.) *Handbuch der biologischen Arbeitsmethoden.* Berlin, 1922, Urban & Schwarzenberg. Vol. 6, pp. 477–546.

115. Die Topik der Grosshirnrinde. *Schweizer Archiv für Neurologie und Psychiatrie,* 1922, *11*, 289–298.

116. Über Agraphie. (Discussion of paper by A. Boettiger). *Deutsche Zeitschrift für Nervenheilkunde,* 1922, *74*, 194.

117. Über anatomische Veränderungen (Atrophie der Substantia nigra) bei postencephalitischem Parkinsonismus. *Zeitschrift für die gesamte Neurologie und Psychiatrie,* 1922, *76*, 627–632.

118. Über den Einfluss von Sprachstörungen auf das Verhalten gegenüber Farben. *Deutsche Zeitschrift für Nervenheilkunde*, 1922, *74*, 260–262.
119. Über den Einfluss von Sprachstörungen auf das Verhalten gegenüber Farben. *Bericht über den VII. Kongress für experimentelle Psychologie*, Marburg, April 20–23, 1921. Jena, 1922, Fischer. Pp. 118–120.
120. With A. Gelb. Psychologische Analysen hirnpathologischer Fälle auf Grund von Untersuchungen Hirnverletzter. VII. Über Gesichtsfeldbefunde bei abnormer "Ermüdbarkeit" des Auges (sog. "Ringskotome"). *Albrecht von Graefes Archiv für Ophthalmologie*, 1922, *109*, 387–403.

1923

121. Die Bedeutung des menschlichen Stirnhirns und die Diagnose seiner Erkrankungen. *Klinische Wochenschrift*, 1923, *2*, 1240.
122. Demonstration von Halsreflexen. *Klinische Wochenschrift*, 1923, *2*, 1623.
123. Die Funktionen des Stirnhirnes und ihre Bedeutung für die Diagnose von Stirnhirnerkrankungen. *Medizinische Klinik*, 1923, *19*, 965–969; 1006–1010.
124. Lokalisation der sensorischen Störungen. *Klinische Wochenschrift*, 1923, *2*, 227.
125. Die Pathologie des Kleinhirns. (Discussion of G. Mingazzini's paper). *Zentralblatt für die gesamte Neurologie und Psychiatrie*, 1923, *33*, 482.
126. Die Topik der Grosshirnrinde in ihrer klinischen Bedeutung. *Deutsche Zeitschrift für Nervenheilkunde*, 1923, *77*, 7–124.
127. Die Topik der Grosshirnrinde. *Klinische Wochenschrift*, 1923, *2*, 227.
128. Über die Abhängigkeit der Bewegungen von optischen Vorgängen. (Bewegungsstörungen bei Seelenblinden). *Monatsschrift für Psychiatrie und Neurologie*, 1923, *54*, 141–194.
129. Über Halsreflexe bein Menschen. *Deutsche Zeitschrift für Nervenheilkunde*, 1923, *77*, 298–302.
130. Über Halsreflexe beim Menschen. *Klinische Wochenschrift*, 1923, *2*, 276.
131. Über induzierte Tonusveränderungen. *Klinische Wochenschrift*, 1923, *2*, 1524.
132. Über induzierte Tonusveränderungen. *Zentralblatt für die gesamte Neurologie und Psychiatrie*, 1923, *33*, 171–175.
133. Über die Störungen des Gewichtsschätzens bei Kleinhirnerkrankungen und ihre Beziehung zu den Veränderungen des Tonus. *Klinische Wochenschrift*, 1923, *2*, 2103–2104.
134. Über die Störungen des Gewichtsschätzens bei Kleinhirnerkrankungen und ihre Beziehung zu den Veränderungen des Tonus. *Zentralblatt für die gesamte Neurologie und Psychiatrie*, 1923, *33*, 485–486.
135. Zur Frage der Restitution nach umschriebenem Hirndefekt. *Schweizer Archiv für Neurologie und Psychiatrie*, 1923, *13*, 283–296.
136. Zur Klinik der Kleinhirngeschwülste. (Discussion of paper by Borgherini). *Zentralblatt für die gesamte Neurologie und Psychiatrie*, 1923, *33*, 491.
137. Book review: Pick, A. Die neurologische Forschungsrichtung in der Psychopathologie. *Psychologische Forschung*, 1923, *3*, 182–185.
138. With W. Riese. Über induzierte Veränderungen des Tonus. (Halsreflexe, Labyrinthreflexe und ähnliche Erscheinungen.) I. Induzierte Veränderungen beim normalen Menschen. (Vorläufige Mitteilung). *Klinische Wochenschrift*, 1923, *2*, 1201–1206.

139. With W. Riese. Über induzierte Veränderungen des Tonus. (Halsreflexe, Labyrinthreflexe und ähnliche Erscheinungen). III. Blickrichtung und Zeigeversuch. *Klinische Wochenschrift*, 1923, *2*, 2338–2340.
140. With R. Cassirer, M. Nonne and B. Pfeiffer (joint editors).
H. Oppenheim, *Lehrbuch der Nervenkrankheiten für Ärzte und Studierende*. Berlin 1923, Karger. 7th edition. 2 vols. Pp. 2270.
Includes the following chapters and sections by Goldstein:
141. Zur Pathologie und Physiologie des Rückenmarks. Vol. I, 121–180.
142. Zur Anatomie und Physiologie des Gehirns, Lokalisationslehre. Vol. II, 927–1025.
143. Allgemeine Symptomatologie der Hirnkrankheiten. Vol. II, 1025–1152.
144. Die Krankheiten der Brücke und des verlängerten Marks. Vol. II, 1592–1653.
145. Die Erkrankungen des Kleinhirns. Vol. II, 1653–1678.
146. Die Tetanie. Vol. II, 2011–2028.
147. Die Chorea minor. Vol. II, 2028–2044.
148. Die Chorea electrica. Vol. II, 2045.
149. Die Erkrankungen des Systems der Stammganglien. Vol. II, 2045–2099.
150. Die Basedowsche Krankheit. Vol. II, 2175–2205.
151. Das Myxödem. Vol. II, 2205–2221.
152. Die Akromegalie (Marie), Pachyakrie (Recklinghausen). Vol. II, 2221–2238.

1924

153. Die Topik der Hirnrinde in ihrer Bedeutung für die Klinik.
Psychiatrisch-Neurologische Wochenschrift, 1924, *26*, 43–46; 55–60.
154. Über den Einfluss motorischer Störungen auf die Psyche. (Vorläufige Mitteilung.)
Deutsche Zeitschrift für Nervenheilkunde, 1924, *83*, 119–133.
155. Über den Einfluss der Motorik auf die Psyche.
Klinische Wochenschrift, 1924, *3*, 427–428.
156. Über die Funktion des Kleinhirnes. (Vorläufige Mitteilung.)
Klinische Wochenschrift, 1924, *3*, 1255–1260.
157. Über gleichartige funktionelle Bedingtheit der Symptome bei organischen und psychischen Krankheiten; im besonderen über den funktionellen Mechanismus der Zwangsvorgänge.
Monatsschrift für Psychiatrie und Neurologie, 1924, *57*, 191–209.
158. Über induzierte Tonus-Veränderungen beim Menschen (sog. Halsreflexe, Labyrinthreflexe usw.) II. Über induzierte Tonus-Veränderungen beim Kranken. 1. Über Lageveränderungen in einem Gliede durch bestimmte Stellungen des Gliedes selbst. 2. Über Lageveränderungen durch Veränderung der Stellung anderer Glieder. *Zeitschrift für die gesamte Neurologie und Psychiatrie*, 1924, *89*, 383–428.
159. Über die Pathologie des Kleinhirns. (Discussion of paper by G. Mingazzini).
Deutsche Zeitschrift für Nervenheilkunde, 1924, *81*, 56–57.
160. Über die Störungen des Gewichtsschätzen bei Kleinhirnerkrankungen und ihre Beziehung zu den Veränderungen des Tonus.
Deutsche Zeitschrift für Nervenheilkunde, 1924, *81*, 68–71; 89–90.
161. Das Wesen der amnestischen Aphasie. (Vorläufige Mitteilung gemeinsamer Untersuchungen mit A. Gelb.)
Schweizer Archiv für Neurologie und Psychiatrie, 1924, *15*, 163–175.
162. Book review: Magnus, R. Körperstellung. Experimentell-physiologische Unter-

suchungen über die einzelnen bei der Körperstellung in Tätigkeit tretenden Reflexe, über ihr Zusammenwirken und ihre Störungen. *Klinische Wochenschrift*, 1924, *3*, 1977–1978.

163. With W. Riese. Über induzierte Veränderungen des Tonus. (Halsreflexe, Labyrinthreflexe und ähnliche Erscheinungen.) V. Kritisches und Experimentelles zur Auffassung des Vorbeizeigens. *Monatsschrift für Ohrenheilkunde*, 1924, *58*, 931–940.
164. With A. Wallenberg (Eds.). L. Edinger's Anatomisch-physiologische Einleitung der Nervenkrankheiten. In F. Kraus and T. Brugsch (Eds.) *Spezielle Pathologie und Therapie innerer Krankheiten*. Berlin & Wien, 1924, Urban & Schwarzenberg. Pp. 1–98.

1925

165. Die Erkrankung des Gehirns und seiner Häute. In L. Mohr and R. Stähelin (Eds.), *Handbuch der inneren Medizin*. Berlin, 1925, Springer. 2nd edition, vol. 5, 147–363.
166. Über den Einfluss motorischer Störungen auf die Psyche. *Allgemeine Zeitschrift für Psychiatrie und psychisch-gerichtliche Medizin*, 1925, *82*, 164–177.
167. Über induzierte Tonusveränderungen beim Menschen (sog. Halsreflexe, Labyrinthreflexe, usw.). VIII. (Vorläufige Mitteilung) Über den Einfluss unbewusster Bewegungen resp. Tendenzen zu Bewegungen auf die taktile und optische Raumwahrnehmung. *Klinische Wochenschrift*, 1925, *4*, 294–299.
168. Das Wesen der amnestischen Aphasie. (Nach gemeinsamen Untersuchungen mit A. Gelb). *Deutsche Zeitschrift für Nervenheilkunde*, 1925, *83*, 324–339.
169. Zur Theorie der Funktion des Nervensystems. *Archiv für Psychiatrie und Nervenkrankheiten*, 1925, *74*, 370–405.
170. With W. Börnstein. Über sich in pseudospontanen Bewegungen äussernde Spasmen und über eigentümliche Stellungen bei "striären" Erkrankungen. *Deutsche Zeitschrift für Nervenheilkunde*, 1925, *84*, 234–275.
171. With A. Gelb. Psychologische Analysen hirnpathologischer Fälle. X. Über Farbennamenamnesie, nebst Bemerkungen über das Wesen der amnestischen Aphasie überhaupt und die Beziehung zwischen Sprache und dem Verhalten zur Umwelt. *Psychologische Forschung*, 1925, *6*, 127-186.
172. With A. Gelb. Psychologische Analysen hirnpathologischer Fälle. XI. Zur Frage nach der gegenseitigen funktionellen Beziehung der geschädigten und der ungeschädigten Sehsphäre bei Hemianopsie. (Mikropsie infolge der Vorherrschaft der Vorgänge in der geschädigten Sehsphäre.) *Psychologische Forschung*, 1925, *6*, 187–199.
173. With W. Riese. Über induzierte Veränderungen des Tonus. (Halsreflexe, Labyrinthreflexe und ähnliche Erscheinungen.) IX. Über den Einfluss sensibler Hautreize auf die sogenannten vestibulären Reaktionsbewegungen. Zugleich ein weiterer Beitrag zur Kenntnis der tonischen Erscheinungen. *Klinische Wochenschrift*, 1925, *4*, 1201–1204.
174. With P. Schwartz. Die embolische Striatumapoplexie. *Münchener medizinische Wochenschrift*, 1925, *72*, 2154–2155.

1926

175. Neue Erfahrungen zum Problem der sogenannten induzierten Tonusveränderun-

gen. Gleichzeitig ein Beitrag zur Symptomatologie der Zerebellar- und Frontalerkrankungen. *Deutsche Zeitschrift für Nervenheilkunde*, 1926, *89*, 72–77.

176. Das Symptom, seine Entstehung und Bedeutung für unsere Auffassung vom Bau und von der Funktion des Nervensystems.
Archiv für Psychiatrie und Nervenkrankheiten, 1926, *76*, 84–108.

177. Über Aphasie.
Schweizer Archiv für Neurologie und Psychiatrie, 1926, *19*, 3–38; 292–322.

178. Über die augenblickliche Lage der Lehre von der Aphasie.
Schweizer Archiv für Neurologie und Psychiatrie, 1926, *18*, 324–328.

179. Über induzierte Veränderungen des "Tonus." X. 1. Über Störungen der akustischen Lokalisation bei Cerebellar- und Frontalhirnkranken. 2. Über den Einfluss des Abweichens auf die Lokalisation von Wahrnehmungen. 3. Über den Einfluss von Augenbewegungen auf die Tonlokalisation. 4. Über den Einfluss sensorischer Reize auf motorische Vorgänge. 5. Über den Einfluss von Sinnesreizen auf gleichzeitige Wahrnehmungen auf anderen Sinnesgebieten.
Schweizer Archiv für Neurologie und Psychiatrie, 1926, *17*, 203–228.

180. With W. Riese. Klinische und anatomische Beobachtungen an einem vierjährigen riechhirnlosen Kinde. *Journal für Psychologie und Neurologie*, 1926, *32*, 291–311.

181. With O. Rosenthal-Veit. Über akustische Lokalisation und deren Beeinflussbarkeit durch andere Sinnesreize. *Psychologische Forschung*, 1926, *8*, 318–335.

182. With P. Schwartz. Studien zur Morphologie und Genese der apoplektischen Hirninsulte Erwachsener. 1. Mitteilung: Anatomische und klinische Beiträge zur embolischen Striatumapoplexie.
Journal für Psychologie und Neurologie, 1926, *32*, 312–328.

1927

183. Die Beziehungen der Psychoanalyse zur Biologie.
Bericht über den II. allgemeinen ärztlichen Kongress für Psychotherapie in Bad Nauheim, April 1927. Leipzig, 1927, Hirzel. Pp. 15–52.

184. Beziehungen zwischen Psychoanalyse und Physiologie.
Zentralblatt für die gesamte Neurologie und Psychiatrie, 1927, *47*, 160–161.

185. Das Kleinhirn. In A. Bethe (Ed.), *Handbuch der normalen und pathologischen Physiologie*. Berlin, 1927, Springer. Vol. 10, pp. 222–317.

186. Die Lokalisation in der Grosshirnrinde. Nach Erfahrungen am kranken Menschen. In A. Bethe (Ed.), *Handbuch der normalen und pathologischen Physiologie*. Berlin, 1927, Springer. Vol. 10, pp. 600–842.

187. Über Aphasie. *Neurologische und Psychiatrische Abhandlungen aus dem Schweizer Archiv für Neurologie und Psychiatrie*. Zurich, 1927, Orell Füssli. Pp. 68.

1928

188. Beobachtungen über die Veränderungen des Gesamtverhaltens bei Gehirnschädigung. *Monatsschrift für Psychiatrie und Neurologie*, 1928, *68*, 217–242.

189. Betrachtungen über den vorklinischen Unterricht.
Klinische Wochenschrift, 1928, *7*, 2399–2402.

190. Über den gegenseitigen Einfluss motorischer und sensorischer Vorgänge. Mit kinematographischen Vorführungen. *Bericht über den X. Kongress für experimentelle Psychologie in Bonn, April 1927*. Jena, 1928, Fischer. Pp. 116–118.

191. With H. Cohn. Kasuistische Mitteilungen zur Klinik und pathologischen Anatomie der Nervenkrankheiten. I. Zur Klinik und Pathologie hypophysärer Erkrankungen, im besonderen der Tumoren der Hypophysengegend. *Deutsche Zeitschrift für Nervenheilkunde,* 1928, *103,* 225–274.

192. With A. Gelb. Die Bedeutung von Beobachtungen am hirngeschädigten Menschen für die Lehre vom Wesen des Menschen. *Davoser Revue* (Switzerland), 1928, 9–12.

1929

193. Einige prinzipielle Bemerkungen zur Psychotherapie. *Allgemeine ärztliche Zeitschrift für Psychotherapie und psychische Hygiene,* 1929, *2,* 146.

194. Zur Methodik des Zeigeversuches. *Nervenarzt,* 1929, *2,* 449–457.

195. Zum Problem der Angst. *Allgemeine ärztliche Zeitschrift für Psychotherapie und psychische Hygiene,* 1929, *2,* 409–437.

196. Zum Problem der Tendenz zum ausgezeichneten Verhalten. Zugleich ein Beitrag zur Symptomatologie der Kleinhirn- und Stirnhirnläsion. *Deutsche Zeitschrift für Nervenheilkunde,* 1929, *109,* 1–61.

197. With H. Cohn. Zur Diagnostik extracerebraler umschriebener Tumoren und tumorähnlicher Affektionen im Gebiete des Stirnhirns und der Uebergangsregion zur vorderen Zentralwindung. II. Kasuistische Mitteilung zur Klinik und pathologischen Anatomie der Nervenkrankheiten. *Deutsche Zeitschrift für Nervenheilkunde,* 1929, *108,* 161–208.

1930

198. Die Restitution bei Schädigungen der Hirnrinde. *Deutsche Zeitschrift für Nervenheilkunde,* 1930, *116,* 2–26.

199. With O. Rosenthal. 1. Zum Problem der Wirkung der Farben auf den Organismus. (Auf Grund von Untersuchungen der Farbeinwirkung auf Abweichen, Grössen- und Zeitschätzung, etc., bei Cerebellar-und Frontalhirnerkrankung. *Schweizer Archiv für Neurologie und Psychiatrie,* 1930, *26,* 3–26.

1931

200. Konstantin von Monakow. *Deutsche Zeitschrift für Nervenheilkunde,* 1931, *120,* 1–7.

201. Die Neuroregulation. Referat. *Verhandlungen der Deutschen Gesellschaft für innere Medizin,* 1931, *43,* 9–13.

202. Die pathologischen Tatsachen in ihrer Bedeutung für das Problem der Sprache. *Sitzungsbericht über den 12. Kongress der Deutschen Gesellschaft für Psychologie,* Hamburg, 1931, pp. 145–164.

203. Das psychophysische Problem in seiner Bedeutung für ärztliches Handeln. *Therapie der Gegenwart,* 1931, *72,* 1–11.

204. Sobre las anomalías de la personalidad causadas por lesiones cerebrales. *Revista médica germano-ibero-americana,* 1931, *4,* 215–225.

205. Über die Plastizität des Organismus auf Grund von Erfahrungen am nervenkranken Menschen. In A. Bethe (Ed.), *Handbuch der normalen und pathologischen Physiologie.* Berlin, 1931, Springer. Vol. 15, 1133–1174.

206. Über Zeigen und Greifen. *Nervenarzt,* 1931, 4, 453–466.

207. Die zwei Formen der Störungsmöglichkeit der Sprache durch Hirnschädigung. *Archiv für Psychiatrie und Nervenkrankheiten,* 1931, *95,* 730–743.

1932

208. Auslösung epileptischer Anfälle durch Musik. (Demonstration).
Zentralblatt für die gesamte Neurologie und Psychiatrie, 1932, *63*, 281–282.
209. Über Neuroregulation.
Ergebnisse der Inneren Medizin und Kinderheilkunde, 1932, *42*, 741–774.
210. Zur Differentialdiagnose zwischen Parkinsonismus und Hysterie. (Demonstration).
Zentralblatt für die gesamte Neurologie und Psychiatrie, 1932, *63*, 733–734.
211. Die zwei Formen der Störungsmöglichkeit der Sprache.
Zentralblatt für die gesamte Neurologie und Psychiatrie, 1932, *61*, 267–273.
212. With H. Cohn. Die Allgemeinerscheinungen bei Hirngeschwülsten in ihrer Bedeutung für die Diagnostik. *Ergebnisse der gesamten Medizin*, 1932, *17*, 257–330.
213. With H. Cohn. *Diagnostik der Hirngeschwülste.*
Berlin, 1932, Urban & Schwarzenberg. Pp. 138.

1933

214. L'analyse de l'aphasie et l'étude de l'essence du langage.
Journal de psychologie normale et pathologique, 1933, *30*, 430–496.
215. Die ganzheitliche Betrachtung in der Medizin. In T. Brugsch (Ed.), *Einheitsbestrebungen in der Medizin.* Dresden, 1933, Steinkopff. Pp. 144–158.
216. Principle of totality of the organism in medicine. (Russian)
Sovetskaya psikhonevrologiya, 1933, *3*, 5–18.
217. Über Täuschungen des Tastsinnes unter pathologischen Umständen.
Zeitschrift für Psychologie und Physiologie der Sinnesorgane. 1. Abteilung. Zeitschrift für Psychologie, 1933, *129*, 282–290.
218. With W. Jablonski. Über den Einfluss des Tonus auf Refraktion und Sehleistung.
Albrecht von Graefes Archiv für Ophthalmologie, 1933, *130*, 395–410.

1934

219. *Der Aufbau des Organismus. Einführung in die Biologie unter besonderer Berücksichtigung der Erfahrungen am kranken Menschen.* Haag, 1934, Martinus Nijhoff. Pp. xi & 363. (For translations see #242, #297, #309; paperback edition, #326.)
220. Der autoptische Befund in einem Fall von Störungen verschiedenster Leistungsgebiete bei Herderkrankung.
Schweizer Archiv für Neurologie und Psychiatrie, 1934, *33*, 242–249.
221. Die Erfahrungen der Psychopathologie der Sprache in ihrer Bedeutung für die Anthropologie.
Congrès International des Sciences Anthropologiques et Ethnologiques. Comptes-rendu, 1. session. London, 1934, Royal Institute of Anthropology. Pp. 316–318.
222. Kritisches und Tatsächliches zu einigen Grundfragen der Psychopathologie, im besonderen zum Aphasieproblem.
Schweizer Archiv für Neurologie und Psychiatrie, 1934, *34*, 69–93; 230–243.
223. Das Problem der Lokalisation vom klinischen Standpunkt.
Congrès International des Sciences Anthropologiques et Ethnologiques. Comptes-rendu, 1. session. London, 1934, Royal Institute of Anthropology, 108–111.
224. Über monokuläre Doppelbilder.
Jahrbücher für Psychiatrie und Neurologie, 1934, *51*, 16–38.

225. Über das Phänomen der Angst.
Nederlandsch Tijdschrift voor Psychologie, 1934, *1*, 434–454.

1935

226. Les relations entre les lobes frontaux et les fonctions psychiques.
Revue neurologique, 1935, *64*, 538–539.

1936

227. Bemerkungen über die Bedeutung der Biologie für die Soziologie anlässlich des Autoritätsproblems. In M. Horkheimer (Ed.), *Studien über Autorität und Familie.* Paris, 1936, Alcan. Pp. 656–668.
228. The function of the cerebellum from a clinical standpoint.
Journal of nervous and mental Disease, 1936, *83*, 1–12.
229. The modification of behavior consequent to cerebral lesions.
Psychiatric Quarterly, 1936, *10*, 586–610.
230. Personality studies of cases with lesions of the frontal lobes. I. The psychopathology of Pick's disease. *Rorschach Research Exchange*, 1936, *1*, 57–64.
231. The problem of the meaning of words based upon observations of aphasic patients. *Journal of Psychology*, 1936, *2*, 301–316.
232. The significance of the frontal lobes for mental performances.
Journal of Neurology and Psychopathology, 1936, *17*, 27–40.

1937

233. Sigmund Freud as a neurologist.
Archives of Neurology and Psychiatry, 1937, *38*, 656–657.
234. With S. Katz. The psychopathology of Pick's disease.
Archives of Neurology and Psychiatry, 1937, *38*, 473–490.

1938

235. A further comparison of the Moro reflex and startle pattern.
Journal of Psychology, 1938, *6*, 33–42.
236. The tonic foot response to stimulation of the sole: its physiological significance and diagnostic value. *Brain*, 1938, *61*, 269–283.
237. With M. Bolles. A study of the impairment of "abstract behavior" in schizophrenic patients. *Psychiatric Quarterly*, 1938, *12*, 42–65.
238. With A. Gelb. Analysis of a case ot figural blindness.
In W. D. Ellis (Ed.) *Sourcebook of Gestalt Psychology*. London, 1938, Routledge, Kegan Paul. Pp. 315–325. Partial translation of #99.
239. With C. Landis, W. A. Hunt and F. M. Clarke. Moro reflex and startle pattern. *Archives of Neurology and Psychiatry*, 1938, *40*, 322–327.
240. With J. Marmor. A case of aphasia, with special reference to the problem of repetition and word finding.
Journal of Neurology and Psychiatry, 1938, *1*, 329–341.

1939

241. Clinical and theoretic aspects of lesions of the frontal lobes.
Archives of Neurology and Psychiatry, 1939, *41*, 865–867.

242. *The Organism. A Holistic Approach to Biology derived from Pathological Data in Man.* With a foreword by K. S. Lashley. New York, N. Y., 1939, American Book Co. Pp. vii & 533. Translation of #219.
243. The significance of special mental tests for diagnosis and prognosis in schizophrenia. *American Journal of Psychiatry,* 1939, *96,* 575–587.

1940

244. *Human Nature in the Light of Psychopathology.* Cambridge, Massachusetts, 1940, Harvard University Press. Pp. viii & 258. (For translation see #308; paperback edition, #325.)
245. On two forms of adaptation to defects. (Russian). *Nevropatologiya i Psikhiatriya,* 1940, *9,* 116–124.
246. Significance of speech disturbances for normal psychology. *Transactions of the New York Academy of Sciences,* 1940, Series II, Vol. 2, 159–163.
247. With S. Schlezinger. Friedreich's ataxia associated with diabetes mellitus. *New York State Journal of Medicine,* 1940, *40,* 415–423.

1941

248. Neuroses in wartime: from personal experience. *Tufts medical Journal,* 1941, *8,* 1–7.
249. The psychosomatic problem: its significance for the physician. *Bulletin of the New England medical Center,* 1941, *3,* 145–147.
250. The sign of Babinski. *Journal of nervous and mental Disease,* 1941, *93,* 281–296.
251. With C. Landis (Eds.). E. Weigl. On the psychology of so-called processes of abstraction. Translated by M. J. Rioch. *Journal of abnormal and social Psychology,* 1941, *36,* 3–33.
252. With M. Scheerer. Abstract and concrete behavior: an experimental study with special tests. *Psychological Monographs,* 1941, *53,* 2, Whole number 239. Pp. 151.
253. With M. Scheerer and E. G. Boring. A demonstration of insight: the Horse-and-Rider puzzle. *American Journal of Psychology,* 1941, *54,* 437–438.

1942

254. *Aftereffects of Brain Injuries in War. Their Evaluation and Treatment.* Foreword by D. Denny-Brown. New York, N.Y., 1942, Grune & Stratton. Pp. 244.
255. Analogous mechanism in the formation of symptoms in organic and functional disorders. (With special consideration of the compulsive phenomena). *Bulletin of the Forest Sanitarium,* Des Plaines, Illinois, 1942, *1,* 28–36.
256. Ottfried Foerster, M.D. (Obituary). *Journal of nervous and mental Disease,* 1942, *95,* 112–113.
257. The problem of cerebral localization from a clinical point of view. In R. D. Halloran and P. I. Yakovlev (Eds.), *Collected lectures of the seventh post-graduate seminar in neurology and psychiatry. Third semester. General Neurology —Jan. 5-April 10, 1942.* Waltham, Massachusetts, 1942, Metropolitan State Hospital. Pp. 155–169.
258. Some experimental observations concerning the influence of colors on the function of the organism. *Occupational Therapy and Rehabilitation,* 1942, *21,* 147–151.
259. The two ways of adjustment of the organism to cerebral defects. *Journal of the Mount Sinai Hospital, New York,* 1942, *9,* 504–513.

260. Book review: P. Schilder, Goals and Desires of Man. A psychological survey. *American Journal of Psychology*, 1942, *55*, 601–603.

261. With J. I. Steinfeld. The conditioning of sexual behavior by visual agnosia. *Bulletin of the Forest Sanitarium*, Des Plaines, Illinois, 1942, *1*, 37–45.

1943

262. Brain concussion: evaluation of the aftereffects by special tests. *Diseases of the nervous System*, 1943, *4*, 325–334.

263. Carl Bonhoeffer, M.D. (Obituary.) *Journal of nervous and mental Disease*, 1943, *98*, 683.

264. The clinical significance of electroencephalography. *Bulletin of the New England Medical Center*, 1943, *5*, 22–24.

265. Concerning rigidity. *Character and Personality*, 1943, *11*, 209–226.

266. Constriction of the visual fields. *Archives of Neurology and Psychiatry*, 1943, *50*, 486–487.

267. Constriction of the visual fields. *Journal of nervous and mental Disease*, 1943, *98*, 196–198.

268. On so-called war neuroses. *Psychosomatic Medicine*, 1943, *5*, 376–383.

269. The significance of psychological research in schizophrenia. *Journal of nervous and mental Disease*, 1943, *97*, 261–279. Reprinted in S. S. Tomkins (Ed.), *Contemporary Psychopathology*. Cambridge, Massachusetts, 1943, Harvard University Press. Pp. 302–318.

270. Some remarks on Russell Brain's article concerning visual object agnosia. *Journal of nervous and mental Disease*, 1943, *98*, 148–153.

1944

271. Frontal lobectomy. *Bulletin of the New England medical Center*, 1944, *6*, 167–169.

272. The mental changes due to frontal lobe damage. *Journal of Psychology*, 1944, *17*, 187–208.

273. Methodological approach to the study of schizophrenic thought disorder. In J. S. Kasanin (Ed.), *Language and Thought in Schizophrenia*. Berkeley, California, 1944, University of California Press. Pp. 17–40.

274. Physiological aspects of convalescence and rehabilitation following central nervous system injuries. *Federation of American Societies for Experimental Biology. Federation Proceedings*, 1944, *3*, 255–265.

275. The significance of mental disturbances in rehabilitation of soldiers with brain injury. *Transactions of the American Neurological Association*, 1944, *70*, 22–24.

276. Special institutions for rehabilitation of soldiers with brain injuries. *Occupational Therapy and Rehabilitation*, 1944, *23*, 115–118.

277. With E. Hanfmann and M. Rickers-Ovsiankina. Case Lanuti: Extreme concretization of behavior due to damage of the brain cortex. *Psychological Monographs*, 1944, *57*, 4, Whole #264. Pp. 72.

1945

278. Frontal lobotomy as therapeutic attempt in mental disease. *Proceedings of the Rudolf Virchow Medical Society, New York*, 1945, *4*, 94–96.

279. With E. Rothmann. Physiognomic phenomena in Rorschach responses. *Rorschach Research Exchange*, 1945, *9*, 1–7.

280. With M. Scheerer. *The Goldstein-Scheerer Tests of Abstract and Concrete Thinking.* New York, N.Y., 1945, The Psychological Corporation. Kit containing reprint of #252 and test materials.

281. With M. Scheerer and E. Rothmann. A case of "Idiot Savant": An experimental study of personality organization. *Psychological Monographs*, 1945, *58*, 4, Whole #269. Pp. 63.

1946

282. On naming and pseudonaming. *Word*, 1946, *2*, 1–7.

283. Remarks on localization. *Confinia Neurologica*, 1946, *7*, 25–34.

1947

284. An organismic approach to the problem of motivation. *Transactions of the New York Academy of Sciences*, 1947, Series II, vol. 9, 218–230.

1948

285. *Language and Language Disturbances. Aphasic Symptom Complexes and their Significance for Medicine and Theory of Language.* (For translation see #293.) New York, N.Y., 1948, Grune & Stratton. Pp. xii & 374.

286. On naming and pseudonaming. *ETC: A Review of general semantics*, 1948, *5*, 191–197. Reprint of #282.

1949

287. Bemerkung zum Vortrag von Prof. Otto Meyerhof: Über Goethes Methoden der Naturforschung. *Proceedings of the Rudolf Virchow Medical Society, New York*, 1949, *8*, 110–112.

288. Einige Bemerkungen zum Schizophrenenproblem. *Monatsschrift für Psychologie und Neurologie*, 1949, *117*, 215–223.

289. Frontal lobotomy and impairment of abstract attitude. *Journal of nervous and mental Disease*, 1949, *110*, 93–111.

290. The idea of disease and therapy. *Review of Religion*, 1949, *13*, 229–240.

1950

291. Address of the president of the Rudolf Virchow Medical Society, New York: 90th anniversary of the society. *Proceedings of the Rudolf Virchow Medical Society, New York*, 1950, *9*, 95–100.

292. Prefrontal lobotomy: analysis and warning. *Scientific American*, 1950, *182*, 44–47.

293. *Trastornos del lenguaje: las afasias.* Translated by E. Sierra Ruiz. Barcelona & Madrid, 1950, Editorial Cientifice Medica. Spanish translation of #285.

294. With W. Riese. The brain of Ludwig Edinger: an inquiry into the cerebral morphology of mental ability and left-handedness. *Journal of comparative Neurology*, 1950, *92*, 133–168.

1951

295. On emotions: considerations from the organismic point of view. *Journal of Psychology*, 1951, *31*, 37–49.

296. Remarques sur le problème épistémologique de la biologie. Translated by S. and G. Canguilhem. *Actes du congrès international de philosophie scientifique, 1949. I. Epistémologie.* Paris, 1951, Herman. Pp. 141–143.

297. *La structure de l'organisme. Introduction à la biologie à partir de la pathologie humaine.* Texte augmenté de fragments inédits. Translated by E. Burckhardt and J. Kuntz. Paris, 1951, Gallimard. Pp. 446. French translation of #219.

1952

298. The effect of brain damage on the personality. *Psychiatry*, 1952, *15*, 245–260.

1953

299. With M. Scheerer. Tests of abstract and concrete thinking. In A. Weider (Ed.), *Contributions toward medical psychology.* New York, N.Y., 1953, Ronald Press. Vol. II. Pp. 702–730.

1954

300. Bemerkungen zum Problem "Sprechen und Denken" auf Grund hirnpathologischer Erfahrungen. *Acta Psychologica*, 1954, *10*, 175–196. Published simultaneously in G. Révész (Ed.), *Thinking and Speaking. A Symposium.* Amsterdam, 1954, North Holland Publishing Co. Pp. 175–196.

301. The brain-injured child. In H. Michael-Smith (Ed.), *Pediatric problems in clinical practice.* New York, N.Y., 1954, Grune & Stratton. Pp. 97–120.

302. The concept of health, disease and therapy. Basic ideas for an organismic psychotherapy. *American Journal of Psychotherapy*, 1954, *8*, 745–764.

303. The concept of transference in treatment of organic and functional nervous disease. *Acta psychotherapeutica, psychosomatica et orthopaedagogica*, 1954, *2*, 334–353.

1956

304. Bemerkungen zur Methodik der Untersuchung psychopathologischer Fälle.— Im Anschluss an die Nachuntersuchung des "seelenblinden" Patienten Schneider, mehr als 30 Jahre nach dem Auftreten der Störung. *Monatsschrift für Psychiatrie und Neurologie*, 1956, *131*, 309–336.

1957

305. Das Lächeln des Kindes und das Problem des Verstehens des Anderen Ich. In M. J. Langeveld (Ed.), *Rencontre—Encounter—Begegnung: contributions à une psychologie humaine, dédiées au Professeur J. J. Buytendijk.* Utrecht & Antwerp, 1957, Spectrum. Pp. 181–197.

306. The nature of language. In R. N. Anshen (Ed.), *Language: an inquiry into its meaning and function.* New York, N.Y., 1957, Harper. Pp. 18–40.

307. New ideas on mental health. In J. Fairchild (Ed.), *Personal problems and psychological frontiers.* New York, N.Y., 1957, Sheridan House. Pp. 96–119.

308. *Ningen.* Translated by Sanshiro Nishitani. Tokyo, 1957, Seishin-Shobe. Japanese translation of #244.

309. *Seitajno kino.* Translated by Masashi Murakami and Shoshire Kuromaru. Tokyo, 1957, Misuzu Shobe. Japanese translation of #219.

310. The smiling of the infant and the problem of understanding the "other." *Journal of Psychology*, 1957, *44*, 175–191.

311. The structure of anxiety. In J. H. Masserman and J. L. Moreno (Eds.), *Progress in psychotherapy*. New York, N.Y., 1957, Grune & Stratton. Vol. II, pp. 61–70.

1959

312. Abnormal mental conditions in infancy.
Journal of nervous and mental Disease, 1959, *128*, 538–557.
313. Aus K. Goldstein's Nachruf.
In *Ludwig Edinger, 1855-1918. Gedenkschrift zu seinem 100. Geburtstag und zum 50 jährigen Bestehen des Neurologischen Institutes (Edinger-Institut) der Universität Frankfurt am Main*. Wiesbaden, 1959, Franz Steiner Verlag. Pp. 26–30. Partial reprint of #93.
314. Concerning the concreteness in schizophrenia.
Journal of abnormal and social Psychology, 1959, *59*, 146–148.
315. Functional disturbances in brain damage. In S. Arieti (Ed.), *American Handbook of Psychiatry*. New York, N.Y., 1959, Basic Books. Vol. I, pp. 770–794.
316. Individuality—the psychological process.
In Associates of Bank Street College of Education (Eds.), *Individuality and education*. New York, N.Y., Bank Street College of Education. Pp. 5–13.
317. Notes on the development of my concepts.
Journal of Individual Psychology, 1959, *15*, 5–14.
318. Health as value. In A. H. Maslow (Ed.), *New knowledge in human values*. New York, N.Y., 1959, Harper. Pp. 178–188.
319. The organismic approach. In S. Arieti (Ed.), *American Handbook of Psychiatry*. New York, N.Y., 1959, Basic Books. Vol. II, pp. 1333–1347.

1960

320. Concerning the concept of "primitivity."
In S. Diamond (Ed.), *Culture in history; essays in honor of Paul Radin*. New York, N.Y., 1960, Columbia University Press. Pp. 99–117.
321. Disease, health and therapy.
Proceedings of the Rudolf Virchow Medical Society, New York, 1960, *19*, 180–191.
322. Sensoritonic theory and the concept of self-realization.
In B. Kaplan and S. Wapner (Eds.), *Perspectives in Psychological Theory*. New York, N.Y., 1960, International Universities Press. Pp. 115–123.
323. Thinking and speaking.
Annals of the New York Academy of Sciences, 1960, *91*, 38–51.
324. What we can learn from pathology for normal psychology.
In G. Leviton (Ed.), *The relationship between rehabilitation and psychology. Conference held at the Institute of Human Development, Clark University, June 11–13, 1959*. Worcester, Massachusetts, 1960, Clark University, Institute of Human Development. Mimeo. Pp. 36–61; 131–135.

1963

325. *Human Nature in the Light of Psychopathology*.
New York, N.Y., 1963, Schocken Books. Pp. xiii & 258. Paperback edition of #244 with a new foreword by the author.

326. *The Organism. A Holistic Approach to Biology derived from Pathological Data in Man.* Boston, Massachusetts, 1963, Beacon Press. Pp. xx & 533. Paperback edition of #219 with a new preface by the author.

1965

327. Stress and the concept of self-realization. In S. Z. Klausner (Ed.), *The quest for self-control.* New York, N.Y., 1965, The Free Press. Pp. 341–355.

1967

328. Autobiography.
In E. G. Boring and G. Lindzey (Eds.), *A History of Psychology in Autobiography. Vol. 5.* New York, N.Y., 1967, Appleton-Century-Crofts. Pp. 145–166.

FILMS

distributed by the Psychological Cinema Register,
The Pennsylvania State University
University Park, Pennsylvania.

Goldstein, K. and Scheerer, M. *Impairment of the Abstract Attitude as shown on the Cube Test.* 1950. 19 min., silent, color (PCR-523K)

Goldstein, K. and Scheerer, M. *Impairment of the Abstract Attitude as shown on the Stick Test.* 1950. 9 min., silent, black and white. (PCR-524)

PART II: SELECTED WRITINGS ABOUT KURT GOLDSTEIN IN ORDER OF THEIR PUBLICATION

Hartmann, H. Review of K. Goldstein, Die Beziehungen der Psychoanalyse zur Biologie. *Allgemeine ärztliche Zeitschrift für Psychotherapie*, 1928, *1*, 183–184.

Gal'perin, P. Remarks on the principle of totality. *Sovetskaya psikhonevrologiya*, 1933, *9*, 19–34. Comments on #216.

Purdy, D. M. The biological psychology of Kurt Goldstein. *Character and Personality*, 1936–1937, *5*, 321–330.

Mourgue, R. La conception de la neurologie dans l'oeuvre de Kurt Goldstein. L'Encéphale, 1937, *32*, 32–56.

Riese, W. Goldstein's Auffassung vom Organismus und ihre Beziehungen zu C. v. Monakow's Neurobiologie. *Schweizer Archiv für Neurologie und Psychiatrie*, 1938, *41*, 257–262.

Gurwitsch, A. Le fonctionnement de l'organisme d'après K. Goldstein. *Journal de Psychologie normale et pathologique*, 1939, *36*, 107–138.

Gurwitsch, A. La science biologique d'après M. K. Goldstein. *Revue philosophique de la France et de l'étranger*, 1940, *129*, 244–265.

Meiers, J. *Forty-five years of Kurt Goldstein's publications. The organismic approach.* New York, 1948, mimeo.

Riese, W. Kurt Goldstein's Stellung in der Geschichte der Neurologie. Versuch einer Würdigung aus Anlass seines 70. Geburtstages: 6. November 1948.
Schweizer Archiv für Neurologie und Psychiatrie, 1948, *62*, 2–10.

Bach, I. Interview with K. Goldstein, June 1958. In L. Besch (Ed.), *Auszug des Geistes. Bericht über eine Sendereihe*. Bremen, 1962, B. C. Heye. Pp. 93–94; 223.

Geschwind, N. The paradoxical position of Kurt Goldstein in the history of aphasia. *Cortex*, 1964, *1*, 214–224.

Berberich, J. Kurt Goldstein. *Proceedings of the Rudolf Virchow Medical Society, New York*, 1965, *24*, 195–198.

Eliasberg, W. In memoriam Kurt Goldstein. *Proceedings of the Rudolf Virchow Medical Society, New York*, 1965, *24*, 185–194.

Jonas, H. In memoriam: Kurt Goldstein, 1878–1965. *Social Research*, 1965, *32*, 351–356.

Schapiro, M. In Memoriam—Kurt Goldstein. *Journal of Philosophy and Phenomenological Research*, 1965, *26*, 302–303.

Wilde, G. Kurt Goldstein ha muerte.
Psicologia—Psiquiatria—Psicoanalisis (Bogota, Columbia), 1965, *1*, 1–2.

Meiers, J. Kurt Goldstein, 1878–1965.
Journal of Individual Psychology, 1966, *22*, 116–125.

Shakow, D. Kurt Goldstein: 1878–1965. *American Journal of Psychology*, 1966, *79*, 150–154.

Simmel, M. L. Kurt Goldstein. *International Encyclopedia of the Social Sciences*, New York, 1968, Crowell-Collier and Macmillan (in press).

Special journal issues dedicated in whole or in part to Kurt Goldstein

Confinia Neurologica, 1949, *9*, Fasc. 1–4, pp. 1–272.
Goldstein Anniversary Number. *Contributors:* A. Bethe; T. Edinger; E. Fischer; J. Lhermitte; O. Loewi; W. Riese; A. Wallenberg; V. v. Weizsäcker; J. C. Yaskin, R. A. Groff and H. A. Shenkin; D. I. Arbuse; M. B. Bender; L. T. Furlow and H. L. Teuber; F. Fromm-Reichmann; E. C. Hoff; L. Van der Horst; M. A. Kennard; F. H. Lewey; O. Marburg; W. Riese; N. Savitsky and S. P. Elpern; M. Scheerer; H. Werner; H. T. Wycis, A. J. Lee and E. A. Spiegel.

American Journal of Psychoanalysis, 1959, *19*, 143–164.
Kurt Goldstein 80th Birthday Tribute.
Contributors: F. A. Weiss; H. Kelman; G. Pankow; H. Jonas.

American Journal of Psychotherapy, 1959, *13*, 537–613.
Five articles presented as a tribute to Kurt Goldstein on the occasion of his eightieth birthday.
Contributors: S. Arieti; Z. A. Piotrowski; C. Bühler; R. E. Shor; M. L. Simmel.

Journal of individual Psychology, 1959, *15*, 3–99.
Kurt Goldstein 80th Anniversary issue. E. Hanfmann & N. L. Mintz (Eds.)
Contributors: A. Adler; F. J. J. Buytendijk; L. H. Chiappo; K. Goldstein; W. Goody;

Note also articles in the following journals, and the reprints of earlier articles by A. Gurwitsch (pp. 119–142) and M. L. Simmel (pp. 3–11) in this volume.

E. Hanfmann; R. Jakobson; A. H. Maslow; J. Meiers; N. L. Mintz; O. H. Mowrer; M. Scheerer; E. J. Thomas; P. Tillich; L. Van der Horst; W. Van Dusen; A. L. van Kaam; H. Winthrop; A. Zander.

Neuropsychologia, 1966, *4*, 297–363.
Special Issue Dedicated to the Memory of Professor Kurt Goldstein (1878–1965). *Contributors:* D. Denny-Brown; H. L. Teuber; A. R. Luria; R. L'Hermitte, H. Hécaen, J. Dubois, A. Culioli and A. Tabouret-Keller; M. L. Simmel; R. G. Rudel, H. L. Teuber and T. E. Twitchell; M. Scheerer and G. Goldstein.

Index

GPSR Compliance

The European Union's (EU) General Product Safety Regulation (GPSR) is a set of rules that requires consumer products to be safe and our obligations to ensure this.

If you have any concerns about our products, you can contact us on ProductSafety@springernature.com

In case Publisher is established outside the EU, the EU authorized representative is:

Springer Nature Customer Service Center GmbH
Europaplatz 3
69115 Heidelberg, Germany

Batch number: 10844669

Printed by Printforce, the Netherlands